L. Wille M. Obladen

Neonatal Intensive Care

Principles and Guidelines

With a Section on Neonatal Cardiology
by H. E. Ulmer

Foreword by A. Merritt

With 49 Figures and 76 Tables

Springer-Verlag
Berlin Heidelberg New York 1981

Prof. Dr. Lutz Wille
Leiter der Sektion für Pädiatrische Intensivmedizin, Universitäts-Kinderklinik, Im Neuenheimer Feld 150, D-6900 Heidelberg

Prof. Dr. Michael Obladen
Oberarzt der Abteilung Neonatologie, Universitäts-Kinderklinik, Rümelinstraße 23, D-7400 Tübingen

PD Dr. Herbert E. Ulmer
Oberarzt der Abteilung Pädiatrische Kardiologie, Universitäts-Kinderklinik, Im Neuenheimer Feld 150, D-6900 Heidelberg

Translator: Terry Telger
3054 Vaughn Avenue, Marina, CA 93933 (USA)

Title of the original German edition:
Neugeborenen-Intensivpflege, 2nd Edition (Kliniktaschenbücher)

ISBN-13: 978-3-540-10462-9 e-ISBN-13: 978-3-642-67903-2
DOI: 10.1007/ 978-3-642-67903-2

Library of Congress Cataloging in Publication Data. Wille, Lutz, 1939 – Neonatal intensive care. Translation of Neugeborenen-Intensivpflege. Includes bibliographies and index. 1. Neonatal intensive care. 2. Infants (Newborn) – Diseases. I. Obladen, Michael, 1944- joint author. II. Ulmer, Herbert E., joint author. III. Title. [DNLM: 1. Critical care – In infancy and childhood. 2. Infant, Newborn, Diseases – Therapy. WS 420 W698n] RJ253.5.W5413 618.92'OL 80-26493

Typesetting, printing, and binding: Oscar Brandstetter Druckerei KG, 6200 Wiesbaden. 2121/3140-543210

Foreword

The significant strides made during the past decade in neonatal medicine are based largely upon the provision of intensive perinatal care to the parturient, her fetus, and the newborn. In addition to technologic advances in the bioelectronic monitoring of the fetus and newborn, the introduction of noninvasive methods to monitor oxygenation, the pharmacologic manipulation of the ductus arteriosus and pulmonary vasculature, and the use of ultrasonographic diagnosis of congenital heart defects and other lesions, intensive efforts by neonatal specialists throughout the world have also contributed to the decline in neonatal and infant mortality.
Professors Wille and Obladen have provided an authoritative manual outlining intensive care of newborns and the ways in which the science of neonatal medicine, the technology of the 1980 s, and the art of application have resulted in the practice of neonatal intensive care at the Kinderklinik of the University of Heidelberg. The English translation resulted from the success of the German edition and will serve well the needs of the English-speaking student and practitioner of neonatal intensive care.

T. Allen Merrit, M. D.
Assistant Professor of Pediatrics,
Obstetrics, and Gynecology
University of Rochester

Preface to the English Edition

The unexpectedly friendly reception accorded our book and the further development of neonatal intensive care have necessitated revision of the first edition only one year after its publication. Our readers have made many critical proposals as to possible improvements for which we would like to thank them. Those chapters on patient supervision, oxygen therapy, artifical ventilation, pulmonary diseases, and cardiological problems have been particularly modified and expanded; new sections dealing with acute renal failure and long-term prognosis following neonatal intensive care have been added, as have tables concerning instruments and pharmacotherapy. The positive response and great demand which these guidelines on clinical practice have met within such a short space of time gave rise to the present English version, designed to make the original book accessible to neonatologists and nurses working within the field of neonatal intensive care in English-speaking countries. The task of translation was kindly accepted by T. C. Telger. Special thanks are extended to T. Allen Merritt, who undertook the difficult assignment of critically examining the text from the point of view of an experienced specialist in perinatal care. Exceptional support in the preparation of the manuscript was provided by our secretary, Mrs. Engelhorn.

Heidelberg, November 1980

Lutz Wille
Michael Obladen
Herbert Ulmer

Preface to the First German Edition

Neonatal intensive care is inseparably linked with neonatology. An understanding of the physiology and pathophysiology of the first four weeks of life, knowledge of the symptoms and differential diagnosis of acute neonatal diseases and dysmorphic syndromes, and a familiarity with advanced medical technology and equipment, combined with extensive clinical experience and manual dexterity, are important elements in the clinical care of critically ill newborns.

The stimulus for this book was the desire of the residents and nurses in our neonatal intensive care unit (NICU) for a revised version of our NICU "bible": a collection of brief, specific guidelines for everyday clinical practice at the University of Heidelberg. Their skillful observations and enthusiasm served as the resource for the present material. This book is concerned primarily with therapeutic modalities, the practical and technical aspects of mechanical ventilation, and the techniques of intensive care. For the study of basic clinical pediatrics, neonatology, neonatal physiology and pathophysiology, the reader is referred to the extensive standard texts in these fields.

Our book represents a summary of therapeutic practices in *one* intensive care facility. It cannot be complete and will have to be continuously modified in accordance with the rapid developments in our discipline. We are also certain that different methods of treatment can be employed with equal success at different intensive care units.

The "working guidelines" presented here must be regarded as simplified suggestions which can be modified as circumstances warrant. They are not intended as a "cookbook" to be followed uncritically: Schemata are no substitute for thoughtful initiative and thorough discussions among those caring for the sick newborn.

Neonatal intensive care cannot be learned from the literature. We are therefore grateful to Prof. H. Bickel, who gave us the opportunity to gain our own experience at the intensive care facilities in Lausanne (L. S. Prod'hom), Copenhagen (B. Friis-Hansen), Helsinki (N. Hallman), and San Diego (L. Gluck). Prof. H. Plückthun has shared with us his extensive knowledge and experience in the field of neonatology, and his thoughtful discussions remain a constant stimulus for us to analyze and find practical solutions for clinical problems in neonatology. We are also grateful to the staff of Springer Verlag for their patient cooperation during preparation of the manuscript and for bringing it so quickly to press.

Heidelberg, September 1977

Lutz Wille
Michael Obladen

Contents

Part II. Diagnosis and Treatment of Respiratory Disorders

Part III. Acute Neonatal Diseases

Part IV. Appendix

Abbreviations

ACD	Acid-Citrate-Dextrose Anticoagulant
ACG	Angiocardiography
ADH	Antidiuretic Hormone
AGA	Appropriate for Gestational Age
BAS	Ballon Artioseptostomy
BE	Base Excess
BPD	Bronchopulmonary Dysplasia
BPM	Beat per Minute
BVH	Biventricular Hypertrophy
BW	Body Weight
CC	Cardiac Catheterization
CCMP	Cardiomyopathy of the Congestive Type
CDP	Continuous Distending Pressure
CNP	Continuous Negative Pressure
CNPV	Continuous Negative Pressure Ventilation
COA	Coarctation of the Aorta
CPAP	Continuous Positive Airway Pressure
CTG	Cardiotocography
CVP	Central Venous Pressure
DDAVP	I-Deamino-8-D-Arginine Vasopressin
DIC	Disseminated Intravascular Coagulation
DOCA	Deoxycorticosterone Acetate
ECG	Electrocardiography
EEG	Electroencephalography
EFE	Endocardial Fibroelastosis
ET	Exchange Transfusion
FiO_2	Fractional Concentration of O_2 in Inspired Air
Hb	Hemoglobin Concentration
HCMP	Cardiomyopathy of the Hypertrophic Type
HK	Hematocrit
HLHS	Hypoplastic Left Heart Syndrome
HOT	Hyperoxia Test
HTSI	Human Thyroid Stimulating Immunglobulin
ICS	Intercostal Space
I:E Ratio	Inspiratory Time-Expiratory Time Ratio

IM	Intramuscular
IMV	Intermittent Mandatory Ventilation
IPPV	Intermittend Positive Pressure Ventilation
IV	Intravenous
ICU	Intensive Care Unit
LA	Left Atrium
LA/Ao	Left Atrial-Aortic Diameter Ratio
LAD	Left-Axis Deviation
LATS	Long Acting Thyroid Stimulator
LD	Loading Dose
LGA	Large for Gestational Age
LV	Left Ventricle
MD	Maintenance Dose per Day
NICU	Neonatal Intensive Care Unit
NP	Neonatal Period
PaO_2	Arterial Oxygen Partial Pressure
PCG	Phonocardiography
PCO_2	Carbon Dioxide Partial Pressure
PDA	Patent Ductus Arteriosus
PEEP	Positiv End-Expiratory Pressure
PFC	Persistence of Fetal Circulation
PO_2	Arterial Oxygen Partial Pressure
PT	Prothrombin Time
PTT	Partial Thromboplastin Time
RA	Right Atrium
RDS	Respiratory Distress Syndrome
RV	Right Ventricle
RVH	Right Ventricular Hypertrophy
SaO_2	Aterial Oxygen Partial Saturation
SC	Subcutaneous
SGA	Small for Gestational Age
StB	Standard Bicarbonate
TV	Tidal Volume
$tcPO_2$	Transcutannous Aterial Oxygen Partial Pressure
TGA	Transposition of the Great Arteries
THAM	Trometamol
UAC	Umbilical Artery Catheter
UVC	Umbilical Vein Catheter
VSD	Ventricular Septual Defect

Part 1
Practical Management of High-Risk Newborns

1 Evaluation and Treatment of the Newborn Immediately After Birth

L. Wille

Within a few minutes after birth, the newborn must assume for itself all critical functions, such as cardiorespiratory adaptation, temperature regulation, and metabolism. To evaluate the newborn properly, the physician must be familiar with the physiologic mechanisms of adaptation and potential risks during the perinatal period. He must determine the gestational age of the infant; classify the status of intrauterine growth; differentiate between the preterm, appropriate, and small-for-gestational-age infant; determine the stage of dysmaturity and its morbidity; and, finally, diagnose the condition of the neonate, institute resuscitation, and implement primary care. A prompt and thorough postpartum examination with consideration for possible risk factors (Tables 1–3) can significantly reduce the high rate of neonatal morbidity and mortality.

1.1 Predisposing Risk Factors

Table 1. Known risk factors before pregnancy (21)

Social factors	
Low income level strenuous physical labor, illegitimacy, emotional stress	Potential danger to fetus/newborn due to inadequate prenatal care, undiscovered maternal disease, unrecognized abnormalities of fetal development, placental insufficiency, antepartum hemorrhage; increased incidence of prematurity and intrauterine malnutrition
Metabolism	
Obesity or weight gain >15 kg	Prematurity, increased perinatal mortality,
Diabetes mellitus	Stillbirth, prematurity, congenital malformations, macrosomia, respiratory distress syndrome, hyperbilirubinemia, hypoglycemia, hypocalcemia, renal venous thrombosis, hydrops fetalis
Malnutrition	Prematurity, intrauterine growth retardation

Table 1. (continued)

Endocrinology	
Primary hyperparathyroidism	Hypocalcemia, neonatal tetany, hypomagnesemia
Hyperthyroidism	Prematurity, neonatal goiter, thyrotoxicosis (LATS, HTSI)
Hypothyroidism	Abortion, prematurity, congenital malformations, retarded psychomotor development in utero, CNS defects, hypothyroidism
Cardiovascular system	
Cardiac insufficiency	Prematurity, hypoxia
Low cardiac output	Prematurity
Vascular disease	Prematurity, intrauterine growth retardation
Lungs	
Asthma, diseases with hypoxia and hypercapnia	Hypoxia, prematurity, intrauterine growth retardation
Gastrointestinal tract	
Regional ileitis	Prematurity
Neurology	
Myasthenia gravis	Myasthenia gravis (transitory), decreased sensitivity to medications
Status epilepticus	Hypoxia
Hematology	
Blood group incompatibility (Rh, ABO)	Erythroblastosis fetalis: hydrops fetalis, anemia neonatorum, hyperbilirubinemia, hypoglycemia, fetal asphyxia
Werlhof's disease	Thrombocytopenic purpura (transitory)
Anemia (iron deficiency, vitamin B12 deficiency) <9 g% Hb	Prematurity, intrauterine growth retardation
Hereditary diseases	E. g., cystic fibrosis of the pancreas, meconium ileus; Tay-Sachs
Obstetrics/gynecology	
<16 or >40 years of age	Potential danger to fetus: abortion, malformations
Primiparas >30 years of age	Potential danger to mother and child
Multiparas >3	Increased perinatal mortality, pre- and postpartum hemorrhage
Prehistory	
Abortion, dead fetus, preterm baby, low birth weight newborn (<2500 g), large birth weight newborn (>4500 g), birth trauma, multiple pregnancies	Potential danger to fetus or newborn

Table 2. Risk factors during pregnancy [21]

Infections	
Toxoplasmosis	Congenial toxoplasmosis
Listeriosis	Granulomatosis infantiseptica
Cytomegalovirus	Microcephaly, cerebral calcifications, hydrocephalus, encephalitis, chorioretinitis, hepatitis, jaundice, hepatosplenomegaly, thrombocytopenia, purpura, anemia
Rubella	Embryopathia rubeolaris, congenital rubella syndrome
Syphilis	Abortion, congenital syphilis
Tuberculosis	Intrauterine (very rare) or neonatal infection (isolation immediately after birth!)
Coxsackie B	Meningoencephalitis, myocarditis, jaundice, thrombocytopenia, hepatitis
Herpes simplex	Groups of reddish-brown vesicles, microcephaly, cerebral calcifications meningoencephalitis, jaundice, hepatitis, thrombocytopenia, anemia, coagulopathy, keratoconjunctivitis, chorioretinitis
Candidiasis (vaginal)	Stomatitis
Acute pyelonephritis	Prematurity, bacterial infection
Enteropathogenic *E. coli* (secretors)	Vomiting and diarrhea
Bacterial infection (fever)	Sepsis, meningitis
Drugs	
Fenoterol bromide	Hypoglycemia, hyperbilirubinemia, hyperexcitability, hypotension
Cephalothin	Positive direct Coombs' test
Chloramphenicol	Gray syndrome
Cigarette abuse	Intrauterine growth retardation
Magnesium sulfate	Hypermagnesemia
Morphine, heroin	Withdrawal syndromes (tremor, dyspnea cyanosis, convulsions)
Reserpine	Apathy, stuffy nose
Alcohol abuse	Fetal alcohol syndrome
Anticonvulsive therapy	Hydantoin embryopathy, hemorrhagic disease of the newborn
Falling estriol values (urine)	Placental insufficiency
Unusual maternal medications	Congenital malformations
Preeclampsia	Prematurity
Hypertension	Danger to fetus

Table 3. Risk factors during labor [21]

Birth complications	
Multiple birth	Prematurity, fetofetal transfusion, hypotrophic newborns, increased perinatal mortality, hypoxia (second twin), hypoglycemia (smaller twin)
Precipitate labor	Hypoxia, tentorial tears
Prolonged labor	Fetal hypoxia, birth trauma (intracranial), increased risk of infection
Fetal heart aberrations	Hypoxia, paroxysmal tachycardia
Fever	Prematurity, neonatal infection
Breech presentation	Hypoxia, intracranial hemorrhage, visceral hemorrhage (adrenal glands, kidneys, spleen), spinal trauma, plexal paresis, fractures
Face presentation	Edema, facial ecchymoses, hypoxia
Transverse presentation	Hypoxia, trauma
Uterine rupture/tetany	Hypoxia
Manual version/extraction	Hypoxia, plexal paresis, spinal trauma
Forceps (high)	Hypoxia, cephalhematoma, intracranial hemorrhage
Amniotic membranes/amniotic fluid	
Amnionitis	Bacterial infection
Premature rupture of the membranes (>24 h)	Bacterial infection, prematurity, prolapse of umbilical cord, hypoxia, postasphyxial syndrome, aspiration of meconium, pneumonia
Oligohydramnios	Postmaturity, renal agenesis, polycystic kidneys, urethral obstruction, fetal death
Polyhydramnios	Abnormal presentation, premature rupture of amnion, cord prolapse, prematurity, atresia of gastrointestinal tract (esophagus), CNS anomalies, hydrops fetalis
Placenta	
Placenta previa	Prematurity, hypoxia, cord prolapse, fetal blood loss
Abruption placentae	Prematurity, hypoxia, fetal blood loss
Fetomaternal transfusion	Fetal blood loss, hypoxia, shock
Placental insufficiency	Hypoxia, intrauterine dystrophy
Circumvallate placenta	Abortion, intrauterine growth retardation
Velamentous insertion	Hypoxia, increased perinatal mortality, fetal blood loss
Umbilical cord	
Inflammation	Bacterial infection, umbilical venous thrombosis (hypoxia)
Prolapse	Hypoxia
Single umbilical artery	Congenital anomalies, intrauterine growth retardation
True knot	Hypoxia
Umbilical cord rupture, aneurysms, etc.	Fetal blood loss
Postmaturity >7 days	Increased fetal mortality
Eclampsia	Prematurity, intrauterine dystrophy, hypoxia

1.2 Diagnosis of Postpartum Condition

Neonatal intensive care is in many cases emergency medicine which calls for the prompt institution of specific diagnostic and therapeutic measures in the delivery room. The Apgar score has proved a useful means for evaluating the newborn infant (Table 4) (1).

Table 4. Apgar system for evaluating newborns [1][a]

Symptom	Apgar score 0	1	2
Skin color	Blue or pale	Cyanosis	Pink
Respiratory effort	Absent	Slow, irregular	Good
Heart rate	Absent	<100/min	>100
Muscle tone	Flaccid	Hypotonic	Active motion
Reflexes irritability	No response	Grimacing	Vigorous cry

[a] Score is assessed after 1′, 5′, X′; X = after recovery without further improvement

The Apgar score at 5 min is of particular prognostic significance. Prospective longitudinal studies have shown a significant correlation with neurologic abnormalities at 1 year of age [3, 5, 6].
An important aspect of the early laboratory evaluation is the determination of the pH of blood from the umbilical vessels [4].

Normal Values
Umbilical artery: pH 7.12–7.42
Umbilical vein: pH 7.20–7.46.

If the pH of the umbilical arterial blood is less than 7.10, or the scalp blood is less than 7.20, severe perinatal acidosis is present. Low Apgar scores combined with low pH values are indicative of marked depression. Neonatal depression without intrauterine acidosis may occur in cases of maternal sedation, cesarean section (anesthetic), and neonatal shock. During the shock state, lactic acid accumulates in the peripheral tissue until adequate perfusion is reestablished and adequate perfusion occurs [2, 14]. The umbilical and scalp pHs reflect the degree of asphyxia (hypoxemia) during labor and delivery.
Due to the grave consequences of marked perinatal acidosis (see p 148), a correction is desirable. However, the infusion of an isotonic solution of $NaHCO_3$ should be reserved for infants who fail to respond to oxygenation and ventilation!
Other parameters of interest in the postpartum evaluation of high-risk infants are the *systolic blood pressure* (Ultrasonic Doppler Flow Detector, Model 811; Parks Electronics Laboratories) and the *oxygen cardiorespirogram* [16, 19]. Risk factors associated with the development of neonatal shock are prematurity, hypothermia,

asphyxia, prolapsed cord, maternal sepsis, and maternal bleeding or fetomaternal hemorrhage. The clinical signs are pallor, tachycardia, and a low systolic blood pressure, which results in diminished cerebral blood flow and possible cerebral ischemia or renal insufficiency [15].
The *oxygen cardiorespirogram* is useful in the recognition of asphyxia or hypoxia with cerebral damage, as well as adaptive difficulties, imminent cardiovascular collapse, peripheral vasoconstriction, and acute cardiorespiratory distress [19].

1.3 Classification of Asphyxia (Table 5)

Indications of Intrapartum Asphyxia [20]
Fetal scalp blood sampling: pH <7.20
Meconium stained amniotic fluid
Pathologic cardiotocography
Recurrent pathologic heart rate on routine ausculation

Table 5. Clinical classification postpartum

Classification		Apgar score	Heart rate/ respiration/min.	Clinical terminology
I	Normal	8–10	120	Unremarkable neonate
II	Moderate depression	5–7	80–120; irregular respiration	Asphyxia livida
III	Severe depression	0–4	<80; absent or gasping respirations	Asphyxia pallida

In addition to the Apgar score and pH measurements of umbilical blood, heelstick pH <7.10 15–30 min postpartum is interpreted as a sign of neonatal asphyxia [4].

1.4 Primary Care and Resuscitation

Every delivery room must be equipped for the diagnostic and therapeutic needs of newborn infants (e.g., surgical instruments, incubator, resuscitation table with a radiant warmer; laboratory: blood count, blood gas analysis, bilirubin, blood sugar). Based on our own experience, the Ohio neonatal intensive care radiant warmer offers particular advantages in the acute treatment of high-risk newborns, owing to its versatility, roominess, good access, ease of visibility, servocontrolled thermoregulation, X-ray cassette, capability for Trendelenburg's and Fowler's positions, connections for oxygen, air, and vacuum, suction apparatus, and audible and visual high-low temperature alarm.

Primary resuscitation cannot be improvised! Its success depends upon thorough preparation for every contingency in the delivery room *before* birth:

a) Checking resuscitation equipment for completeness and working order
b) Presence of experienced personnel
c) Systematic procedure based on a protocol
d) A clock with audible time signals should be used.

Technique of Primary Lung Expansion. The lungs are expanded by applying a peak inspiratory pressure of 25–30 cm H_2O for 10–15 s during the first four to five breaths. Higher pressures can lead to focal overexpansion [20, 24]. After expansion is achieved, but no later than after the first five respiratory cycles, the peak inspiratory pressure is limited to 15–20 cm H_2O, and an inspiratory-expiratory ratio of 1 : 2–1 : 1 is set (for special form of ventilation for respiratory distress syndrome, see p 113).

This ventilation technique can also be performed by bag and mask (Penlon, Ambu). If spontaneous respiration is not established, intubation and mechanical ventilation are necessary (Tables 6, 7).

Technique of External Cardiac Massage. If there is no heart beat, or the heart rate is 50 or less, with no response to intravenous or intracardial injection of orciprenaline and calcium gluconate, external cardiac massage is performed: The thorax is grasped with both hands, while the thumbs press the midsternum toward the spinal column (Fig. 1). Three ventilation cycles with 100% oxygen are followed by 15 cardiac compressions. Cardiac compression rate: 80–100/min; ventilation cycles: 25–30/min.

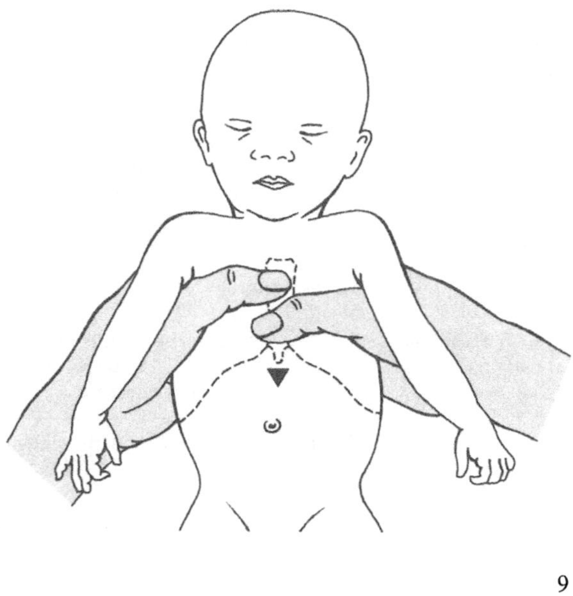

Fig. 1. External cardiac massage of the newborn infant

Table 6. Procedure according to clinical classification. *Avoid heat loss*! Use overhead radiant heater!

Class I	Airways are suctioned and kept clear
Class II	First oropharyngeal, then nasal suctioning (beware of vagal stimulation); administration of oxygen by mask (Penlon). Intubation and endotracheal suctioning only for inadequate pulmonary ventilation based upon thoracic excursion (retractions immediately after birth, inadequate inspiration), suspected laryngeal malformations with airway obstruction. Buffer administration (puncture of umbilical vein, catheterization)
Class III	Orotracheal suctioning under direct visualization, intubation, ventilation, specific therapy (e. g., orciprenaline, buffer administration, volume replacement), cardiac massage

Table 7. Medications commonly used for resuscitation

Medication	Indication	Dosage
Sodium bicarbonate 8.4%	Severe metabolic acidosis	3 mEq/kg IV via umbilical vein; use only in 1 : 1 mixture with 5% glucose. Infusion time should be at least 2 min[a]
Orciprenaline	Severe bradycardia	0.1 mg/dose (0.2 ml IV or intracardiac)
Calcium gluconate 10%	Severe bradycardia	1 mg/kg IV or intracardiac (do not mix with bicarbonate!)
Human albumin 20%	Severe shock	10 ml/kg IV by infusion
Dextran 40 Na-free	Shock with peripheral vasoconstriction	3–7 ml/kg by infusion
Dextran 60	Hypovolemia	5–10 ml/kg by infusion
Glucose 10%	Hypoglycemia	4 ml/kg IV (low birth weight infants, hypoglycemia suspected from Dextrostix findings)
Levallorphan	Depression due to maternal use of Dolantin	0.1–0.25 mg/kg/(IM or IV; repeat as needed)
Furosemide	Severe edema, pulmonary edema	1 mg/kg IV
Digoxin	Cardiac insuffiency	0.03 mg/kg/day, half immediately, half after 12 h; maintenance dose 0.005–0.01 mg/kg/day
Phytomenadione (vitamin K_1)	Prematurity, infants of clinical class II/III, suspected hemorrhagic disease	1 mg/kg IM

[a] The risk of cerebral hemorrhage depends on the volume, concentration and rate of the $NaHCO_3$ infusion!

The practical management of the newborn can be summarized as follows:

1. 1–5 min postpartum
   - Cord is clamped and cut; cord blood pH is measured, while blood samples are drawn from the placental portion of the cord for infant blood typing, direct Coombs' test and serology
   - Airways are suctioned, cleared, and kept clear
   - Stomach contents are aspirated: impaired passage → esophageal atresia. Stomach contents > 20 ml: atresia in upper gastrointestinal region
   - Condition is assessed: Apgar score, blood gas analysis, blood pressure, $tcPO_2$
   - Clinical classification is made with institution of necessary measures
   - Further continuous clinical and instrumental supervision (oxygen cardiorespirogram, Dextrostix, hematocrit) if necessary.

2. After adaptation or resuscitation (about 10 min postpartum)
   - Temperature is checked (patency of anus and rectum)
   - Nasal patency is checked by passing nasal catheter (choanal atresia). Credé's eye prophylaxis is administered (1% $AgNO_3$)
   - Vitamin K is given (preterm infants, class II and III infants, or suspected hemorrhagic disease of the newborn).

3. Initial examination in the delivery room
   - Quality of intrauterine growth
   - Capability for postnatal adaptation
   - Absence or presence of fetal/neonatal disease symptoms or syndromes
   - Suspicion or presence of malformations (Fig. 2, s. S. 12).

1.5 Assessment of Gestational Age

1.5.1 Definitions [25]

Neonatal Period. First-28th day of life (1st–7th day, early neonatal period; 8th–28th day, late neonatal period).

Perinatal Period. Twentieth-eighth week of gestation through the 7th full day of life.

Gestational Age. Age timed from the 1st day of the last normal menstrual period. If in rare cases the date of conception is known, but not the last menstrual period, the gestational age is timed from the date of conception, plus 14 days.

Maturity. The full degree of development of a neonate following a normal pregnancy, which enables it to make the normal transition from an intrauterine to extrauterine existence [10].

Maturity is dependent on gestational age of the infant and other factors (e.g., biologic variation) and encompasses morphological and functional criteria [10].

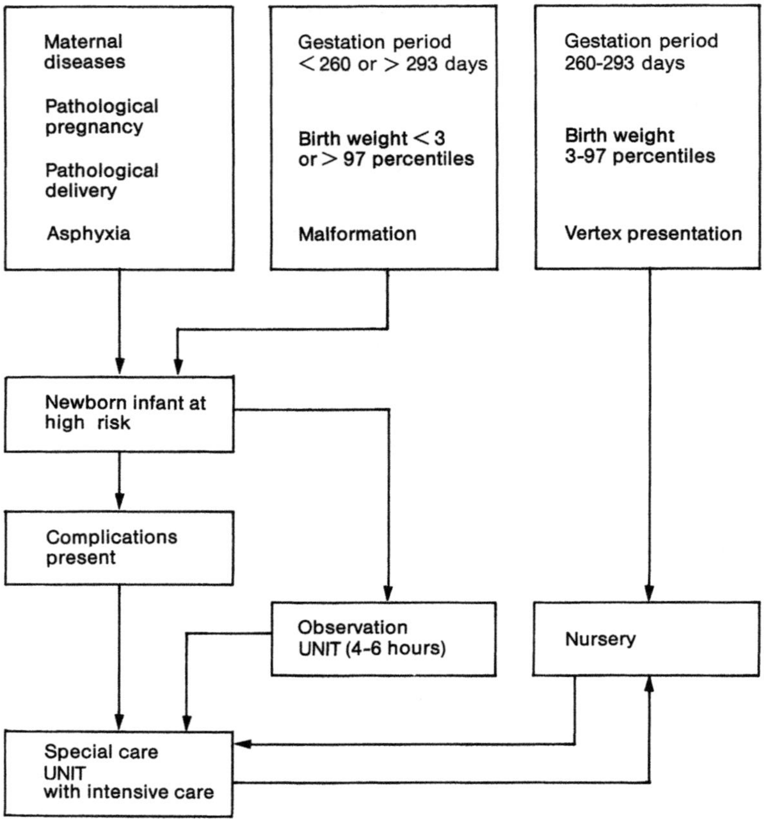

Fig. 2. Postpartum management of high-risk infants (see Prod'hom, 1972 [17])

Preterm Infant. Gestational age <260 days (<37 weeks).

Term Infant. Gestational age 260–293 days (37–41 weeks).

Postterm Infant. Gestational age >293 days (>41 weeks).

The following definitions are based on the relation between birth weight and gestational age:

Appropriate-for-Gestational-Age (*AGA*) *Infant.* Infant with a birth weight between the 3rd and 97th percentile [23 a].

Small-for-Gestational-Age (*SGA*) *Infant.* Infant with a birth weight <3rd percentile.

Large-for-Gestational-Age (*LGA*) *Infant.* Infant with a birth weight >97th percentile.

1.5.2 Requirements for Assessment of Gestational Age [11, 12]

The assessment of gestational age must:
- Be in good agreement with obstetric data (Nägele's rule, ultrasound measurement: biparietal)
- Be simple to perform
- Be done without injury to sick infants
- Be independent of the infant's state of health
- Be based on precisely defined criteria
- Have multi-examiner reliability.

Based on years of personal experience, we believe these conditions are best met by Finnström's clinical criteria for assessing the gestational age [8].

1.5.3 Criteria for Assessment of Gestational Age

Breast Tissue (Diameter). The horizontal diameter is measured bilaterally with a centimeter rule, and the largest diameter is registered. The circumference of the palpable and measurable breast tissue increases with gestational age.

Nipple Formation. Estimated by inspection. As gestational age increases, the mamilla becomes more clearly demarcated from the surrounding skin, and the areola becomes raised about its edge above the general skin level.

Skin Opacity. Estimated by inspection of the trunk. The transparency of the skin of the trunk, especially in the region of the abdomen above the navel, is observed, and the number and distinctness of large and small blood vessels are recorded.

Scalp Hair. Examined by inspection. As gestational age increases, the hair loses its cotton-wool quality; it becomes thicker, with individual strands of hair.

Ear Cartilage. Both auricles are palpated in order to determine the distribution of cartilage. In case of lateral disparity, the "more mature" ear is taken (Fig. 3). Palpable auricular cartilage is found first at the tragus and antitragus. The helix and anthelix are felt as flaps of skin in very immature preterm infants; the cartilaginous lamellae, while present, are extremely delicate and as yet impalpable. By the 32nd week of pregnancy a distinct cartilaginous framework is present and is most easily detected by compressing the anthelix in a longitudinal direction, thus giving rise to elastic resistance. The helical cartilage develops from the ventral and caudal directions (see *arrows*). When it is also palpable in the dorsal and cranial quadrants, it is considered that a complete cartilaginous framework is present [10].

Fingernails. The fingernails are inspected and the fingertip palpated by stroking or scratching the nail over the hand of the examiner. "In the very immature fetus the curve of the fingertips may be so slight that the extremely thin, almost skin-like nails, appear almost to reach the tips. Thus, two maturity points may be assigned when the nail reaches the fingertips and when the margin of the nail is distinct" [10].

Plantar Skin Creases. The sole of the foot is inspected. Only the relatively broad creases are analyzed. Fine superficial lines may be present, especially if the skin is dry, but usually disappear if the sole is stretched from toes to heel.
The creases become more marked with increasing gestational age, and their posterior distribution increases (Fig. 4 a–c) (Table 8 a, b).

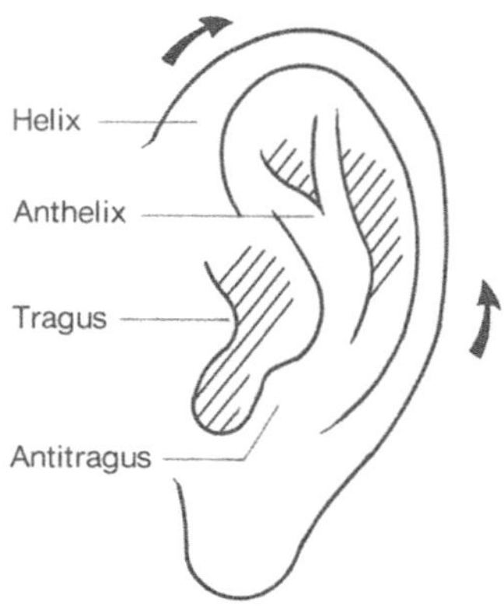

Fig. 3. Development of the auricular cartilage (after v. Harnack, 1971 [10])

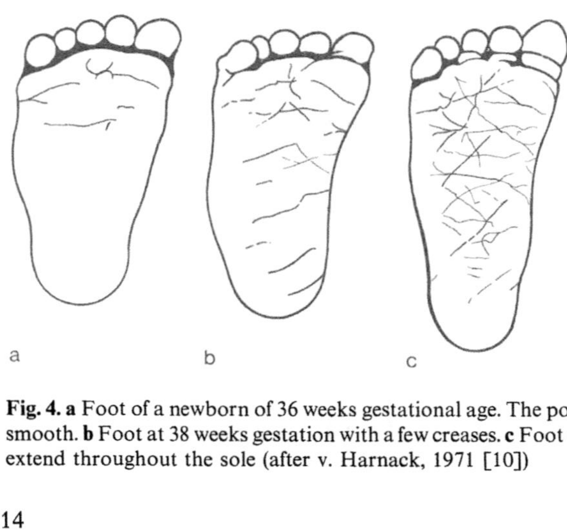

Fig. 4. a Foot of a newborn of 36 weeks gestational age. The posterior three-fourths of the foot is smooth. **b** Foot at 38 weeks gestation with a few creases. **c** Foot at 40 weeks gestation. The creases extend throughout the sole (after v. Harnack, 1971 [10])

Table 8 a. Assessment of the gestational age [8]

Clinical features	1	2	3	4
Skin opacity	Numerous veins, tributaries, and venules are clearly seen, particularly over the abdomen	Veins and tributaries are seen	A few large blood vessels are clearly seen over the abdomen	A few large blood vessels are indistinctly seen over the abdomen, or no blood vessels are seen.
Ear cartilage	No cartilage is felt in antitragus	Cartilage is felt in antitragus	Cartilage is present in anthelix	Cartilage formation is completed in helix
Plantar skin creases	No skin creases are present	Anterior transverse creases only are present	Occasional creases are seen on the anterior two-thirds of the sole	The whole sole is covered with creases, i.e., also the heel
Breast size Nipple formation	Below 5 mm Nipple barely visible, no areola	5–10 mm Nipple well defined, areola present but not raised	More than 10 mm Nipple well defined, edge of the areola raised above the skin	
Fingernails	Nails do not reach the finger tips	Nails reach the finger tips	Nails reach or pass the fingertips, distal edge of the nail is distinct and relatively firm	
Scalp hair	Hair fine, woolly, or fuzzy. Individual strands difficult to distinguish	Hair coarse and silky. Each hair appears as a single strand		

Table 8 b. Calculation of the gestational age [9]

Maturity score (Seven criteria)	Gestational age (days)	Weeks
7	191	27+2
8	198	28+2
9	204	29+1
10	211	30+1
11	217	31
12	224	32
13	230	32+6
14	237	33+6
15	243	34+5
16	250	34+5
17	256	36+4
18	263	37+4
19	269	38+3
20	276	39+3
21	282	40+2
22	289	41+2
23	295	42+1

1.6 Intrauterine Growth Curves [22] (Fig. 5 a–d)

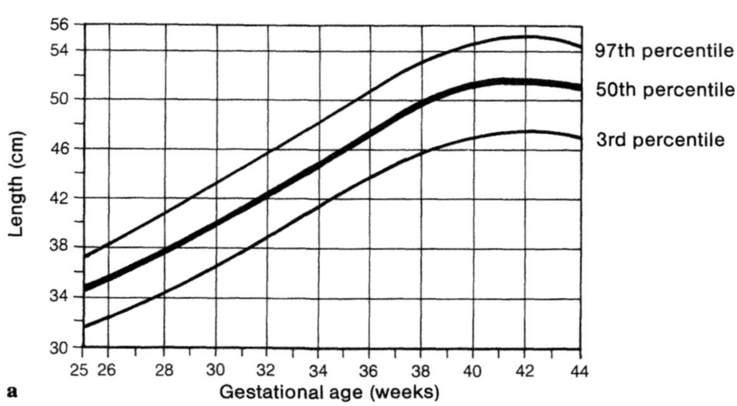

a

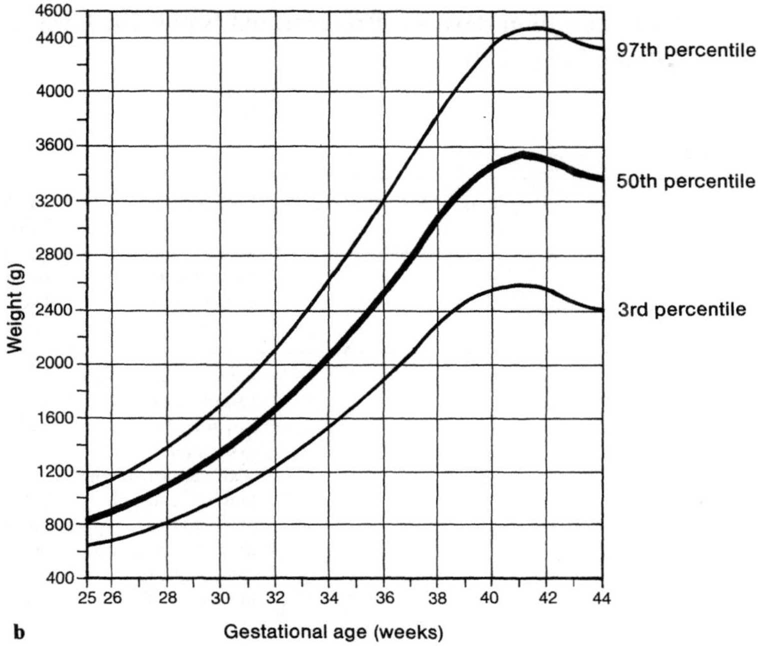

b

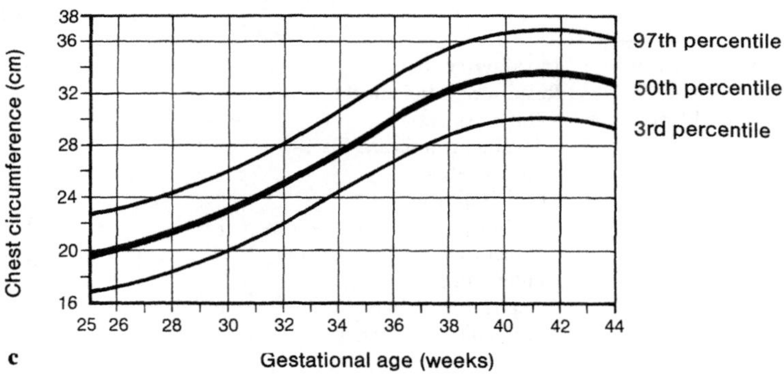

c

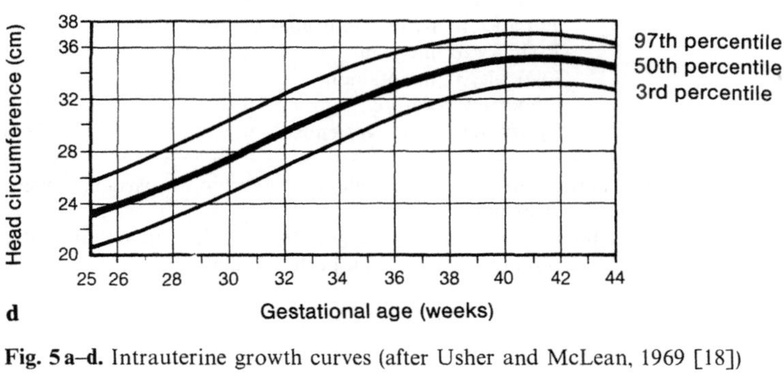

d

Fig. 5a–d. Intrauterine growth curves (after Usher and McLean, 1969 [18])

1.7 Differentiation Between Preterm and Small-for-Gestational-Age Infants [18] (Table 9)

Table 9

	Problems	Preterm baby	Small-for-dates baby
Definition		Born before 37 weeks' gestation	Birth weight below 10th percentile for gestational age
Etiology		Cause of early birth usually unknown, but may be associated with cervical incompetence, multiple pregnancy, antepartum hemorrhage, or early induction of labor	1. Impaired fetal growth potential with or without congenital malformation. 2. Intrauterine undernutrition, possibly due to placental insufficiency
Cause of problems		Immaturity	Often intrauterine undernutrition
Frequency of occurrence of problems	Intrauterine hypoxia	+	+ + +
	Respiratory difficulties:		
	Birth asphyxia	+	+ + +
	Hyaline membrane disease	+ + +	0
	Apneic attacks	+ + +	+
	Feeding difficulties:		
	Inability to suck or swallow	+ + +	0
	Functional obstruction and enterocolitis	+ +	+ +
	Aspiration of feeds	+ +	+
	Intracranial hemorrhage:		
	Intraventricular	+ + +	0
	Subdural	+	+
	Jaundice (hyperbilirubinemia)	+ + +	+
	Liability to infection	+ + +	+ +
	Difficulty in maintaining body temperature	+ + +	+ +
	Symptomatic hypoglycemia	+	+ + +

The plus signs indicate the relative likelihood of developing particular problems in the two kinds of low-birth-weight baby:
+ + +, Very common; + +, Fairly common; +, A little more common than in the normal term baby; and 0, No more common than in the normal term baby

1.8 Determining the Stage of Dysmaturity [23 b]

Table 10

	Placental insufficiency[a]		
	Acute	Subacute	Chronic
Mechanism	Impairment of respiratory function predominant	Impairment of nutritive function predominant	
Rate of outset	Rapid	Fairly slow	Slow
Intensity	Variable	Medium	Severe
Weight gain	Slightly retarded	Slightly/considerably retarded	Considerably retarded
Growth in stature	Normal	Normal	Considerably retarded
Cerebral growth	Normal	Normal	Slightly retarded
Appearance of newborn	Thin; desquamation of skin; meconial staining	Thin, long with large head	Small, short, with relatively large head
Neonatal complications	Asphyxia; respiratory distress, postasphyxial syndrome with inhalation of amniotic (meconial) fluid	Hypoglycemia (the higher the head: birth weight ratio, the more serious the hypoglycemia)	
		Hypothermia	

[a] The different forms of placental insufficiency may occur in various combinations

1.9 Main Symptoms During the First Days of Life [13]

Respiratory difficulties
Cyanosis or pallor
Early or pronounced jaundice
Conspicuous, nonphysiologic skin eruptions
Rectal temperatures $>37.5°$ C
Constant subnormal rectal temperature $<36.5°$ C
Pyoderma, umbilical, or other infections
Hemorrhage or edema

Vomiting
Distended or severely retracted abdomen
Impaired urination or defecation
Feeding difficulties
Apathy, hyperexcitability, convulsions, tremors, jitteriness
Birth injuries
Bulging of the fontanel.

References

1. APGAR, V.: A proposal for a new method of evaluation of the newborn infant. Curr. Res. Anesth. *32*, 4 (1953)
2. BANCALERI, E., BERLIN, J. A.: Meconium aspiration and other asphyxial disorders. Clin. Perinatal. *5* (2), 317 (1978)
3. BERENDES, H. W.: Cerebrale Spätschäden nach perinataler Asphyxie. Gynäkologie *1*, 89 (1968)
4. BRETSCHER, J., SALING, E.: pH values in the human fetus during labor. Amer. J. Obstet. Gynec. *97*, 906 (1967)
5. DRAGE, J. S., BERENDES, H. W.: Apgar score and outcome of the newborn. Pediatr. Clin. North. Am. *13*, 635 (1966)
6. DRAGE, J. S., KENNEDY, C., BERENDES, H., SCHWARZ, B. K., WEISS, W.: The Apgar score as an index of infant mortality. Develop. Med. Child. Neurol. *8*, 141 (1966)
7. EIDELMAN, A. B., HOBBS, J. F.: Bicarbonate therapy revisited. Am. J. Dis. Child. *132*, 847 (1978)
8. FINNSTRÖM, O.: Studies on maturity in newborn infants. II External characteristics. Acta Paediat. Scand. *61*, 24 (1972)
9. FINNSTRÖM, O.: Studies on maturity in newborn infants. IX Further observations on the use of external characteristics in estimating gestational age. Acta Paediatr. Scand. *66*, 601 (1977)
10. v. HARNACK, G.-A.: Kennzeichen mangelnder Reife. In: Handbuch der Kinderheilkunde. OPITZ, H., SCHMID, F. (ed.), Band 1/2, S. 333. Berlin-Heidelberg-New-York: Springer 1971
11. JÜRS, G.: Die Zweckmäßigkeit der Gestationsalterbestimmung mittels Ultraschall in der Frühschwangerschaft. Inaugural-Dissertation, Heidelberg, 1977
12. KEMMER, A.: Bestimmung des Gestationsalters an reifen Neugeborenen nach der Methode von FINNSTRÖM. Inaugural-Dissertation, Heidelberg, 1977
13. KEUTH, U.: Probleme der Erfassung und Versorgung von Risikokindern einschließlich Frühgeborener, pädiat. prax. *13*, 29 (1973/74)
14. LITSCHGI, M.: Neonatale Depression ohne intrauterine Azidose Z. Geburtshilfe. Perinatol. *181*, 329 (1978)
15. LOU, H. C., LASSEN, N. H., FRIIS-HANSEN, B.: Low cerebral flow in hypotensive perinatal distress. Acta Neurol. Scand. *56*, 343, (1977)
16. PAXSON, Ch. L.: Neonatal shock in the first day. Am. J. Dis. Child. *132*, 509 (1978)
17. PROD'HOM, L. S.: Die Erkrankungen des Fetus und Neugeborenen. In: Lehrbuch der Pädiatrie. FANCONI, G. (Hrsg.). S. 343. Basel-Stuttgart: Schwabe 1972
18. ROBINSON, R. R.: The pre-term body. Brit. med. J. *4*, 416 (1971)
19. SCHACHINGER, H.: Das Sauerstoff-Kardiorespirogramm, technische Grundlagen und klinische Bedeutung bei der Überwachung Neugeborener. Med. Tech. *99*, 16 (1979)
20. STOLL, W.: Die primäre Reanimation des Neugeborenen. Stuttgart: Enke, 1975
21. SWYER, R. P.: The organization of perinatal care with particular reference to the newborn. In: Neonatology. AVERY, G. B. (ed.). p. 15 Philadelphia-Toronto: Lipincott 1975

22. USHER, R., MCLEAN, F.: Intrauterine growth of live-born caucasian infants at sea level: Standards obtained from measurements in 7 dimensions of infants born between 25 and 44 weeks of gestational. J. Pediat. *74*, 901 (1969)
23 a. WHO: The prevention of perinatal mortality. Public health paper Nr. *42*, p. 47, Geneva 1972
23 b. loc. cit., p. 46
24. WOLFART, M., LOSKANT, G.: Primärversorgung des Neugeborenen. Dtsch. Ärztebl. *72*, 503 (1975)
25. Working party to discuss nomenclature based on gestational age and birth weight. Proc. 2nd Europ. Congr. Perinatal Medicine, London 1970. p. 172. Basel: Karger 1971

2 Transport of High-Risk Newborns

L. Wille

2.1 Indications for Transfer

High-risk pregnancies and deliveries should be promptly referred to a tertiary care facility to provide optimal care utilizing all the facilities of modern perinatology. The fetus and newborn requiring treatment must rely upon a high level of cooperation among obstetrical and pediatric perinatologists [3, 4]. In some cases, unforeseen risks or complications may occur immediately before, during, or after the delivery which place the neonate in jeopardy. The condition of the mother during pregnancy or labor and unforeseen urgencies may make maternal transfer inadvisable. In such cases a safe, reliable means of transporting the compromised infant from the delivery room to the intensive care facility must be available [6]. The safe transport of newborns manifesting or with anticipated impairments of vital function requires special preparations. The professional expertise for such an undertaking is found in the realm of neonatal intensive medicine [4]. The goal of the transport of high-risk newborns is to extend the facilities of neonatal intensive medicine into the maternity clinic.

The following recommendations apply to the transport of high-risk newborns [6]:

- Term infants after primary resuscitation and intubation with Apgar 1′ <7, Apgar 5′ <6
- Preterm and term infants with cardiorespiratory problems (e. g., respiratory distress, cyanosis, cardiac insufficiency)
- Very immature preterm infants (<35 weeks gestation, <2000 g)
- Preterm and term Infants with anemia or symptoms of shock
- Preterm and term infants with neurologic impairment (e. g., convulsions, apnea, meningitis, hemorrhage)
- Infants of diabetic mothers, infants of preeclamptic mothers
- Preterm and term infants with malformations (e. g., diaphragmatic hernia, myelomeningocele, gastrointestinal atresias)
- SGA infants <2000 g.

2.2 Informations Prior to Transport

As a rule, the transport of high-risk newborns should be decided only by the responsible physicians at the clinics involved. The telephone numbers of the neonatal intensive care unit must be posted in the delivery rooms of the maternity clinics which it serves. It is essential that all pertinent information be given during telephone contact so that the receiving unit is fully briefed as to the situation:

- Single or multiple birth
- Apgar score at 1 and 5 min
- Birth weight, gestational age
- Predisposing risk factors (pregnancy, delivery)
- Current findings
- Ventilatory status
- Tentative diagnosis of the referring physician.

On the basis of these data, a rapid decision can be made on the urgency of the transport, the need for dispatching personnel and equipment, and necessary preparations at the intensive care unit [2]. Preliminary therapeutic measures can be discussed by telephone. In cases where doubt exists, transport should be undertaken. Until the transport personnel arrive, the infant remains under the care of the referring physician. A transport system for compromised infants in no way lessens the responsibility of the maternity clinic (personnel, equipment) for primary resuscitation [3]!

2.3 Organization and Conduct of the Transport [2, 4, 6]

The conduct of an intensive-care transport depends upon the possibility of cooperation with local rescue services (Red Cross, fire department, etc.). The prime consideration is the rapid availability of the transport vehicle. An ambulance is generally used, but a helicopter may be employed in exceptional cases e. g., long distances, mountainous terrain). Travel time to the maternity clinic should not exceed 30–45 min [4]. Unhampered communication between the intensive care unit and transport service is essential. A doctor and nurse from the intensive care unit should be available for conducting the transport. The transport personnel must be well trained in primary resuscitation, possess adequate skills in the clinical evaluation, supervision, and treatment of high-risk newborns, and be experienced in the transport of sick infants.

On arrival at the maternity clinic, the accompanying personnel assume the responsibility for the infant and for transport preparations. The referring physician must orient them with regard to the course of the pregnancy and delivery, the status of the infant and any therapeutic measures already taken. Based on the findings of a thorough examination, a therapeutic plan is formed. The rectal temperature and blood glucose ((Dextrostix) are checked. A blood gas analysis is performed when possible, and the blood count and hematocrit are determined if necessary. An infusion of 10% glucose via a peripheral vein or the umbilicial vein should be started. When in doubt the infant should be intubated and ventilated before transport is begun to avoid incidents during transit. Nasotracheal intubation is advantageous owing to its stable placement. A gastric tube is used to remove air and fluid from the stomach. The goal of all preliminary measures is to stabilize the cardiorespiratory status of the infant prior to transport, or to improve it to the extent that transport can be undertaken with minimal risk.

Prior to transport the parents are informed about their infant's illness and the necessity of transferring it to a special care unit. It is advisable to maintain telephone contact with the intensive care unit to keep abreast of clinical development.

During transport, the condition of the infant is continuously monitored by clinical observation (skin color, peripheral circulation, pallor, cutis marmorata, cold extremities, sweating, and respiration rate). Facilities should be available for both the audible and visual recoding of the heart rate, mechanical ventilation, continuous monitoring of body temperature and $tcPO_2$. If trained personnel are present, the transport can be carried out slowly and atraumatically.

A written record of data on the course of the pregnancy and the delivery is essential for the complete evaluation of the infant at the intensive care unit. Ten-ml specimens of maternal and umbilical cord blood, properly labeled, must accompany the infant for serologic and blood-type analysis of the mother and infant.

A transport record should be kept which details all diagnostic and therapeutic measures taken before and during transport. It should begin with the date and time of referral and conclude with admission to the ICU [4, 6] and is included in the infant's medical records.

2.4 Equipment of a Mobile Intensive Care Unit

All transfer of high-risk infants require facilities for close clinical observation, constant electronic monitoring, and intensive-therapeutic measures. Accordingly, the transport vehicle, transport incubator, and accessory equipment must form a functional unit and must be adapted to traffic conditions [4].

Based on recommendations of the Study Group on Neonatal Transport and Resuscitation [1], the vehicle must be equipped in accordance with the transport requirements of critically ill infants (Table II, Fig. 6).

It is economocally unfeasible to outfit an ambulance specifically for neonatal use. It has proved practical therefore, to design the intensive-care transport incubator and its accessories so that they can operate independently of the vehicle. The mobile intensive care unit used by us is described in Table 12 [5]:

Table 11. Equipment of the infant transport ambulance

Two 12-V automobile batteries, connected in parallel
Adequate interior lighting
Electric ventilation system
Interior heating, independent of engine
Adjustable suction device
Mount for securing transport incubator
Battery hookup for transport incubator
Working area for two persons
Working surface with radiant heater
Standard built-in cabinets with accessory materials
Wash basin
Disinfectant dispenser
Tower dispenser
Waste receptacle
Safety belts for accompanying personnel

Special measures are necessary when the transport is performed by helicopter or aircraft:
Call civilian or military flight dispatcher
Clear landing site, prepare empty vehicle
Protect personnel from noise (ear muffs)
Use monitor in helicopter, since auscultation is impossible
Take extra measures against radiant heat loss (aluminum swaddler)
Infuse fluids only by pump or syringe, not by drip (due to vibration)
Use flexible venous catheters
Check cabin pressure (expansion of trapped gas, decreased oxygen tension).

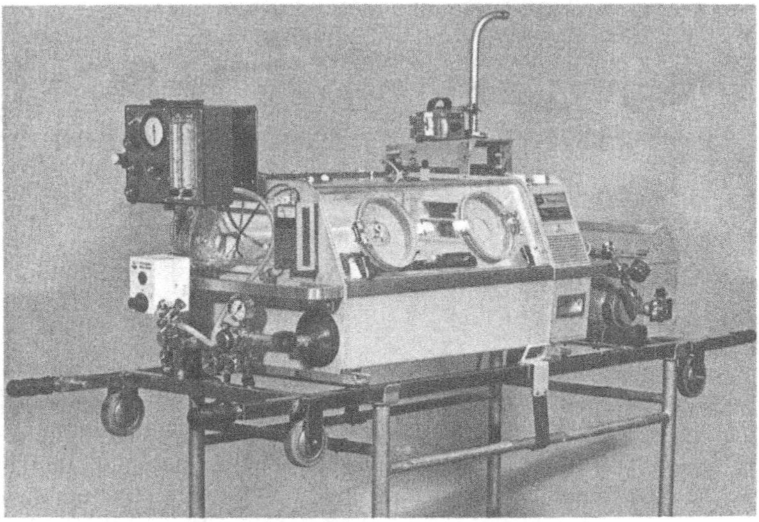

Fig. 6. Mobile intensive care unit for the transport of high-risk neonates

Table 12. Equipment of the mobile intensive care unit[a]

1. Incubator
Ohio Transport Incubator with battery, mounted on a standard litter.
Operation: 220 V, 50 Hz; 12 V/24 V; 12-V output for monitoring equipment.
Vital support unit: Thermostatically controlled heater, overheat protection, blower and control unit. The gas mixture is warmed in the heating unit, filtered, humidified (40–60 r. h.) and vented into the incubator.
Oxygen supply: Two inlets, one for up to 40%, one for up to 100%; slide-in rack for O_2 cylinder.
Access: Tilt-up Plexiglas hood with two iris entry ports and a large head-access door.
IV pole
Mount for respirator
Securing devices for travel: Restraining straps, hood latch, clamps on mobile stand
2. Monitoring equipment
Visicard-8 ECG Monitor, independent of main electrical system with connecting cable for 12-V power supply and patient cable, equipped with audible and visual signal: mounted on the vital support unit. Battery-tcPO_2-unit (Roche, Draeger).
3. Respirator
Cavitron Model PV-10 pediatric ventilator with oxygen blender; this unit has CPAP, IPPV with or without PEPP, and IMV capability); brackets to mount on incubator. Penlon bag with Rendell-Baker masks (Nos. 0 and 1) for manual ventilation in the incubator.
4. Infusions therapy
Battery-Injectomat 50 (Fa. Fresenius) with nickel-cadmium battery (internal supply for about 8 h) and charger for 220-V power source, equipped with 50-ml syringe and infusion set (infusion rate 1 ml/h–100 ml/h); attached to the vital support unit.
Other accessory equipment
One 4-l steel oxygen cylinder
One 5-l steel air cylinder mounted on the litter
One oxygen reducing valve: one high-pressure manometer, one flowmeter, two exhausts with regulating valve (Weinmann).
One suction device: Draeger-Laerdal jet suction unit
One oxygen analyzer: Draeger-Bio Marine

[a] The mobile intensive care unit is checked daily with the aid of a checklist for operational readiness

2.5 Contents of the Emergency Kit

Essential to the successful conduct of an intensive-care transport is a complete array of accessory equipment corresponding to the medical needs of the critically ill newborn. For this purpose we employ two emergency kits which contain everything needed for intubation, ventilation, infusion therapy, and umbilical vessel characterization, as well as the most important medications [3, 4, 6]. This kit makes the accompanying personnel independent of the varying resources of different maternity hospitals and enables them to administer intensive therapy during transit (Table 13).

Table 13. Transport equipment (emergency kit)

I. Medications
Glucose 5%, 20%
Sodium bicarbonate 8.4%
Orciprenaline
Calcium gluconate 10%
Furosemide
Digoxin
Diazepam
Phenobarbital
Phytomenadione
Pyridoxine
Prednisolone
Heparin
Levallorphan
Alcuroniumdichloride
Chloral hydrate (supp.)
Atropine
Verapamil
Pethidine
Clonazepam
Dopamine

II. Infusions
Glucose 5%, 10%
Dextran 40, Na-free
Dextran 60
NaCl 0.9%
Aqua bidest.
Human albumin 5%, salt-poor

III. Resuscitation/intubation
Negus laryngoscope, ∅ 18 mm
Negus blade, 75 mm
Negus blade, 105 mm
Spare batteries
Spare bulbs
Magill infant forceps
Bacterial filters
Infusion set
Leukoflex, 1.25/2.5 cm
Leukoplast, 1.25/5 cm
Elastic bandages, 4 cm
Elastoplast, 6 cm
Narrow arm splint
Plaster bandage
Ampule files
Single-use scalpel, lancets
Surgical gloves, sizes 7/8
Surgical smock
Steri drape, 40 × 40 cm
Catgut 2-0
Ethibond 3-0
Centimeter rule (metal)
Guedel tubes no. 0/00/000
Xylocaine gel 2%
Silicone spray

IV. Umbilical vessel catheter set
Umbilical vessel catheters Fr 3.5/5
Sterile surgical set

V. Ascites puncture set
Trocar catheter Fr 12 (Argyle)
Sterile surgical set

VI. Pneumothorax set
Trocar catheter Fr 10 (Argyle)
Two-way suction valve (Heimlich type)
Sterile surgical set

VII. Miscellaneous
Hand disinfectant
Skin disinfectant
Aluminium swaddler
Injection needles no. 1/17
Perfusion set 25/23
Abboven no. 16/18
Medicat G 22
Syringes: Tuberculin, 2, 5 and 20 ml
Luer-Record adapter
Marking tape, 1 cm (red and blue)
Clamps for arterial catheters
Antibiotic powder
Dextrostix
Exchange transfusion set
Urine collecting system
Blood culture medium
Table for umbilical catheter tube length
Thermometer (metal case)
Stopwatch
Flashlight
Cuff fixation
Fibrin plate

2.6 Measures Following Transport

After arrival at the intensive care unit, the temperature of the transport incubator is determined, the infant's boy temperature is measured, a blood gas analysis is performed, and the blood glucose is tested. The quality of the transport can be judged by these parameters.

References

1. AHNEFELD, F. W., EWERBECK, H., SALING, E.: Neugeborenen-Notfallwagen. Zusatzausrüstungen für Notarztwagen zur Versorgung von Neugeborenen. In: Perinatale Medizin Bd. IV, S. 413. Dudenhausen, J. W., Saling, E. (Hrsg.) Stuttgart: Thieme 1973
2. Bossi, E.: Notfalltransporte von Neugeborenen. Schweiz. med. Wschr. *105*, 1210 (1975)
3. DANGEL, P.: Der Transport von Risiko-Neugeborenen. Pädiat. Fortbk. Praxis, *41*, 59 (1975)
4. LEMBURG, P.: Der Transport von Neugeborenen. Z. Geburtsh. und Perinat. *180*, 375 (1976)
5. WILLE, L., OBLADEN, M., SCHLUNK, P., WEISSER, J.: Mobile Intensivpflegeeinheit für den Transport gefährdeter Früh- und Neugeborener. 1. Technische Mitteilung. Mschr. Kinderheil. *123*, 49 (1975)
6. WILLE, L., WEISSER, J.: Zum Transport von Risikoneugeborenen. Z. Geburtsh. und Perinat. *180*, 388 (1976)

3 Patient Supervision

M. Obladen

The best "monitor" is the intelligent, concerned, and experienced nurse who is in constant attendance with the critically ill infant. She should be completely informed about the condition of the neonate for whom she is caring in regard to course of illness, physical findings, diagnosis, and therapeutic plans [8]. Besides caring for the infant and administering the prescribed therapy, her duties include observation of the infant and the documentation of changes in his condition. Only in her hands do the various electronic monitoring devices become valuable tools in the treatment of the critically ill neonate. The number and quality of the nursing staff are the limiting factors for all intensive care efforts [2]. A monitor does nothing of its own volition. It is both detached and uncritical, and it is not a labor-saving device.

In our opinion, a central monitoring system is of little value in pediatric intensive care: Monitor alarm and patient condition are not identical.

- At least half the alarms sounded by the monitor are artifactual in nature (due to crying or movement of the infant, faulty electrode contact, inadequate calibration of the device, etc,); thus, the nurse must still be present at the infant's bedside to determine whether the disturbance is patient or instrument related.
- When the alarm is "real," it is particularly important that the nurse react to the situation at the infant's bedside. Hence, the *only* surveillance method in pediatrics is *bedside monitoring.*

3.1 Pulse and Heart Rate

Range of variation. 70–170/min, depending on resting state. *But* a heart rate below 100 is almost always pathologic. Regardless of the absolute level of the heart rate, any rapid rise or fall in the heart rate is a warning sign.

Recording Method. R-wave analysis from the ECG [14]. The simultaneous, continuous display of the ECG on an oscilloscope screen makes it considerably easier to recognize instrument artifacts, faulty electrode contact, or artifacts resulting from the inclusion of a high T-wave. It also facilitates the recognition of electrolyte disturbances and cardiac arrhythmias.

Best Electrode Placement. Generally, left-precordial to obtain a high positive R-wave and flat T-wave. Extremity leads for continuous monitoring are used only if special cardiological problems are present. Pointer instruments usually give the nurse a better and faster idea of the level of readings than do devices with a digital display. We have found audible signals to be particularly useful. Even without looking at the monitor, the nurse is alerted to impending bradycardia long before the alarm threshold of the monitor is reached. The monitor should have an output for at least a single-channel recorder. The regular recording of the ECG trace with measurement of the PQ interval makes it much easier to digitalize the infant and also provides documentation for electrolyte disturbances and arrythmias. This can also be accomplished by using an oscilloscope with a "freeze" display capacity.

3.2 Variance of the Heart Rate

Within the framework of cardiorespirography (Fig. 1), the beat-to-beat variance of the heart rate represents a powerful new diagnostic technique in pediatric monitoring [18]. By simultaneously recording the respiratory curve, correlations can be established between cardiac and respiratory activity [17]. Combined with transcutaneous measurement of the PO_2 (oxygen-cardiorespirogram), this technique can quickly reveal almost any change in the infant's condition [12]. The variability of the

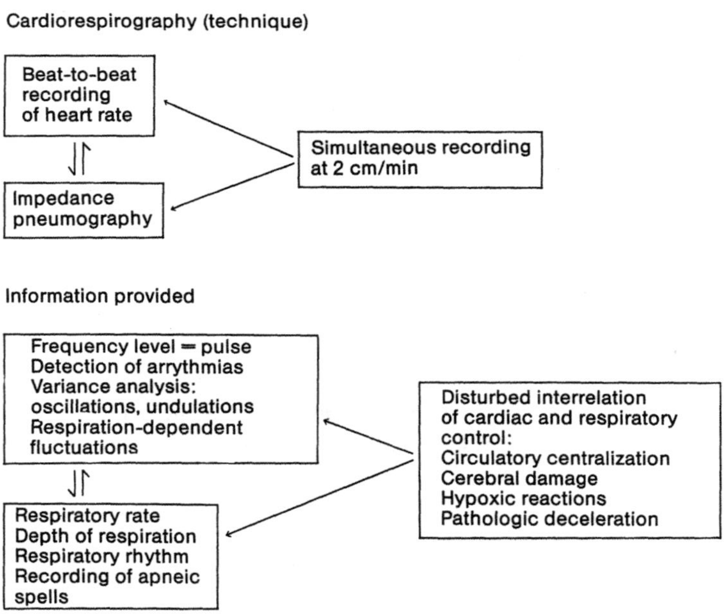

Fig. 7. Schematic representation of the recording technique of cardiorespirography and the information provided

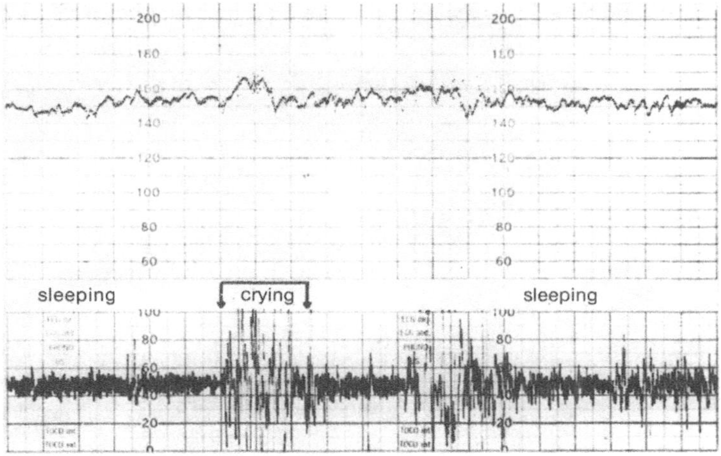

Fig. 8 a. Normal cardiorespirogram: 1400 g/31st week of gestation: 10th day of life. No respiratory difficulties, marked short-term variability and long-term variability of heart-rate. The heart rate increases during crying

heart rate is often diminished in seriously ill newborns with acidosis or circulatory centralization. Silent or sinusoidal curves, found in cerebral hemorrhage or cardiac decompensation (see p 34), imply a poor prognosis [4, 5] (Fig. 8 a–h).

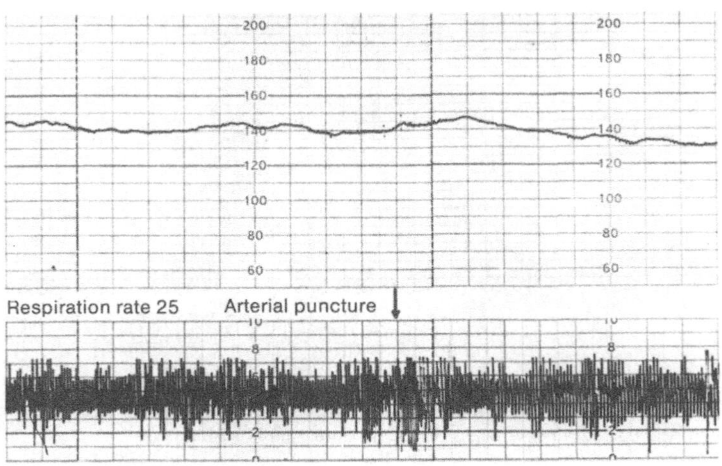

Fig. 8 b. Diminished heart-rate variability in early stage of respiratory distress syndrome: 920 g/28th week of gestation, 1st day of life. Controlled ventilation with FiO_2 0.6 at a rate of 25/min

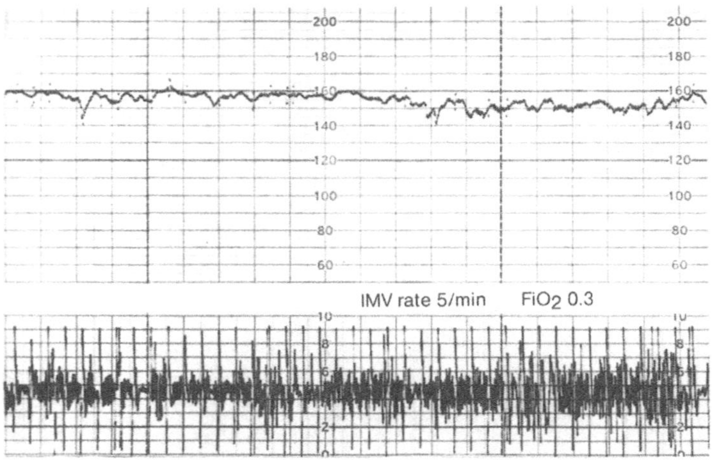

Fig. 8c. Near-normal variability in the IMV respiratory curve. Recovery stage of respiratory distress syndrome. Same infant as in Fig. 8 b.; 5th day of life, after clinical stabilization; FiO_2 0.3 and IMV at a rate of 5/min

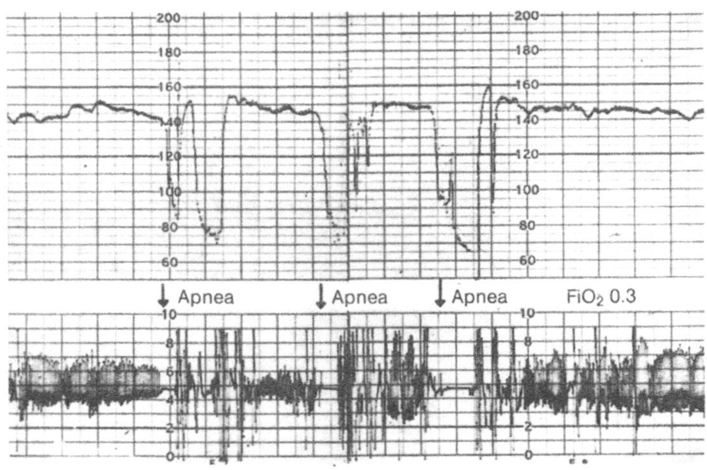

Fig. 8d. Apneic episodes in immature infant. Same infant as in Fig. 8 b.; 10th day of life, good general condition, spontaneous respiration; recording made 1 h after CPAP was withdrawn. The apneic episodes cease when the infant is manually stimulated

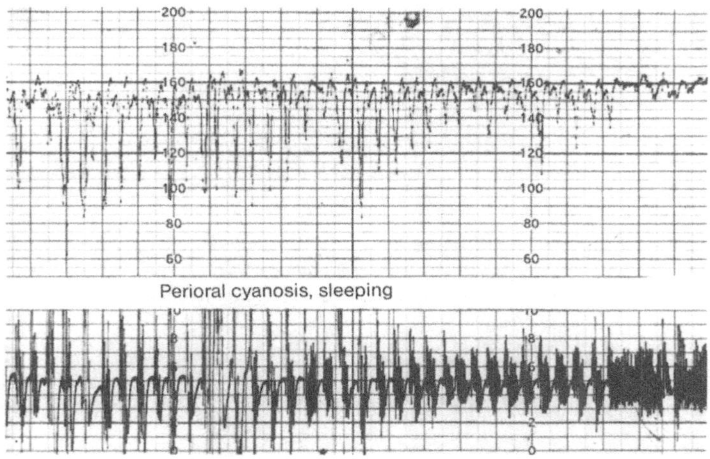

Fig. 8 e. Periodic respiration in the preterm infant. 1300 g/31st week of gestation, 28th day of life. Condition after RDS and recurrent pneumothorax. Brief, regular apneic episodes, with heart rate deceleration, which cease spontaneously

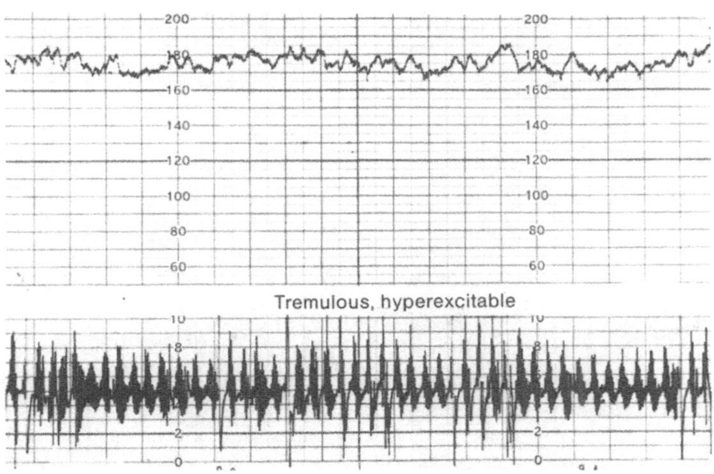

Fig. 8 f. Pathologic rhythm: Cheyne-Stokes respiration. 3500 g/39th week of gestation, 7th day of life. Meningitis from group B streptococci. Spasms, general hyperexcitability. The heart rate variability is normal

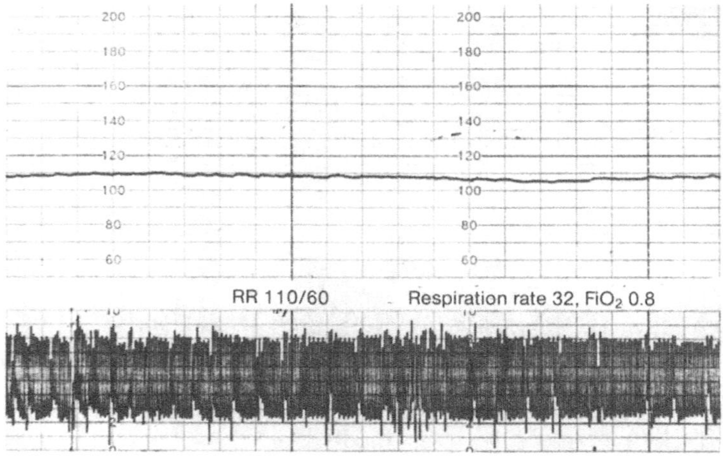

Fig. 8 g. Silent heart rate (no short- or long-term variability): 2890 g/40th week of gestation, 4 weeks old. Aortic isthmus stenosis, 5th postoperative day, condition 20 h after electrical defibrillations, "shock" kidney, oliguria

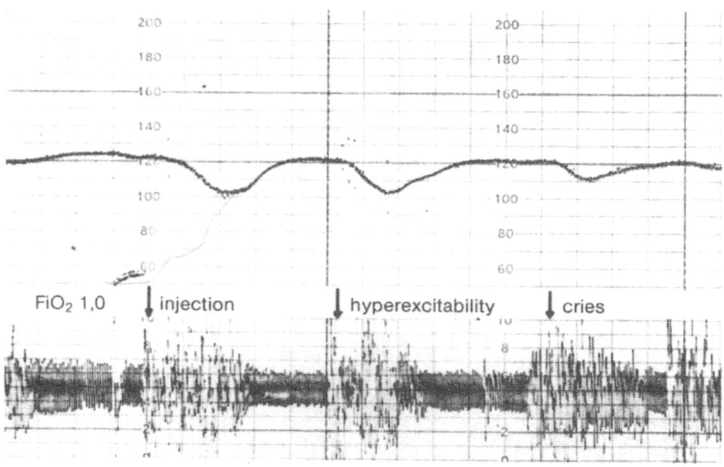

Fig. 8 h. Minimal or absent variability with sinusoidal deceleration during activity: 3850 g/39th week of gestation, 3rd day of life. Hypoplastic left-heart syndrome, controlled ventilation with FiO_2 1.0 Death occurred 1 day later

3.3 Respiration

There are two basic techniques of respiratory monitoring [14]:

1. Recording of respiratory gas movements
   - Differential thermistor at the nostrils (unsuitable for preterm infants in incubators)
   - Preheated sensor at the nostrils (responds to cooling; danger of burns).
2. Recording of respiratory movements.
   - Chambered air mattress with pressure sensor
   - Magnetic field induction (generation of electric current)
   - Impedance pneumography (changes in resistance).

We employ impedance pneumography exclusively at our clinic for monitoring the respiratory activity of newborns. The anterior axillary line at the level of the breasts has proved to be the most favorable electrode placement for preterm infants. The sensitivity of the impedance monitor should be adjusted so that a shallow breath is barely registered. If the setting is too low, there is a danger that thoracic movements associated with cardiac activity will also be recorded. The apnea alarm should be set to sound if breathing stops for more than 20 s. The normal respiration rate of the newborn is 40–60/min, with considerable fluctuations depending on the resting state. As with the heart rate, a rapid change in the respiration rate, especially an increase, is a more important warning sign than the absolute level.

Note. Switching off the monitor alarm is no substitute for proper calibration of the device!

3.4 Temperature

3.4.1 Servocontrol

In servocontrol systems the temperature is continuously measured by a skin electrode which is connected via a control switch to the incubator heating system or radiant heater. An alarm is necessary; there is a danger of overheating if the thermocouple becomes detached from the skin. Disadvantage: Fever may be overlooked in the septic infant.

3.4.2 Temperature Monitoring

The temperature is measured continuously by a skin or rectal probe. Continuous temperature monitoring is required for:

- Preterm infants below 1500 g, whose body temperature may fall if the incubator is opened
- Newborns with severe hypothermia below 34° C [10]
- Postoperative and septic states
- Prolonged states of shock.

3.4.3 Intermittent Manual Measurement

Much time is saved by using an electronic fever thermometer (IVAC 820, 821). However, such instruments have a lower temperature limit of only 33° or 34° C. For hypothermic preterm infants, the use of a special premature thermometer with an extended lower range is still required.

3.4.4 Incubator Temperature

The incubator temperature for seriously ill infants should correspond as closely as possible to the neutral temperature, that is, the temperature at which the infant's oxygen consumption and CO_2 production are lowest [10, 11]. The basal metabolism is lowest at an ambient temperature of 34°–36° C [16, 19]. The most favorable incubator temperatures for sick term and preterm infants are shown in Table 14. For preterm infants <1500 g, an additional plastic hood can be used in the incubator to prevent radiant heat loss.

Table 14. External temperature for the care of unclothed high-risk infants in incubators (modified from [21])

Birth weight	0–24 H	2nd–3rd day	4th–7th day	8 Days or more
<1500 g	34–36° C	33–35° C	33–34° C	32–33° C
1501–2000 g	33–34° C	33° C	33–32° C	32° C
2001–2500 g	33° C	32–33° C	32° C	32° C
>2500 g	32–33° C	32° C	31–32° C	31–30° C
Humidity	60–80%	50–60%	50%	50%
Measurement of infant's temperature	Every hour until stabilized between 36.5° and 37° C	8 times in 24 h	6 times in 24 h	4 times in 24 h

3.5 Blood Pressure

Blood pressure should be routinely measured in neonatal intensive care:
- On admission
- In states of shock
- During any unusual administration of parenteral fluids
- In cases of cardiac insufficiency (i. e., generally weak pulse) or
- During postoperative supervision.

The systolic blood pressure of the newborn is directly proportional to its gestational and postnatal age. Infants with respiratory distress syndrome and asphyxia often suffer from hypotension [1]. The blood pressure can be measured by the following various means

3.5.1 Flush Method [9]

After manual compression of the arm, a suitable cuff on the upper arm is quickly inflated to 100 mm Hg. The extremities are white. Now the cuff is slowly deflated; the pressure at which the arm suddenly turns red (flushes) is registered as the systolic blood pressure.

3.5.2 Detection of Pulse Waves or Vascular Movements with Ultrasound

(Arteriosonde, Infrasonde) Measured with an Inflatable Cuff
The transducer is located on the inside upper arm or the popliteal fossa. The value measured by the Doppler method correlates well with direct arterial measurements [3]. The proper cuff width for newborns is 2.5–4 cm, depending on the infant's size. A disparity between the arm and leg blood pressure, with a weak femoral pulse, is of diagnostic significance in aortic isthmus stenosis.

3.5.3 Direct Measurement

Done with an electronic pressure transducer (Statham), especially if an umbilical artery catheter is in place. Direct blood pressure monitoring of the newborn is not necessary as a matter of routine (Table 15, see p. 38).

Table 15. Normal arterial blood pressure values of newborns (Doppler method) (modified from [7] and [13])

Day of life	1	2	3	4	5	6	7	14	21
Preterm infants <2000 g Brachial artery	53/29	56/30	59/31	62/33	61/30	60/30	65/32	70/36	72/36
Preterm infants 2000–2500 g Brachial artery	57/28	61/31	64/32	68/37	68/36	69/34	71/37	70/34	72/31
Term infants Brachial artery	60/	65/	67/	69/	67/	74/	79/		
Term infants Popliteal artery	74/	78/	80/	80/	80/	88/	91/		

3.6 Central Venous Pressure

The normal range of the central venous pressure is 0–8 cm H_2O, but it can very considerably depending on cardiopulmonary status. The central venous pressure is elevated in the respiratory distress syndrome [6]. The indications for central venous pressure monitoring in neonatal intensive care are as follows:

- Hydrops fetalis
- Congenital heart disease and cardiogenic shock
- Postoperative supervision.

The central venous pressure can be measured by the following methods:

3.6.1 Umbilical Vein Catheter

Position in right atrium. The end of the open catheter is raised, and the level to which the fluid in the catheter rises or falls is measured.

3.6.2 Continuous Measurement with Electronic Pressure Transducer

(Statham, Hewlett-Packard 1280c). Particularly useful postoperatively. It is important that the zero of the instrument be checked regularly. The pressure transducer should be placed at the level of the xyphoid process for calibration. The calibration is rechecked hourly.

3.7 Computer-Assisted Patient Monitoring

Conventional monitors are designed to indicate situations in which a preset limit is reached, that is, to show that an acute situation already exists. By contrast, a continuous trend analysis of vital parameters by a process computer makes it possible to quickly recognize or even predict an impending problem. The necessary hardware is already available [22], and special infant monitoring programs are being tested and developed [23, 25]. The monitor provides the input data on vital parameters. Using a bedside video display terminal, the nurse or physician can interrogate the computer with regard to pertinent data, laboratory findings, and trends. This information is then displayed graphically on a viewing screen. We use the Hewlett Packard 5600 A automated monitoring system with 64 channels, disk storage system, and thermo-printer [27] to serve eight beds. The following parameters are continuously and simultaneously recorded, stored, and evaluated for each patient:

- Temperature
- Respiration rate
- Heart rate
- Systolic blood pressure
- Central venous pressure
- $tcPO_2$
- FiO_2
- Monitor malfunctions.

Historical data, laboratory data, and blood gas analyses are entered manually. Trends can be displayed visually on a screen, and 8-h shift reports can be printed out at selected intervals. Specially developed programs can be used to analyze the heart rate variability (cardiorespirography) and differentiate apnea and bradycardia.

The high costs of such a system are justified only if:

- The intensive care unit is large and adequately staffed
- Increased quantitative or qualitative information on the patient is ensured [26]
- The system is simple to use and can be operated by any nurse [24]
- The system is installed with software tailored to the special needs of the facility, and the dialogue with the viewing screen is conducted in the language familiar to the staff.

References

1. Bucci, G., Scalamandré, A., Savignoni, P. G., Mendicini, M., Picece-Bucci, S., Piccinato, L.: The systemic systolic blood pressure of newborns with low weight. A multiple regression analysis. Acta paed. scand. Suppl. *229*, 1–26 (1972)
2. Dangel, P., Nüssli, R., Duc, G.: Intensivbehandlung für das Neugeborene. Therapeut. Umschau *31*, 527 (1974)
3. Dweck, H. S., Reynolds, D. W., Cassady, G.: Indirect blood pressure measurements in newborns. Am. J. Dis. Child. *127*, 492 (1974)
4. Ekert, W. D., Schenck, H. W.: Die Kardiorespirographie: Eine Methode zur Überwachung und Zustandsdiagnostik bei gefährdeten Kindern. In: Pädiatrische Intensivmedizin. Band 3, S. 97. Emmrich P. (Hrsg.). Stuttgart: Thieme 1977

5. ELGNER, W., SIMON, B., SCHÖBER, J. G.: Beat-te-Beat Analyse nach Herzoperationen. In: Pädiatrische Intensivmedizin, Band 3, S. 138. EMMRICH, P. (Ed.). Stuttgart: Thieme 1977
6. FENNER, A., v. STOCKHAUSEN, H. B.: Die Bedeutung des zentralen Venendruckes für die Überwachung von Frühgeborenen. In: Pädiatrische Intensivpflege. 1. Symposion (KÖTTGEN, U., JÜNGST, B. K., TOUSSAINT, W., EMMRICH, P. (ed.)). Stuttgart: Enke 1971
7. FUCHSHOFEN, M., METZE, H.: Der Blutdruck von Frühgeborenen in den ersten drei Lebenswochen. Mschr. Kinderheilk. *124*, 596 (1976)
8. GLUCK, L.: Design of a perinatal center. Pediat. Clin. North Amer. *17*, 777 (1970)
9. GOLDRING, D., WOHLTMANN, H.: Flush method for blood pressure determinations in newborn infants. J. Pediat. *40*, 285 (1952)
10. GRAUSZ, J. P.: The effects of environmental temperature on the metabolic rate of newborn babies. Acta Paediatr. Scand. *57*, 98 (1968)
11. HEY, E.: The care of babies in incubators. In: Recent advances in pediatrics. HULL, D., GAIRDNER, D., (Eds.). p. 171. London: Churchill, 1971
12. HUCH, R., HUCH, A.: Zustandsdiagnostik beim Neugeborenen unmittelbar post partum durch das Sauerstoff-Kardiorespirogramm (SCR). In: Pädiatrische Intensivmedizin, Band 3, S. 65. EMMRICH, P. (Ed.). Stuttgart: Thieme 1977
13. KIRKLAND, R. T., KIRKLAND, J. L.: Systolic blood pressure measurement in the newborn infant with the transcutaneous Doppler method. J. Pediat. *80*, 52 (1972)
14. v.LOEWENICH, V.: Apparative Patientenüberwachung in der Pädiatrie. Msch. Kinderheilk. *119*, 474 (1971)
15. MCLAUGHLIN, G. W., KIRBY, R. R., KEMMERER, W. T., de LEMOS, R. A.: Indirect measurement of blood pressure in infants utilizing Doppler ultrasound. J. Pediat. *79*, 300 (1971)
16. RYSER, G., JÉQUIER, E.: Study by direct calorimetry of thermal balance on the first day of life. Europ. J. clin. Invest. *2*, 176 (1972)
17. STEIN, J. M., SHANNON, D. C.: The pediatric pneumogram: A new method for detecting and quantitating apnea in infants. Pediatrics *55*, 595 (1975)
18. STEMMANN, E. A., KOSCHE, F., ICKS, U., ALBRECHT, H., LEMBURG, P., SCHMIDT, E.: Registrierung der momentanen Herzfrequenz, eine neue Methode zur Überwachung gefährdeter Kinder. Mschr. Kinderheilk. *122*, 596 (1974)
19. STERN, L.: Environmental temperature, oxygen consumption and catecholamine excretion in newborn infants. Pediatrics *36*, 367 (1965)
20. TAFARI, N., GENTZ, J.: Aspects on rewarming newborn infants with severe accidental hypothermia. Acta Paediatr. Scand. *63*, 595 (1974)
21. PROD'HOM, L. S.: Die Erkrankungen des Foetus und des Neugeborenen. In: Lehrbuch der Pädiatrie. FANCONI, G., WALLGREN, A. 1972. Basel/Stuttgart: Schwabe
22. ALLEN, L. P., CLIFTON, J. S., INGRAM, D., LeSOUEF, P. N., REYNOLDS, E. O. R., WIMBERLEY, P. D.: Computer system for recording and display of data from newborn infants with respiratory illnesses. Arch. Dis. Child. *53*, 169 (1978)
23. FRANK, H.-D.: Computer-Trendanalyse – ein neuer Weg der elektronischen Patientenüberwachung in der Neugeborenenintensivpflege. Med. Tech. *99*, 26 (1979)
24. HUGENHOLTZ, P., van der VOORDE, L. S., DEUTSCH, F., ZEELENBERG, C.: An overview of recent developments in computerized intensive care monitoring. Biomed. Tech. *22*, 3 (1977)
25. KATONA, P. G., DURAND, D., STERN, K., FLEMING, D. G., and MARTIN, R. J.: Microprocessor-Controlled Memory for Cardiopulmonary Monitoring of High-Risk Infants. IEEE Trans. Biomed. Eng. *24*, 536 (1977)
26. KÖNIG, Ch., KEMTER, B. E., NAGE, M., FAUST, U.: Computergestützte Langzeitüberwachung von Atmung, Herzfrequenz und transcutanem PO_2 bei herzkranken Säuglingen. Biomed. Tech. *22*, 25 (1977)
27. OBLADEN, M., PRANTL, N., NICK, W., WILLE, L.: Prozessorgesteuertes Überwachungssystem für die Neugeborenen-Intensivpflege. 9. Dt. Kongreß f. Perinatale Medizin, Berlin 1979

4 Nutrition During the First Days of Life

L. Wille

4.1 General

At birth the newborn infant loses its continuous supply of nutrients via the placenta. If the postnatal metabolic demand (Table 16) is not met, the limited caloric reserves of the newborn (glycogen, fat) are quickly exhausted. This catabolic state is manifested by hypoglycemia, hyperkalemia, hyperbilirubinemia, and acetonemia. Postnatal malnutrition can lead to a disturbance of cerebral metabolism, with permanent brain damage. The prompt and adequate administration of fluid and calories is essential for optimal postnatal development [21, 22].

4.2 Oral Feeding

There is general agreement that feeding in normal infants should begin early (3–6 h postpartum). With an adequate feeding technique, good observation, and proper positioning, the danger of aspiration is slight.

Table 16. Energy demand

During the first 7–10 days of life [21]	
Basal metabolism	50 cal/kg/day
+30% for physical activity	15 cal/kg/day
+20% for caloric loss in the stool	10 cal/kg/day
+12% for specific dynamic action	8 cal/kg/day
+growth demand	25 cal/kg/day
Total	108 cal/kg/day
During the 10th–20th day of life	
Mature term infants	100–200 cal/kg/day
Preterm infants	120–150 cal/kg/day
SGA infants	120–175 cal/kg/day

4.2.1 Healthy Term Infants

Human breast milk is preferred for healthy term babies, and breast feeding is highly desirable. The nitrogen balance is positive after the 3rd day of life in nursing infants. If human milk is not available, a fully-adapted milk is given [5]. The oral feeding plan is outlined in Table 17.

4.2.2 Preterm Infants

a) During the 1st week of life, the daily fluid and caloric requirements cannot be met by an oral feeding regimen alone. Thus, supplementary intravenous feeding is begun immediately after admission (see p. 45).
b) Feeding behavior is tested by gavage feedings of 5% glucose at half the desired individual feeding volume during the 4th hour of life (danger of aspiration from pharyngeal incoordination).
c) Feeding with 5% glucose is begun during the 6th hour of life (individual volumes in Table 17). Severe respiratory difficulties or gastrointestinal symptoms or selected syndromes may delay the start of regular oral feeding, permitting only partial oral feeding, or prevent it altogether. In such cases the followings procedures for supplementary (see p. 45) or total parenteral nutrition (see p. 46) are followed.
d) After two successful feedings with 5% glucose, the infant is placed on mothers's milk (skimmed if necessary), pooled breast milk (protein content > 1.0 g/100 ml), or a fully adapted premature formula (Table 17). For preterm infants < 1500 g, the gastric contents should be aspirated immediately before the tube feedings to check for residual milk in the stomach.
e) The oral feed is increased to one-sixth the body weight. If human milk is given, the feed is increased to 170–200 ml/kg/day to compensate for the lower caloric and protein content. Recent evidence indicates that human milk is adequate for the rearing of preterm infants and offers various advantages [11, 15, 18].

Table 17. Oral feeding plan for healthy term and preterm infants

Weight groupings (g)	Daily volume increment (g)	Number of feedings	Daily volume increment per feeding (ml)	$^1/_6$ body weight reached with ml
⩾3500	70	5	14	600
3499–3000	70 g	5–6	14–12	585–500
2999–2500	(60)–70 g	5–6	14–12	500–420
2499–2000	50 g	8[a]	6–(7)	420–330
1999–1800	40 g	8[a]	5	330–300
1799–1500	35 g	8[a]	4,5	300–250
1499–1300	30 g	10[a]	3	250–215
1299–1000	(15)–25 g	12	(1)–2	215–165
⩽1000	(10)–20 g	24	(0,5)–1	165–135

[a] Up to 12 feedings, depending on state of health

f) Gavage: A fluid volume of 130–150 ml/kg body wt. should not be exceeded, if this is necessary for the child to thrive (term and preterm SGA infants).
Bottle feeding: Bottle feeding is usually possible after 35 weeks gestation. The infant may choose his volume; supplementary tube feeding may be necessary.
g) Oral feeding is reduced or interrupted if regurgitation, abdominal distension gastric residuals, or diarrhea occurs and is supplemented or replaced by parenteral nutrition.
h) Supplementary intravenous feeding is reduced in accordance with the increase in oral feeding (oral + parenteral = 150 ml/kg body wt.). Intravenous feeding is discontinued as soon as the oral feeding regimen has reached 100 ml/kg/day.
i) Vitamin requirements: Vitamin D: 1000 units/day after 1st week of life, allowing for that supplied by the adapted premature formula.
Vitamin C: 50 mg/day after 3rd day of life, taking into account the protein and vitamin C supplied by the premature formula (avoids tyrosinemia from an increase in tyrosine-oxidase activity).
Vitamin E (tucopherol) 25 IU/day orally until the infant is 38 weeks of age portconception.

4.2.3 Small-for-Gestational-Age Infants

The feeding plan for SGA infants corresponds to that described for preterm infants, with the following modifications:

re b) Immediately after postnatal adaptation, begin feeding with 5% glucose at 2-h intervals.

re c) After the third glucose feeding has been accepted without complications, change to fully adapted term formula. The number of feedings is 12 per day.

Also. Screen for hypoglycemia (Dextrostix).

4.2.4 Sick Infants

The feeding plan corresponds basically to that for healthy infants. As a rule, parenteral nutrition is unnecessary. Exceptions are acute pulmonary, cardiac, or gastrointestinal syndromes which contraindicate the normal start of oral feeding, or certain risk factors (presumed congenital aminoacidopathy). In these cases supplementary or total parenteral nutrition (with or without amino acids) is necessary to avoid a catabolic situation. In our opinion, intubation and controlled ventilation do not contraindicate oral feeding. It is necessary only to interrupt oral feeding for 6 h after extubation.

4.3 Nasojejunal Feeding

Purpose. Enteral nutrition without the difficulties and complications of parenteral nutrition or the risks of stomach tubes (reflux, aspiration).

Advantages
Rapid delivery of fluid and calories
better weight gain [23]
Permits enteral nutrition of seriously ill infants.

Indications
Preterm/SGA infants <1300 g
Extremely weak preterm/SGA infants weighing 1300–1500 g
Term infants with severe respiratory difficulties, disturbances of consciousness, recurrent convulsions or severe cardiac insufficiency.

Apparatus. Regular gastric tube made of polyurethane or polyethylene; polyvinyl chloride is not suitable (necrotizing enterocolitis?). Weighting the tube with a special plug at the tip [7, 19] is unnecessary.

Procedure. The tube is inserted nasally and advanced into the stomach in the usual manner. Length measurement: Earlobe-to-nose, nose-to-epigastrium. The tube position is checked by auscultation while air is insufflated through the tube. The infant is placed in a 60° sitting position, turned onto his right side. After 30 min the tube is advanced to the jejunum. At a given infant body weight of *x* grams, the jejunum should be reached with a total insertion length of *y* cm:

x	y
1000 g	13–21 cm
1000–1500 g	21–26 cm
1500–3500 g	23–34 cm

The patient is kept on his right side for 2–4 h.

Checking Tube Placement. Gastrointestinal secretions are aspirated; if the secretions have a bilious appearance or give a weakly acidic to alkaline reaction (pH 5.0–7.0; litmus paper), the tube is beyond the pylorus.
Tube placement is checked once by X-ray.

Infusion of Formula. After the 6th hour of life.

Composition of Formula. 5% Glucose for 12 h, 5% glucose for another 12 h; 1:1 adapted milk formula (beware of hyperosmolar solution overload of the jejunum). This is followed by fully adapted milk regime.

Feeding Volume
a) 60 ml/kg body wt. during the first 24 h of life.
b) After the 2nd day, the following increments are given:
   Birth weight <1500 g, 30 ml/kg/day
   Birth weight <2200 g, 45 ml/kg/day
   Birth weight >2200 g, 60 ml/kg/day
   Increase to 165 ml/kg/day

Administration Continuous infusion by pump.
Infection prophylaxis: The bottle and system are changed every 8 h. The transition to a regular gastric feeding regimen is made in stages in accordance with the age and tolerance of the individual child.

Complication (Rare) [4, 8].
Perforation
Necrotizing enterocolitis
Focal necrosis of the jejunum
Milk ileus.

4.4 Supplementary Intravenous Feeding

The goal is to supplement the oral feeding regimen of preterm and SGA infants to avoid a catabolic situation. The intake of carbohydrates, electrolytes, L-amino acids, and vitamins is geared toward the daily requirement (Table 18).

Table 18. Oral daily requirements of newborn infants [1, 21]

Protein	3 g/kg
Calories	100–110 kg
Glucose	25.5% of caloric intake
Fat	4–6 g/kg
Fluid volume	150 ml/kg
Sodium	3 mEq/kg
Potassium	2 mEq/kg
Calcium	15 mEq
Phosphorus	5 mEq
Magnesium	1 mg/kg
Vitamin D	400 IU
Vitamin A	1400 IU
Vitamin K	5 µg
Vitamin E	0.5 mg/kg
Vitamin C	35–50 mg
Thiamine	0.3 mg
Riboflavin	0.4 mg
Niacin	5 mg
Pyridoxine	200–400 µg
Pantothenic acid	405 µg
Folic acid	50 µg
Vitamin B12	0.3 µg
Biotin	150–300 µg

Table 19. Supplementary parenteral nutrition

Päd. pfrimmer, 5%, carbohydrate-free	50 ml/day
Glucose 20%	50 ml/day
Multibionta (vitamins)	0.5–1.0 ml/day
Total calories	58 kcal/day
Total fluid volume	100 ml/day

In consideration of these requirements, we employ the following supplementary infusion program (per kg body wt.) (Table 19)
Our own investigations have shown that this pediatric L-amino acid solution employed satisfies the daily requirement for protein and the most important electrolytes [25]. Since the intravenous feeding is supplementary, phosphate and fat need not be given. The daily reduction corresponds to the increase in the oral feeding regimen (oral + parenteral = 150 ml/kg/day).

4.5 Total Parenteral Nutrition

Indications

- Congenital malformations of the gastrointestinal tract
- Massive intestinal resections (short bowel syndrome)
- Repeated abdominal operations
- Severe diarrhea with secondary malabsorption
- Seriously ill term and preterm infants with complex health problems and impaired gastrointestinal functions [26].

Technique

Peripheral Vein. Access on scalp or extremities, using perfusion set or Abboven No. 18.

Central Venous Catheter and Venesection. see p. 236, 241

Daily Requirements (Table 20a, b)

Infusion Program. We recommend a parenteral feeding solution which contains 70–120 kcal/100 ml, 40%–45% of which is provided by carbohydrates, 45%–50% by fat (10% Intralipid) and 10%–15% by a synthetic L-amino acid mixture with all amino acids essential for term and preterm infants (Table 21).

Table 20 a. Daily requirements during parenteral nutrition [3, 6, 15, 17]

Fluid volume	130–150 ml/kg/day
Calories	90–140 kcal/kg/day
Carbohydrates: glucose	5–18 g/kg/day
Fat (Intralipid)	2–4 g/kg/day
Protein (L-amino acids)	2.5 g/kg/day
Electrolytes	
Na	3–4 mEq/kg/day
K	2–3 mEq/kg/day
Cl	2–3 mEq/kg/day
Ca	0.5 mEq/kg/day
P	0.4–0.8 mEq/kg/day
Mg	0.25–0.45 mEq/kg/day

Table 20 b. Daily requirements for vitamins and trace elements during total parenteral nutrition [9, 12, 24, 28]

Vitamins (daily total)		Trace elements[a] (per kg per day)	
A (IU)	600	Iron (μmol)	2.0
D (IU)	400	Manganese (μmol)	1.0
E (mg)	1.5	Zinc (μmol)	0.6
K (mg)	0.1	Copper (μmol)	0.3
B_1 (mg)	0.3	Fluorine (μmol)	3.0
B_2 (mg)	0.4	Iodine (μmol)	0.04
Niacin (mg)	5.0		
B_6 (mg)	0.3		
C (mg)	35		
B_{12} (μg)	0.3		
Folic acid (μg)	50–75		
Biotin (mg)	0.6		
Pantothenic acid (mg)	10.0		

[a] Because the daily requirements for trace elements in the neonate are not precisely known, the weekly infusion of 20 ml plasma/kg is recommended to avoid deficiencies

Remarks. As in oral feeding, the individual nutrients (glucose, Intralipid) should be increased gradually in order to match the nutrient intake to the adaptation of insulin secretion and lipolysis. A full, immediate intake will cause hyperglycemia, osmotic diuresis, and hyperlipemia.

Strict aseptic technique must be followed in preparing the infusion solutions (laminar air flow unit is recommended), as well as in changing the infusion solution, infusion system (every 12 h), and dressings.

The supplementary infusion of electrolytes, vitamins, and trace elements not contained in the infusion solution is determined by the daily requirement. Since calcium and phosphorus cannot both be incorporated into one infusion solution, a two to three bottle system is necessary (allowing for the concurrent infusion of Intralipid).

Table 21. Increase in the infusion program for total parenteral nutrition in term and preterm infants during the first week of Life (ml/kg/day)

	1st day	2nd–3rd Day	4th–5th Day	6th–7th Day
Päd. pfrimmer 5‰, carbohydrate free	50	50	50	50
Intralipid 20%	5	10	15	20
Glucose 20%	25[a]–50[b,c]	62,5	75	90
NaCl 10%	–	0,5	0,5	0,5
K-phosphate 1.0 M	–	1,0	1,0	1,0
Total	105	124	141,5	161,5
Kcal	60,5	80	99,7	121

Vitamins		*Trace elements*
Multivitamines	0.5–(1.0) ml/day	Biseko 10 ml/kg/2 × week (perhaps PED electrolyte solution)
Vitamin B complex	0.5–(1.0) ml/day	
Vitamin K_1	3 mg/2 × week	
Folsan	3 mg/2 × week	
Vitamin D	1 mg/4–6 week, depending on age	

[a] Preterm infants <1500 g during the 1st 12 h
[b] Preterm infants <1500 g during the 2nd 12 h
[c] Preterm infants >1500 g on the 1st day of life

The infusion volume is increased according to the weight gain. Parenteral nutrition is gradually reduced in accordance with the possibilities of oral feeding.

Increase in individual nutrients:

a) *Glucose.* Preterm and SGA infants have a limited glucose tolerance due to an insufficient secretion of insulin. If severe cerebral damage is present (postasphyxia syndrome, cerebral hemorrhage), glucose homeostasis may be impaired. Hyperglycemia, glucosuria, and osmotic diuresis can result.

b) *Sugar alcohols* (sorbitol, xylitol). Not necessary; only the first metabolic steps are insulin independent. May worsen existing acidosis. Beware of fructose intolerance (fructose-1-6-diphosphatase deficiency)!

c) *Fat.* An infusion volume of 2–4 g Intralipid/kg body wt. is recommended [6]. The infusion of fat permits a reduction in glucose concentration and a lower osmolarity of the infusion solution. Metabolic utilization capacity is limited in SGA and seriously ill neonates and in preterm infants <32 weeks gestation. Heparin in a dose of 50–100 IU/kg per day increases the serum lipoprotein lipase activity. Experience in sepsis and respiratory distress is limited; thus reliable recommendations on the use of a fat emulsion in these cases cannot be made. Intralipid is not added to the infusion solution (creaming), but is administered through a bypass. The infusion volume is evenly spaced over 24 h; otherwise an overloading syndrome (fat embolism) may result [2]. The infusion of Intralipid during long-term total parenteral nutrition may impair the pulmonary function and reticuloendothelial system [10].

d) *L-amino acids.* The quantitative and qualitative ratio of the individual amino acids to one another is adapted to the daily requirement of term and preterm infants. The amino acid infusate should contain all amino acids essential for this pediatric age group. According to the recommendations of Ghadimi [9], a complete physiologic mixture should ideally contain up to 70% essential amino acids. Our own investigations have demonstrated no amino acid imbalances in infants receiving infusion of Päd. pfrimmer 5%, carbohydrate free (26).

Supervision (Table 22)

Table 22. Supervision during total parenteral nutrition [13, 20, 27]

		1st Week	Thereafter
I.	Clinical signs Skin turgor, fontanel, oral mucosa, lacrimation	Daily	Daily
II.	Growth parameters		
	Weight	Daily	Daily
	Length	Weekly	Weekly
	Head circumference	Weekly	Weekly
III.	Fluid balance		
	Intake	Daily	Daily
	Output (urine, stool, secretions, drainage, perspiration)	Daily	Daily
IV.	Hematology		
	Hgb, hematocrit Leukocytes Platelet count Differential blood count	3 × weekly	1 × weekly
V.	Serum chemistry		
	Electrolytes (Na, K, Cl)	Daily	3 × weekly
	Ca, P, Mg, total protein	2 × weekly	1 × weekly
	Urea, creatinine, SGOT, SGPT, bilirubin	3 × weekly	2 × weekly
	Electrophoresis, ammonia	1 × weekly	1 × weekly
	Glucose	1–3 × daily	3 × weekly
	Blood gas analysis	Daily	2 × weekly
VI.	Urine		
	Glucose, acetone, specific weight, or osmolarity	2–4 × daily	1 × daily[a]
VII.	Microbial investigations[a] Blood culture Stool Urine Gastric juice Sputum Cerebrospinal fluid Catheter tip	As required	As required

[a] For patients receiving intensive care, smears from the skin, ear, throat, anus, vagina, and ventilator are routinely taken twice a week

Complications (Table 23)

Table 23. Complications of total parenteral nutrition [3, 13, 14, 27]

I.	Mechanical	
	Catheter malposition	
	Catheter dislocation, disconnection, occlusion	
	Thrombophlebitis, thrombosis of large vessels	
	Intracardiac curling or knotting of catheter	
	Pneumo-, hemato-, hydrothorax	
	Embolism (thrombus, air, catheter)	
	Arteriovenous fistula	
	Extravasation	
II.	Infection	
	Catheter entry (local)	
	Contamination during insertion	
	Prolonged duration of catheter placement	
	Systemic infection:	spread from catheter tip
		hematogenous
		remote focus
		diminished resistance (cellular, humoral)
III.	Metabolic	
	Hyperosmolarity: glucose, electrolytes, osmotic diuresis, dehydration	
	Electrolyte imbalance (Na, Cl, Mg, Ca, K)	
	Volume overload: edema formation, cardiac insufficiency	
	Amino acid imbalance	
	Hyperammonemia	
	Metabolic acidosis	
	Deficiency of essential fatty acids, vitamins, trace elements	
	Hypertriglyceridemia, increased free fatty acids	
	Anemia	
	Exanthema	
	Hypoproteinemia	
	Hepatopathy: cholestasis, necrosis	
	Ossification defects	
	Negative nitrogen balance	
	Postinfusional hypoglycemia	
	Glucosuria	

References

1. AVERY, G. B., FLETCHER, A. B.: Nutrition. In: Neonatology, AVERY, G. B. (Ed.). p. 839. Philadelphia-Toronto: Lippincott 1975
2. BARSON, A. J., CHISWICK, M. L., DOIG, C. M.: Fat embolism in infancy after intravenous fat infusion. Arch. Dis. Child. *53*, 218 (1978)
3. BERGER, H., FRISCH, H., KOFLER, J., RESCH, R.: Komplette parenterale Ernährung im Kindesalter. Infusionstherapie *4*, 1 (1977)
4. BOROS, St. J., REYNOLDS, W.: Duodenal perforation: A complication of nasojejunal feeding. J. Pediat. *85*, 107 (1974)

5. BREMER, H. J., DROESE, W., GRÜTTNER, R., KÜBLER, W., SCHMIDT, E.: Einteilung der Säuglingsmilchnahrung auf Kuhmilchbasis. Mschr. Kinderheilk. *122*, 761 (1974)
6. BRYAN, H. SHENNAN, A., GRIFFIN, E., ANGEL, A.: Intralipid: its rational use in parenteral nutrition of the newborn. Pediatrics *58*, 787 (1976)
7. CHEEK, J. A., STAUB, G. F.: Nasojejunal alimentation for premature and full-term newborn infants, J. Pediat. *82*, 955 (1973)
8. CHEN, J. W., WONG, P. W. K.: Intestinal complications of nasojejunal feeding in low-birth-weight infants. J. Pediat. *85*, 109 (1974)
9. GHADIMI, H.: Total parenteral nutrition p. 393. New York-London-Sidney-Toronto: Wiley & Sons 1975
10. FRIEDMAN, Z., MARKS, K. H., MAISELS, M. J., THORSON, R., NAEYE, R.: Effect of parenteral fat emulsion on the pulmonary and reticuloendothelial systems in the newborn infant. Pediatrics *61*, 694 (1978)
11. HANSON, L. A.: Zur immunologischen Bedeutung der Frauenmilch. Padiat. FortbildK. Praxis *37*, 1 (1973)
12. HARRIES, J. T.: Intravenous feeding in infants. Arch. Dis Child. *46*, 855 (1971)
13. HEIRD, W. C., DRISCOLL, J. M., SCHULLINGER, J. N., GREBIN, B., WINTERS, R. W.: Intravenous alimentation in pediatric patients. J. Pediat. *80*, 351 (1972)
14. HEIRD, W. C., WINTERS, R. W.: Total parenteral nutrition. J. Pediat. *86*, 2 (1975)
15. HEIRD, W. C., ANDERSON, Th. L., DRISCOLL, J. M., NASH, M. A.: Nutrition, body fluids and acid-base homeostasis, in: Neonatal-Perinatal Medicine. BEHRMAN, R. E. (Ed.), p. 235. St. Louis: Mosby 1977
16. HERSCHKOWITZ, N.: Effekt der Unterernährung auf die Gehirnentwicklung. Mschr. Kinderheilk. *122*, 240 (1974)
17. LORCH, V., LAY, S. A.: Parenteral alimentation in the neonate. Pediatr. Clin. North. Am. *24*, 547 (1977)
18. RÄIHÄ, N. C. R., HEINONEN, K., RASSIN, D. K., GAULL, G. E.: Milk protein quantity and quality in low birth weight infants. Pediatrics *57*, 659 (1976)
19. RHEA, J. W., GHAZZWI, O., WEIDMAN, W.: Nasojejunal feeding: An improved device and intubation technique. J. Pediat. *82*, 951 (1973)
20. SHAW, J. C. L.: Parenteral nutrition in the management of sick low birthweight infants. Pediat. Clin. N. Amer. *20*, 333 (1973)
21. SINCLAIR, J. C., DRISCOLL, J. M., HEIRD, W. C., WINTERS, R. W.: Supportive management of the sick neonate. Pediat. Clin. N. Amer. *17*, 863 (1970)
22. SWYER, R. P.: The intensive care of the newly born. Basel-München-Paris-London-New York-Sydney: Karger 1975
23. WELLS, D. H., ZACHMANN, R. D.: Nasojejunal feeding in low-birth-weight infants. J. Pediat. *87*, 276 (1975)
24. WHO: Handbook on human nutritional requirements, WHO Monograph. Series No. *61:* Geneva, WHO
25. WILLE, L.: Untersuchungen zur parenteralen Ernährung Frühgeborener in der ersten Lebenswoche. Habilitationsschrift. Heidelberg 1976
26. WILLE, L., LUTZ, P., JÜRGENS, P.: A comparison of oral feeding and total parenteral nutrition in premature infants. Pediat. Res. *10*, 877 (1976)
27. WILLE, L.: Parenterale Ernährung in der Pädiatric Aktuel. Ernährungsmed. 2, 179 (1977)
28. WRETLIND, A.: Ernährungsphysiologische und pharmakologische Gesichtspunkte in der kompletten parenteralen Ernährung, In: Parenterale Ernährung, BERGER, H. (ed.). S. 9. Bern-Stuttgart-Wien: Huber 1972

Part II
Diagnosis and Treatment of Respiratory Disorders

5 Blood Gas Analysis

M. Obladen

5.1 Measuring Techniques

5.1.1 Direct Measurement with Sensitive Electrodes (e.g., Corning, AVL)

The pH is measured with a glass electrode, while the PCO_2 is measured directly with a CO_2-sensitive electrode of the Severinghaus type. Figure 9 shows a modified Severinghaus nomogram for calculating the standard bicarbonate [16].

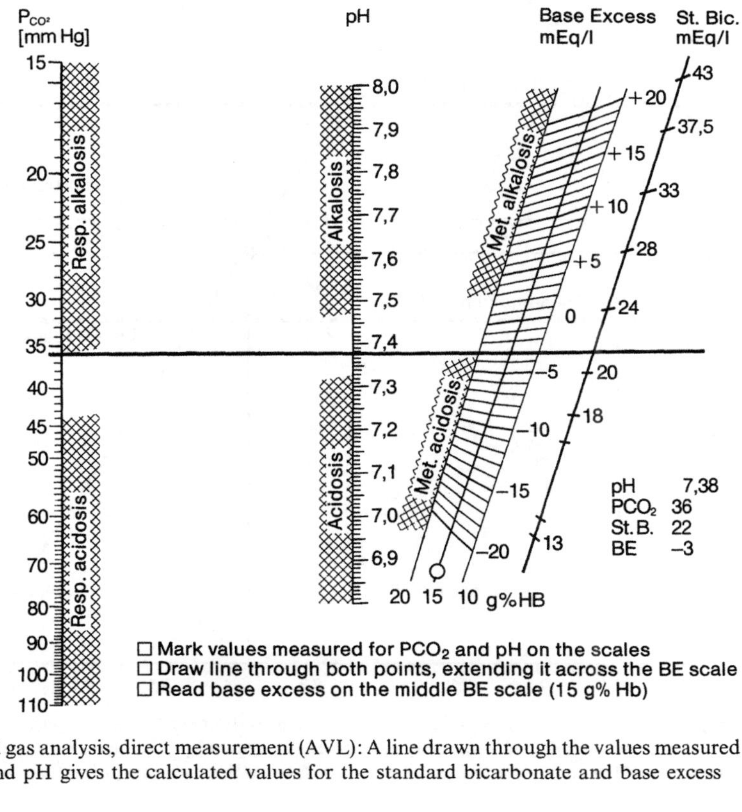

Fig. 9. Blood gas analysis, direct measurement (AVL): A line drawn through the values measured for PCO_2 and pH gives the calculated values for the standard bicarbonate and base excess

5.1.2 Indirect Measurement

The Astrup technique is used [13]. The pH is measured with a glass electrode, and the PCO_2 is calculated for the pH measurement of the blood after it has been equilibrated with two different CO_2 concentrations. A line is drawn through both points (see Fig. 10), and the point where the pH value of the example blood specimen intersects this line horizontally gives the PCO_2.
An additional Clark-type electrode is needed to measure the PO_2. In both techniques the standard bicarbonate is calculated from the pH and PCO_2 with a Severinghaus nomogram. The base deficit or base excess is directly proportional to the standard bicarbonate and facilitates buffer therapy.

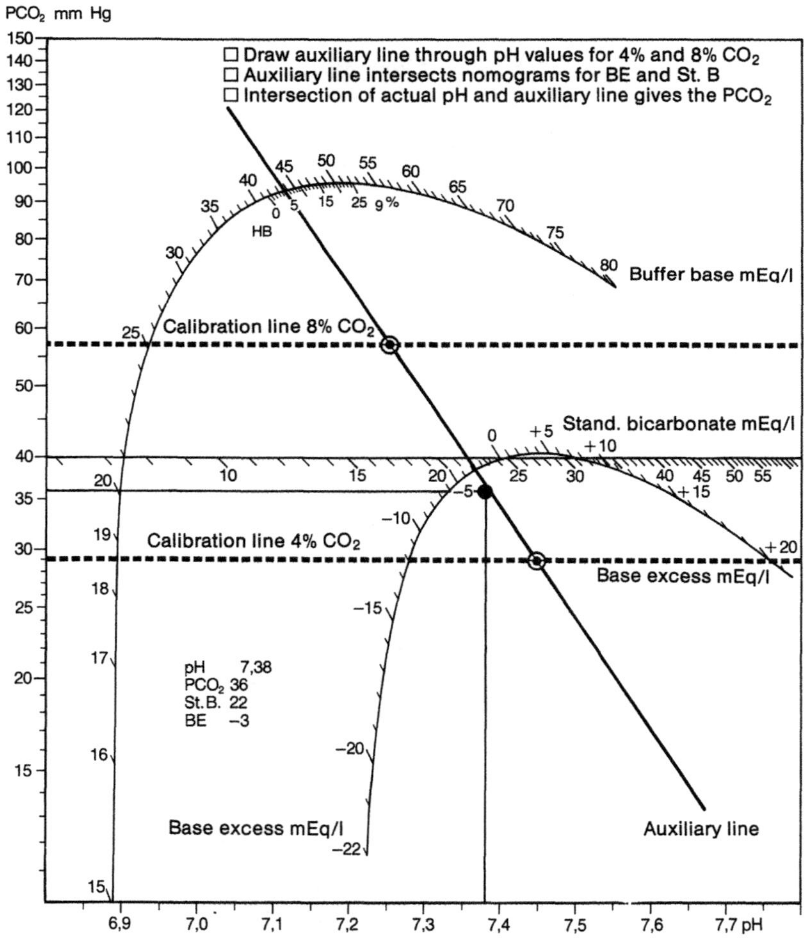

Fig. 10. Blood gas analysis, indirect measurement (radiometer): The sample's pH values after equilibration with 4% and 8% CO_2 are circled. The actual pH is entered on the auxiliary line drawn through these two points. The horizontal line through this point gives the PCO_2

5.1.3 Criteria for Selecting a Blood Gas Analyzer

The blood gas analyzer is a basic tool of the intensive care unit. Neither ventilation nor buffer therapy can be successfully administered without it. A malfunction or series of faulty determinations leads immediately to grave consequences for the patient.

The criteria for selecting a blood gas analyzer are:
- Small blood volume
- Simple operation
- Rapid analysis
- High precision
- Simple cleaning and calibration
- Simple maintenance
- High reliability
- Rapid service.

The staff of the intensive care unit should be familiar enough with the device to perform minor repairs and calibration work whenever necessary. An adequate supply of spare parts should be stocked.

5.2 Transcutaneous Oxygen Measurement

This technique provides information on oxygen tension without the necessity of drawing blood samples. A Clark electrode heated to 44° C is used to measure the oxygen diffusing through the skin. The oxygen tension is graphically recorded, while the electrode's heating power is simultaneously recorded as a measure of blood flow. This technique yields acceptable results, except in states of extreme vasoconstriction, and is described in detail on p 67.

5.3 Collection of Blood Samples

General Preliminary Remarks. Do not fill heparinized capillary tubes to the end, since contact with glass activates clotting. Avoid air bubbles in the tube. Do not seal with clay. Analyze within 5 min if possible; otherwise store sealed tube in ice water.

5.3.1 Capillary Sampling [3, 7, 15]

The heel or thenar eminence is pricked with a lancet, and the free-flowing blood is collected into the heparinized capillary tube.
It is not worthwhile to determine the PO_2 of simple capillary samples!

5.3.2 Warmed Capillary Sampling [2]

The heel is warmed for 5 min to 40°–50° C. The sample is drawn as in 5.3.1. Within limits, this method yields a clinically useful correlation with arterial PO_2 in term and preterm infants with a stable circulatory status. In any case this correlation is useful at PO_2 values below 60 mm Hg: A warmed capillary sample PO_2 below 35 corresponds roughly to an arterial PO_2 below 50 mm Hg; a warmed capillary PO_2 above 50 mm Hg corresponds to an arterial PO_2 above 90 mm Hg. Warmed capillary blood samples from warmed fingers [19] have better correlations with the PaO_2; although only a limited number of digital blood samples can be drawn from preterm infants. Warmed capillary PO_2 values should always be critically judged due to their doubtful reliability.

5.3.3 Arterial Puncture

Suitable arteries: radial, brachial (preferably on the right side = preductal blood) and temporal. Never puncture the femoral artery due to risk of arterial spasm and necrosis. Blood gas analysis by arterial puncture is valid only if sampling is successful within 30 s, otherwise the infant's pain reaction, crying, straining, etc., will cause a rapid fall of the PO_2 (for techniques see p 238).

5.3.4 Umbilical Artery Catheter

Most reliable postductal PO_2 value [6]. Sampling causes no discomfort to the infant, but there is a risk of infection, thrombosis, and necrosis (for technique see p 232).

5.3.5 Indwelling Catheter in Radial or Temporal Artery

A precise and simple method with low complication rates even after several days' catheterization [1]. As a safety precaution before continuous cannulation of the radial artery, this artery should be compressed (Allen test) to determine whether the ulnar artery provides sufficient collateral circulation to the hand [17] (for technique see p 239).

5.4 Interpretation

A blood gas analysis during artificial ventilation can be evaluated only if all ventilator settings are documented! [12]

pH. The negative logarithm of the hydrogen ion concentration. A measure of the overall acidity of the blood.

pH 6.8 = H^+ 125 nEq/l
pH 7.4 = H^+ 40 nEq/l
Acidosis = pH <7.35 = excess of H^+
Alkalosis = pH >7.45 = deficiency of H^+.

PCO_2. Carbon dioxide tension (partial pressure) in mm Hg.
A measure of pulmonary ventilation (respiration rate, depth of respiration, respiratory minute volume) and, to some extent, of the diffusion capacity.

PO_2. Oxygen tension (partial pressure) in mm Hg.
A measure of the diffusion capacity of the lung (total respiratory function) and, to some extent, of ventilation. It is the most important indicator of intra- and extrapulmonary shunts.

HCO_3. The standard bicarbonate in mEq/l is a measure of the metabolic component of the acid-base balance. This determination is important for the assessment of buffering capacity and renal compensation in chronic acidosis. The standard bicarbonate is that value calculated in the plasma at 37° C, with full O_2 saturation and at a PCO_2 of 40 mm Hg. The actual bicarbonate and buffer base (i.e., the sum of all buffers in the blood), not adjusted for standard conditions, is of added value for clinical evaluation in individual cases (8, 11) (Table 24).

BE (Base Excess). The base concentration in the blood (in mEq/l) which corresponds to the titration volume to a pH of 7.40. It is derived from the standard bicarbonate and facilitates buffer therapy.

Table 24. Compensatory mechanisms for acid-base regulation

Compensatory mechanism	Reaction time
Dilution (local effect)	Seconds
Buffers (HCO_3^-, Hb, protein, $H_2PO_4^-$)	Minutes
Respiration (hypo- or hyperventilation)	Hours
Renal (HCO_3^-, HPO_4^-, carbonic anhydrase NH_3 formation)	At least 1 day

5.5 Blood Gas Analysis: Normal Values in the Newborn (Modified from Koch and Wendel [9]) (Table 25)

Table 25

	At birth		Arterial blood, age			
	Umbilical vein	Umbilical artery	10 min	1 h	24 h	5 days
pH	7.32	7.24	7.21	7.33	7.37	7.37
PCO_2	38	49	46	36	33	35
St. B	20	19	17	19	20	21
BE	− 4	− 7	−10	− 7	− 5	− 4
PO_2	27	16	50	63	73	72

5.6 Disturbances of the Acid-Base Balance (Table 26)

Table 26

Disturbance	Dissociation	Clinical condition	Blood gases in acute form	Physiologic compensation	Blood gases in chronic form (compensated)
Respiratory acidosis	$\frac{(HCO_3-)}{(CO_2)\uparrow}$	Atelectasis	pH 7,21 PCO_2 74 StB 22,5 BE −2 PO_2 44	Alkali reabsorption, hypochloremia	pH 7,36 PCO_2 71 StB 33 BE +10 PO_2 46
Respiratory alkalosis	$\frac{(HCO_3-)}{(CO_2)\downarrow}$	Iatrogenic hyperventilation	pH 7,62 PCO_2 19 StB 24,5 BE +1 PO_2 92	Chlorine retention, renal base excretion	pH 7,41 PCO_2 23 StB 18 BE −8 PO_2 98
Metabolic acidosis	$\frac{(HCO_3)\downarrow}{(CO_2)}$	Transposition (lactate acidosis due to hypoxia)	pH 7,03 PCO_2 46 StB 11 BE −20 PO_2 21	Hyperventilation	pH 7,35 PCO_2 24 StB 17 BE −10 PO_2 20
Metabolic alkalosis	$\frac{(HCO_3-)\uparrow}{(CO_2)}$	Pyloric stenosis	pH 7,51 PCO_2 40 StB 31 BE +8 PO_2 78	Hypoventilation	pH 7,42 PCO_2 58 StB 33 BE +10 PO_2 81

5.7 Medicinal Treatment of Acid-Base Disturbances

5.7.1 Indications

- Bicarbonate therapy is almost never curative, and acidosis is almost always a symptom. Respiratory acidosis should be treated primarily by ventilation and hypovolemia by volume replacement. The value of sodium bicarbonate in respiratory distress syndrome has been disputed [18].
- Metabolic acidosis with a pH <7.25 [25].
- Respiratory or mixed acidosis (i.e., administration of base excess) only when ventilation is not indicated.
- Metabolic alkalosis: At a pH >7.50, administer lysine hydrochloride (severe alkalosis is as hazardous to cerebral blood flow and cerebral oxygenation as acidosis due to vasoconstriction).

5.7.2 Dosage

a) 8.4% sodium bicarbonate: base deficit X kg body wt. X 0.3 (correction factor for extracellular volume) = mEq replacement. As a rule, dilute 1 : 1 with 5% glucose.
Side Effects. Hypernatremia, hyperosmolarity, brain damage (see below).
b) 0.3 *M* THAM, which may have stronger intracellular than extracellular action [10], is indicated in hypernatremia when sodium bicarbonate is contraindicated. Administer only with 10% glucose solution! (1 ml THAM: 2 ml 10% glucose)
Dosage. Base deficit X kg body wt.
Side effects. Hypoglycemia, irritation, apnea, local hypokalemia.
c) 3 *M* THAM: only in cardiac insufficiency, when fluid volume must be conserved. Administer only by continuous drip infusion; do not infuse into a peripheral vein (danger of necrosis).
Side effects as with 0.3 *M* THAM. Hypoglycemia hyponatremia, hypokalemia.
d) 18.2% lysine hydrochloride or 21.06% arginine hydrochloride.
Dosage. Base excess X kg body wt. X 0.3 (correction factor for extracellular volume).

Note. Due to the danger of iatrogenic acidosis, lysine hydrochloride should be used both very carefully and sparingly. This is especially true in infants with respiratory insufficiency. We never correct more than one-fourth to one-third of the calculated base excess initially.

5.7.3 Administration

Buffer solutions must be administered slowly due to the risk of hyperosmolar brain hemorrhage (8.4% sodium bicarbonate has an osmolarity of 2000 mosmol) [10]. Do not use bolus injection. If possible, administer by infusion pump over a period of

15–20 min [14]. At a high dosage, divide the dose up into three or four individual doses which are slowly infused every 15 min. Maximum infusion rate for sodium bicarbonate: 0.1 mEq/kg/min. If 10 mEq/kg/4 h is exceeded, sodium levels must be monitored.
In peripheral vasoconstriction and shock, adequate volume replacement often makes buffer therapy unnecessary.

References

1. Adams, J. M., Rudolph, A. J.: The use of indwelling radial artery catheters in neonates. Pediatrics, *55*, 261 (1975)
2. Avery, M. E., Fletcher, B. D.: The lung and its disorders in the newborn infant. Philadelphia, London, Toronto: Saunders 1974
3. Banister, A.: Comparison of arterial and arterialized capillary blood in infants with respiratory distress. Arch. Dis. Child *44*, 726 (1969)
4. Bartels, H., Riegel, K., Wenner, J., Wulf, H.: Perinatale Atmung. Berlin, Heidelberg, New York: Springer 1972
5. Baum, J. D., Robertson, N. R. C.: Immediate effects of alkaline infusion in infants with respiratory distress syndrome. J. Pediatrics *87*, 255 (1975)
6. Brown, D. R., Fenton, L. J., Tsang, R. C.: Blood sampling through umbilical catheters. Pediatrics *55*, 257 (1975)
7. Corbet, A. J. S.: Oxygen tension measurements on digital blood in the newborn. Pediatrics *46*, 780 (1970)
8. Kildeberg, P., Engel, K.: A rational approach to acid-base therapy in the newborn: A commentary. Pediatrics *43*, 827 (1969)
9. Koch, G., Wendel, H.: Adjustment of arterial blood gases and acid base balance in the normal newborn infant during the first week of life. Biol. Neonat. *12*, 136 (1968)
10. Manzke, H.: Therapie Frühgeborener mit Atemnotsyndrom. Verhalten von Serumelektrolyten, Osmolarität und Blutzucker vor und nach Alkali-Glukose-Infusionen. Fortschr. Med. *88*, 519 (1970)
11. Nelson, N. M., Riegel, K. P.: A schematic approach to acid-base therapy in the newborn. Pediatrics *43*, 821 (1969)
12. Shapiro, B. A.: Clinical Application of Blood Gases, Year Book Medical Publishers, Chicago: 1973
13. Siggaard-Andersen, O.: Blood acid-base alignment nomogram. Scand. J. Clin. Lab. Invest. *15*, 211 (1963)
14. Simmons, M. A., Adcock, E. W., Bard, H., Battaglia, F. C.: Hypernatremia, intracranial hemorrhage and $NaHCO_3$ administration in neonates. N. Engl. J. Med. *291*, 6 (1974)
15. Stamm, S. J.: Reliability of capillary blood for the measurement of PO_2 and O_2 saturation, Dis. Chest *52*, 191 (1967)
16. Thews, G.: Nomogramme zum Säure-Basen-Status des Blutes und zum Atemgastransport: In: Anaesthesiologie und Wiederbelebung. Vol. *53*, Frey, R., Kern, F., Mayrhofer, O. (Hrsg.). Berlin, Heidelberg, New York: Springer 1971
17. Todres, D., Rogers, M. C., Shannon, D. C., Moylan, F. M. B., Ryan, J. F.: Percutaneous catheterization of the radial artery in the critically ill neonate. J. Pediatr. *87*, 273 (1975)
18. Eidelmann, A. I., Hobbs, J. F.: Bicarbonate therapy revisited. Am. J. Dis. Child *132*, 847 (1978)
19. Karna, P., Poland, R. L.: Monitoring critically ill newborn infants with digital capillary blood samples: An alternative. J. Pediatr. *92*, 270 (1978)

6 Oxygen Therapy

M. Obladen

6.1 Indication

- Confirmed hypoxemia with PaO_2 <50 mm Hg is the only indication for the administration of oxygen
- Artificial ventilation is not therapeutically synonymous with oxygen administration [5]
- Oxygen is a medication with dangerous side effects and must be prescribed with specific dosages (FiO_2) like any other medication [2].

Table 27 gives the oxygen diffusion conditions in the healthy lung. It can be seen that with good diffusion conditions, even an oxygen concentration of 30%–40% can raise the PO_2 to levels at which retrolental fibroplasia can develop in the neonate [1]. In the diseased lung, no clear correlation can be established between FiO_2 and PaO_2. Since the assessment of oxygen diffusability is uncertain during spontaneous respiration, it is similarly unpredictable during artificial ventilation, especially if CPAP, PEEP, or prolonged inspiration (which greatly increases the PaO_2) are employed [7].

Table 27. Oxygen diffusion during spontaneous respiration in the healthy lung (adults [17])

FiO_2 Oxygen concentration of inspired gas	PaO_2 Arterial oxygen tension in torr (=mm Hg)
0.21	100
0.30	150
0.40	200
0.50	250
0.60	300
0.70	350
0.80	400
0.90	450
1.00	500

6.2 Hypoxia Diagnosis, Hyperoxia Test

We employ the hyperoxia test in two clinical situations:

6.2.1 Indication for Artificial Ventilation

At FiO_2 0.6 for 10 min, the PaO_2 is normally 200–300 mm Hg. Figure 11 shows the hyperoxia test modified from Davies [3] applied as an indication for artificial ventilation in the respiratory distress syndrome.

6.2.2 Differential Diagnosis of Congenital Heart Defects

At FiO_2 1.0 for 10 min, the PaO_2 is normally 400–600 mm Hg. Figure 12 shows the diagram for calculating the right-to-left shunt after the hyperoxia test, modified from Klaus [11].

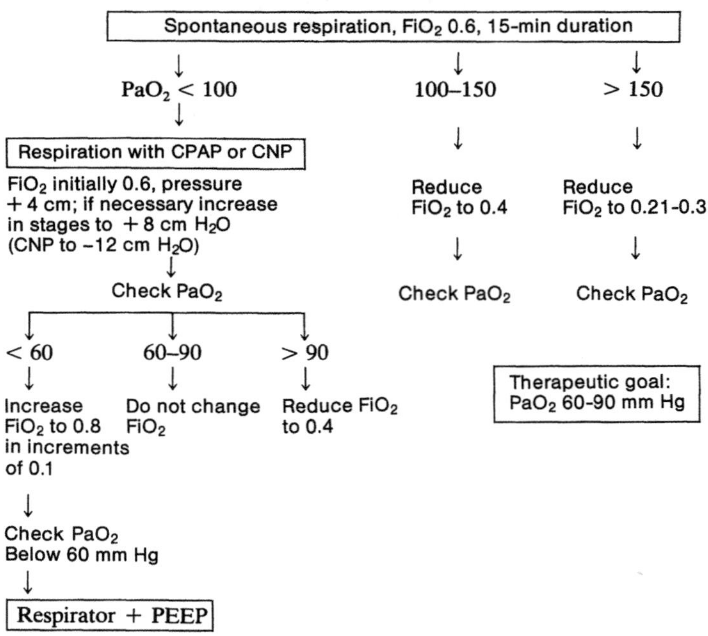

Fig. 11. Hyperoxia test as a guideline in the treatment of respiratory distress syndrome

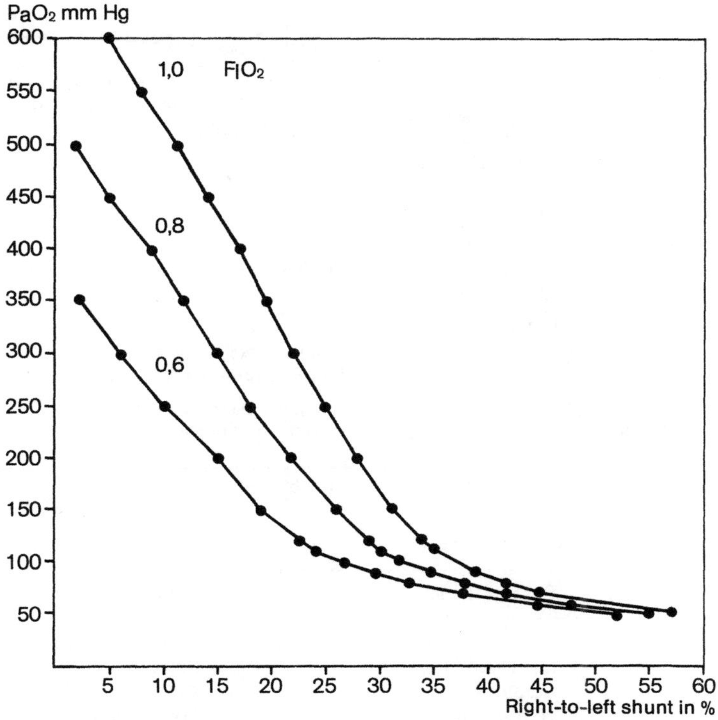

Fig. 12. Graph for calculating the right-to-left shunt at various FiO_2 values. Based on Hb 16 g% and PCO_2 40 mm Hg. (Modified from Klaus, 1966 [11])

6.3 Oxygen Dissociation

Figure 13 shows the oxygen dissociation curve and explains the mechanisms which can shift it to the left or right in newborn infants. Due to the steepness of the slope in the central part of the curve, the skin color of a newborn cannot be considered an index of adequate oxygenation. Hypoxemia may already be present (Fig. 13, see p. 66).

6.4 Causes of Disturbances in Oxygenation

6.4.1 Impaired Ventilation

Central Respiratory Disturbance. Meningitis, sepsis, cerebral hemorrhage, convulsions. Immature respiratory center, apneic spells.
Maldistribution. Aspiration (meconium), atelectasis.

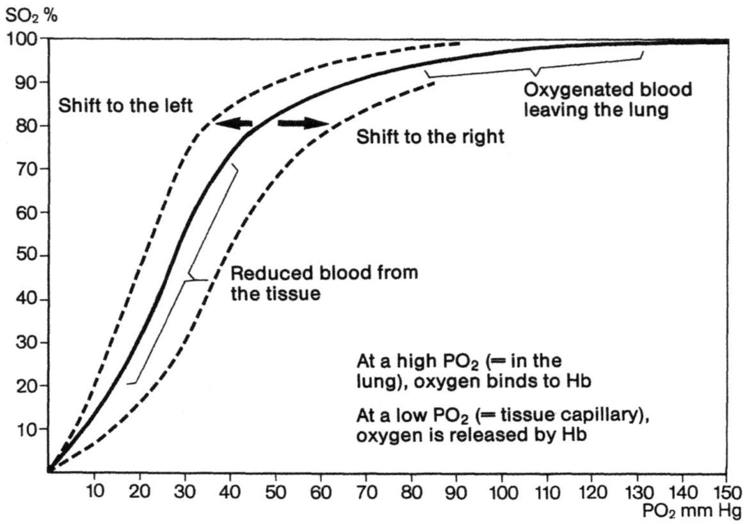

Oxygen Dissociation Curve

	Shift to the left	Shift to the right
Causes	Severe immaturity (increased HbF) Alkalosis Hypocapnia Hypothermia Decrease in 2, 3 DPG (4)	Blood exchange (increased HbA) Acidosis Hypercapnia Fever Increase in 2, 3 DPG
Result	Increased O_2 binding to Hb: O_2 is not released to the tissues as readily (i.e., only at higher tensions).	Decrease in O_2 affinity: More favorable release of O_2 to the tissues, since the tension gradient is greater.

Fig. 13. Oxygen dissociation curve. Significance of left and right shifts of the curve in the newborn infant

6.4.2 Impaired Diffusion

Respiratory distress syndrome, bronchopulmonary dysplasia, pulmonary edema, transitory tachypnea [2].

6.4.3 Impaired Perfusion

Respiratory distress syndrome, intrapulmonary right-to-left shunt in atelectasis, cyanotic defect with extrapulmonary right-to-left shunt, persistent fetal circulation after asphyxia, hypovolemia with hypotension, and right-to-left shunt through the ductus arteriosus.

6.4.4 Disturbances of Oxygen Binding and Oxygen Transport

One gram Hb binds 1.3 ml O_2. The oxygen-transporting capacity of the blood is optimal at an hematocrit of 45. At Hb 15 g%, the O_2 transport capacity is 21 vol.%. At Hb 8 g%, the O_2 transport capacity is 11 vol.%. For disturbances of oxygen binding, see also Fig. 13.

- Anemia (severe erythroblastosis)
- Polycythemia (maternofetal transfusion)
- Methemoglobinemia
- Peripheral vasoconstriction and shock
- Metabolic acidosis.

6.5 Dosage of Oxygen in Respiratory Gas

Oxygen analyzers operate on the basis of thermal conductivity, paramagnetic sensitivity, or with a Clark-type oxygen-sensitive electrode. If the device does not allow continuous measurement, the oxygen content of the respiratory gas must be measured at least hourly. Every oxygen analyzer must be calibrated daily with 21% and 100% oxygen. We use two oxygen analyzers:

1) The Biomarine 202 R operates with a gold-lead electrode as a fuel cell.
   Advantages. Requires no batteries, is very compact and easy to handle.
   Disadvantage. The fuel cell is very expensive and is used up in about 6 months.
2) The Vickers 404 operates with an electrolyte-filled oxygen-sensitive electrode.
   Advantages. Allows cost-saving electrode renewal, has alarm.
   Disadvantage. Requires batteries.

6.5.1 PaO_2 Measurement

Besides an accurate determination of the O_2 in the respiratory gas, oxygen therapy requires constant monitoring of the PaO_2 in the blood (see Chaps. 5.3, 5.4). This can also be done continuously with the aid of suitable electrodes [8].

6.5.2 $tcPO_2$ Measurement

Principle. Continuous measurement of the O_2 diffusing through localized warmed skin with a Clark-type electrode [9, 20]. Active vasodilation is induced by heating the electrode 44° C. The electrode placement must be changed every 2h to avoid second-degree burns. A harmless erythema occurs which may persist for several days. The electrode is calibrated in room air. In case of peripheral vasoconstriction or faulty electrode placement, the correlation with the PaO_2 is poor even in seriously ill infants.

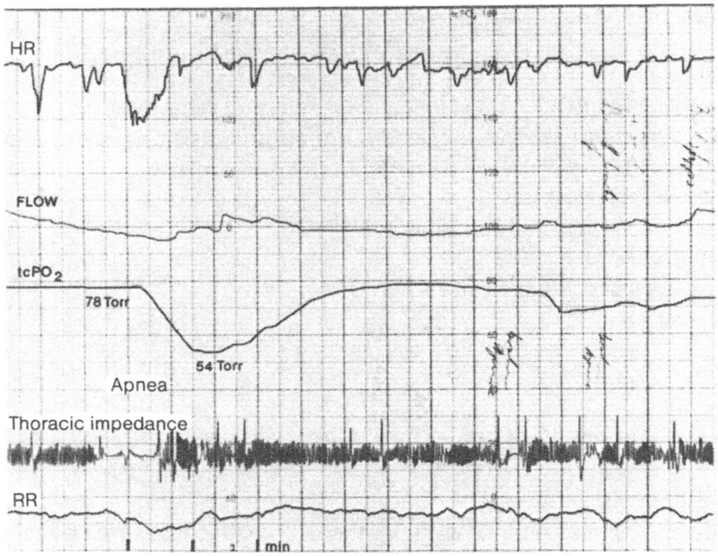

Fig. 14. Oxygen cardiorespirogram, shown here for an apneic spell. After 30 s the heart rate falls from 150/min to below 100/min; after 1 min the $tcPO_2$ falls frcm 78 to 54 mm Hg. (After Schachinger, 1979 [24])

Agreement with an arterial blood gas analysis must be checked once a day [19]. A decade of developmental work has produced several high-quality sensors and devices (Hellige, Radiometer, Roche), which have shown very good correlations between $tcPO_2$ and PaO_2 in clinical trials [22, 23, 25]. We prefer the Roche Oxygen Monitor 632, which is simple to operate and allows simultaneous and continuous recordings from two electrodes on a trend recorder. This makes it possible to monitor two infants simultaneously or to perform a dissociated hyperoxia test on a single infant with one electrode attached to the upper thorax (preductal) and the other to the lower abdomen (postductal). Optimal information is provided by cardiorespirography combined with $tcPO_2$ ("oxygen cardiorespirogram," Fig. 14), which also allows a differentiated hyperoxia test [24]. This noninvasive method can also be used to evaluate immediate postpartum adaptation and facilitates decisions regarding advisability of referral of sick neonates [25]

6.6 Modes of Administration

Oxygen must always be heated and humidified.

6.6.1 Incubator

In the Dräger 6500 intensive care incubator, oxygen can be administered up to an FiO_2 of 0.8. However, the FiO_2 falls immediately when the incubator is opened.

6.6.2 Plastic Head Box (Oxyhood)

Has proved favorable for all oxygen concentrations above FiO_2 0.6, especially when performing the hyperoxia test.

6.6.3. Ventilation

- Mask (Rendell-Baker, size 0–2) with Penlon bag (safety valve, check for free action!) or Kuhn system
- CPAP system (regulated by oxygen blender)
- Respirator (regulated by oxygen blender)

6.7 Side Effects of Oxygen Therapy

6.7.1 Retrolental Fibroplasia

Risk factors are immaturity, PaO_2 over 102–120 mm Hg and oxygen therapy in excess of 6 h duration. Numerous brief, uncontrolled hyperoxic peaks (as in the administration of O_2 by mask during apneic spells) has also been associated with retrolental fibroplasia [1]! The clinical course may be highly variable [14]. Patz [15] has developed the following system for classifying the disease according to degree of severity:

Active Stage
- Vasoconstriction and tortuosity
- Neovascularization
- Proliferation, incipient peripheral retinal detachment
- Increased proliferation and retinal detachment
- Complete retinal detachment.

Cicatricial Stage

- Minor changes, opaque tissue in periphery of the fundus
- Displacement of the optic disk
- Retinal folds, opacity of the vitreous body
- Extensive opacity which covers parts of the pupil
- Complete retrolental opacity.

6.7.2 Bronchopulmonary Dysplasia

Risk Factors. Immaturity, combination of mechanical injury and oxygen toxicity in the pneumocytes, particularly during long-term ventilation with FiO_2 over 0.8 and over 44 h.

Pathogenesis. Inactivation of surfactant leads to damage of the pneumocytes, poor alveolar expansion with unequal alveolar expansion, interstitial proliferation, and fibrosis. Oxygen inhibits the pulmonary synthesis of DNA (13). The deficiency of superoxide dismutase may also be responsible for the increased risk of hyperoxic tissue damage in newborn infants (6). For the stages of bronchopulmonary dysplasia, see p. 106.

6.7.3 Ventilatory Depression

If a high concentration of O_2 is administered suddenly, a ventilatory inhibition of several minutes' duration may result (16). Ventilation is controlled largely by receptors that respond to oxygen deficiency, particularly with hypercapnia (PCO_2 >80 mm Hg). Apnea results if these receptors are inhibited by the sudden administration of oxygen.

References

1. Aranda, J. V., Saheb, N., Stern, L., Avery, M. E.: Arterial Oxygen Tension and Retinal Vasoconstriction in Newborn Infants. Am. J. Dis. Child *122*, 189 (1971)
2. Avery, M. E., Fletcher, B. D.: The lung and its disorders in the newborn infant. Philadelphia-London-Toronto: Saunders, 1974
3. Davies, P. A., Robinson, R. J., Scopes, J. W., Tizard, J. P. M., Wigglesworth, J. S.: Medical Care of Newborn Babies. London-Philadelphia Heinemann-Lippincott 1972
4. Delivoria-Papadopoulos, M., Roncevic, N. P., Oski, F. A.: Postnatal changes in oxygen transport of term, premature, and sick infants: The role of red cell 2,3-diphosphoglycerate and adult hemoglobin. Pediatr. Res. *5*, 235 (1971)
5. Dick, W., Ahnefeld, F. W.: Primäre Neugeborenen-Reanimation. Berlin-Heidelberg-New York: Springer 1975
6. Frank, L., Antor, A. P., Roberts, R. J.: Oxygen therapy and hyaline membrane disease: the effect of hyperoxia on pulmonary superoxide dismutase activity and the mediating role of plasma or serum. J. Pediatrics *90*, 105 (1977)

7. HERMAN, S., REYNOLDS, E. O. R.: Methods for improving arterial oxygen tension in infants mechanically ventilated for severe hyaline membrane disease. Arch. Dis. Child. *48*, 612 (1973)
8. HUCH, A., HUCH, R., NEUMAYER, E., ROOTH, G.: Continuous intra-arterial PO_2 measurements in infants. Acta Paediatr. Scand. *61*, 722 (1972)
9. HUCH, A., LÜBBERS, D. W., HUCH, R.: Patientenüberwachung durch transkutane PO_2-Messung bei gleichzeitiger Kontrolle der relativen lokalen Perfusion. Anaesthesist *22*, 379 (1973)
10. HUCH, A., HUCH, R.: Physiologische und methodische Grundlagen der transkutanen PO_2- und PCO_2-Messungen. In: Pädiatrische Intensivmedizin, Band 3, S. 58. EMMRICH P. (Hrsg.) Stuttgart: Thieme 1977
11. KLAUS, M., MEYER, B.: Oxygen therapy for the newborn. Pediatr. Clin. North. Am. *13*, 731 (1966)
12. METZE, H.: Über den therapeutischen Einsatz von Sauerstoff beim Atemnotsyndrom Früh- und Neugeborener. Klin. Pädiat. *186*, 19 (1974)
13. NORTHWAY, W. H., REZEAU, L., PETRICEKS, R., BENSCH, K. G.: Oxygen toxicity in the newborn lung. Pediatrics *57*, 41 (1976)
14. O'GRADY, G. E., FLYNN, J. T., HERRERA, J. A.: Clinical course of retrolental fibroplasia in premature infants. South. med. J. *65*, 655 (1972)
15. PATZ, A.: Retrolental fibroplasia. Survey Ophthal. *14*, 1 (1969)
16. RIGATTO, R., BRADY, J. P., de la Torre VERDUZCO, R.: Chemoreceptor reflexes in preterm infants. In: The effect of gestational and postnatal age on the ventilatory response to inhalation of 100% and 15% oxygen. Pediatrics *55*, 604 (1975)
17. SHAPIRO, B. A., et al.: Clinical Application of Respiratory Care. Chicago: Year Book Medical Publishers 1975
18. SWANSTRÖM, S., ELISAGA, I. V., CARDONA, L., CARDENES, A., MENDEZ-BAUER, C., ROOTH, G.: Transcutaneous PO_2 measurement in seriously ill newborn infants. Arch. Dis. Child. *50*, 913 (1975)
19. DUC, G., BUCHER, H. U., MICHELI, J., JOHANSON, B.: Is transcutaneous PO_2 reliable for arterial oxygen monitoring in newborn infants? Pediatrics *55*, 566 (1975)
20. EBERHARDT, P., MINDT, W.: Skin Sensors for Continuous Oxygen Monitoring of Newborns. Biotelemetry *4*, 48 (1977)
21. HUCH, R. u. A.: Zustandsdiagnostik beim Neugeborenen unmittelbar post partum durch das Sauerstoff-Kardiorespirogramm (SCR). In: Pädiatrische Intensivmedizin. EMMRICH, P. (Hrsg.), Bd. 3, S. 65. Stuttgart: Thieme 1977
22. LÖFGREN, O., HENRIKSSON, P., JACOBSON, L., JOHANNSSON, Ö.: Transcutaneous PO_2 Monitoring in neonatal intensive care. Acta Paediatr. Scand. *67*, 693 (1978)
23. ROOTH, G.: Transcutaneous oxygen tension measurements newborn infants. Pediatrics *55*, 232 (1975)
24. SCHACHINGER, H.: Das Sauerstoff-Cardiorespirogramm, technische Grundlage und klinische Bedeutung bei der Überwachung Neugeborener. Med. Tech. *99*, 16 (1979)
25. LESOUEF, P. N., MORGAN, A. K., SOUTTER. L. P., REYNOLDS, E. O. R., PARKER, D.: Comparison of transcutaneous oxygen tension with arterial oxygen tension in newborn infants with severe respiratory illnesses. Pediatrics *62*, 692 (1978)

7 Artificial Ventilation

M. Obladen

7.1 Ventilatory Status of the Newborn (Tables 28, 29)

Table 28. Ventilatory failure in the newborn

Definition
PaO_2 <50 mm Hg in FiO_2 0.6, or
PCO_2 >80 mm Hg, or
Apnea >20 s

Symptoms
Tachypnea
Tachycardia
Inspiratory retractions
Expiratory grunting
Nasal flaring
Cyanosis
Apnea

Causes in order of frequency
1. Respiratory distress syndrome
2. Congenital heart defects
3. Aspiration syndrome
4. Central respiratory disturbance (apnea, cerebral hemorrhage, meningitis, sepsis)
5. Maternal sedation (morphine, anesthesia)
6. Pneumonia
7. Pneumothorax
8. Malformation of the upper airways (choanal atresia, Pierre-Robin syndrome, laryngomalacia, stenoses, etc.)
9. Other malformations (lobar emphysema, pulmonary hypoplasia, diaphragmatic hernia, etc.)

Table 29. Comparison of the pulmonary physiology of adults and newborns (modified from Nelson [25] and Doershuk [6])

Quantity measured	Dimension	Adults		Newborns	
		total	Per kg	total	Per kg
Lung weight	g	800	11	50	17
Number of alveoli		$300 \cdot 10^6$	$4{,}3 \cdot 10^6$	$24 \cdot 10^6$	$8 \cdot 10^6$
Alveolar diameter	μ	200–300		50	
Alveolar surface area	m^2	70	1,0	2,8	1,0
Respiration rate	Per min	20		40	
O_2 consumption	ml/min	250	3,5	18	6,0–6,7
Lung compliance (total)	ml/cm H_2O	100	1,4	4,9	1,3
Flow resistance	cmH_2O/ 1/sec	5,5		68	
Alveolar ventilation (respiratory minute volume)	ml/min	4200	60	400	100–150
Tidal volume	ml	450	7	20	6
Anatomical dead space	ml	150	2,2	7,0	2,2
Functional residual capacity	ml	2400	34	90	30
Residual volume	ml	1190	17	60	20

7.2 Indication for Artificial Ventilation

Besides improving the aeration of the lungs, artificial ventilation also increases the oxygenation of the blood by its effect on diffusion. This therapy is indicated for essentially all infants with correctable respiratory failure and should be initiated before systemic damage occurs as a result of hypoxia or acidosis. In recent years the tendency observed toward earlier intervention in respiratory distress syndrome (11, 24, 27) increasingly has reached a level of acceptance with mechanical ventilation instituted at a FiO_2 of 0.6 for respiratory failure (20).

7.2.1 Birth Asphyxia or Emergency

Ventilate immediately for bradycardia below 80/min or if the 1-min Apgar is $\leqq 4$. Ventilate after 1 min if persistent apnea occurs.

7.2.2 Central Respiratory Disturbance and Immaturity

Preterm infants with recurrent or prolonged apneic spells that are irreversible after mask ventilation for 5 min; persistent respiratory acidosis, no response to theophylline [37] and nasal CPAP [17].

7.2.3 Respiratory Distress Syndrome

PaO_2 below 60 mm Hg in the hyperoxia test [5] (see p 64).

7.2.4 Aspiration Syndrome

PaO_2 below 60 mm Hg as indicated in the hyperoxia test (see p 64).
PCO_2 above 80 mm Hg with uncompensated respiratory acidosis $<$pH 7.30.

7.2.5 Cardiac Failure

Respiratory acidosis with PCO_2 above 80 mm Hg and pH below 7.25 with compensated base deficit.

7.3 Technical Essentials

Artificial ventilation is a demanding procedure which requires all the technical resources of the intensive care unit [4]: 3 m wall space per bed, 25 m^2 floor space per patient, including ancillary rooms (workroom, dressing room, laboratory, holding rooms, etc.), wall outlets for oxygen, purified air and suction, equipment for continuous and immediate blood gas analysis, and proximity to laboratory, X-ray, and surgical facilities.
For every child being administered to in the intensive care unit, an ET tube of the proper length and size should be on hand, together with all accessories (see p 255).

7.3.1 Disinfection of Tubing and Equipment

a) *Instrument Cleaning.* (E. g., 1% Edisonite solution for 30–60 min) used for surgical instruments, heavily contaminated tubing and connectors.
b) *Surface Spray.* (E. g., undiluted Buraton liquid = isopropanol-aldehyde mixture) used for transport incubators, telephone receivers, wheels of X-ray unit, etc.
c) *Surface Wipe.* (E. g., 3% Lysoformin = aldehyde derivative) used for respirator control elements, monitors, instrument tables, wash basins, etc.
d) *Soaking.* (E. g., 3% Korsolin = aldehyde derivative) used for oxygen hoses, ventilator tubing systems, vaporizer jars, etc. Objects are soaked for at least 30 min, then rinsed with water for 30 min and dried with a sterile towel or desicator.
e) *Automatic Gas Disinfection.* (E. g., Draeger Aseptor 5400, 8800 = formaldehyde-ammonia).

After cleaning. Open all cavities and covers; expose to formaldehyde vapor for 70 min, then neutralize with ammonia and aerate. Total disinfection time: 2.5 h). Hang a UV lamp in incubators during disinfection.

Used for incubators, cribs, respirators, ventilation bags.

f) *Gas Sterilization.* (E. g., ethylene oxide) used for all ventilator parts, is also suitable for electronic devices.

Advantage. The parts to be sterilized can be sealed beforehand in plastic bags.

In All Methods. The instruments should be packaged aseptically and stored after cleaning, preferably heat-sealed in clear plastic film.

7.3.2 Assembly of Ventilator Tubing

For each tubing set used at the intensive care unit, at least two sets must be disinfected and ready for use at all times:

a) Bird tubing system with PEEP modification and heated humidifier [32] (see Fig. 15).
b) Universal CPAP system with humidifier and manometer (see Fig. 22).
c) IMV system with humidifier and reservoir bag (see Fig. 20).

7.4 Ventilators and Their Operation

7.4.1 Classification of Some Ventilators Suitable for Neonatal Use

Respirators are nothing more than sophisticated air pumps. To make them useful as therapeutic tools, the doctors and nurses must be thoroughly familiar with their technical properties and operation. The type of respirator used is not as important as the *level of training* and experience of the personnel. Next to this criterion, the long and heated debate about volume versus pressure cycling [18, 21] and assisted versus controlled ventilation [15] is of little consequence: The different types of ventilators have shown no differences in terms of survival rate or the frequency of complications [40]. With suitable modifications, all ventilatory support in neonatology can be administered with two or three different types of devices. We use the Bourns BP 200, Bourns LS 104–150, Bird Mark 8, and Cavitron PV 10 in our neonatal intensive care unit. Table 30 lists several ventilators which are suitable for neonatal use, together with their modes of operation.

Table 30. Classification of some ventilators for neonatal use

Working principle (i. e., what is produced by the device?)	Ventilator	Control principle (i. e., what terminates the inspiratory phase?)
1. Constant flow	Bourns LS 104–150	Volume
	Bennett MA 1 B Ped.	Time
	Baby Bird	Time
	Cavitron PV 10	Time
	Biomed MVP 10	Time
	Draeger Babylog 1/2	Time
	Spiromat K	Time
	Loosco AIV	Time
	Roche Baby Control	Volume
2. Sinusoidal flow	Engström ER 314/322	Volume
3. Constant flow or constant pressure	Servo-Ventilator 900	Volume
4. Constant pressure	Bennett PR 2	Flow
	Bird Mark 8	Pressure
	Assistor 644	Pressure
	Bourns BP 200	Time

7.4.2 Bird Mark 8

This is a study pressure-controlled ventilator which is suitable for universal use (Fig. 16). When the inspiratory pressure is reached, the attraction of a magnet to an iron plate is overcome, and a sliding valve shuts off the flow of gas. The flow rate is the main control variable. PEEP can be produced by utilizing the expiratory gas flow of a negative-pressure generator [32] and bypassing the venturi. With this PEEP modification and a heated humidifier [22], the unit is capable of continuous ventilation. Very high ventilation pressures at high flow rates can be achieved if desired. The "assist" mode should not be used in neonates due to the high trigger volume of 1.5 ml and the slow response time of 157 ms [8].

Advantages. The ventilator is independent of electrical outlets and is thus ideal for transport; it is suitable for all age groups.

Disadvantages. Complicated tubing assembly, no alarm capability, nebulizer requires modification for use. We use this ventilator mainly for meconium aspiration and for large infants with severe RDS in the initial stage. The Bird tubing system modified for PEEP ventilation is shown in Fig. 15.

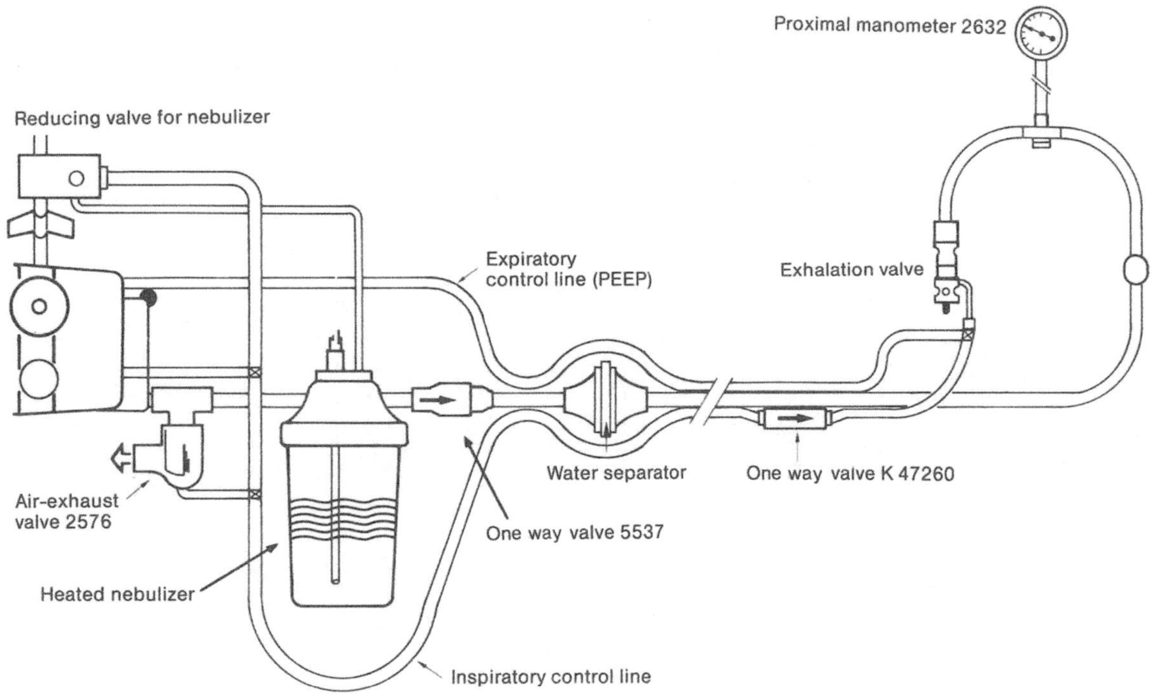

Fig. 15. Modified neonatal tubing system for the Bird Mark 8. The expiratory control line is used for the production of PEEP. The inspiratory control line and patient line must be equipped with one-way check valves

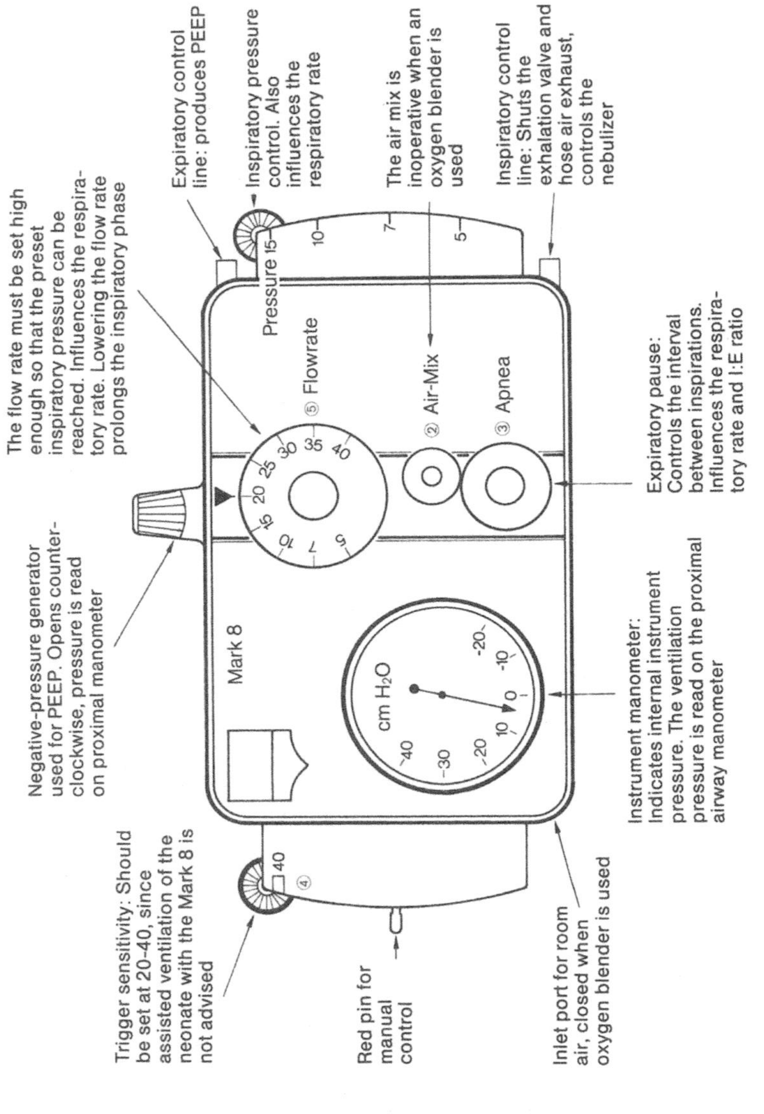

Fig. 16. Diagram of the Bird Mark 8 control panel

7.4.3 Bourns LS 104–150

Volume-controlled ventilator for infants and neonates (Fig. 17). The unit produces a constant volume with an electronically controlled piston pump. A highly sensitive electronic sensor permits operation in the "assist" mode even for neonates; the trigger volume is 0.05 ml, the response time 35 ms [8]. Pressure-limited operation is possible. *Advantages.* Simple operation and assembly; built-in low-pressure alarm.

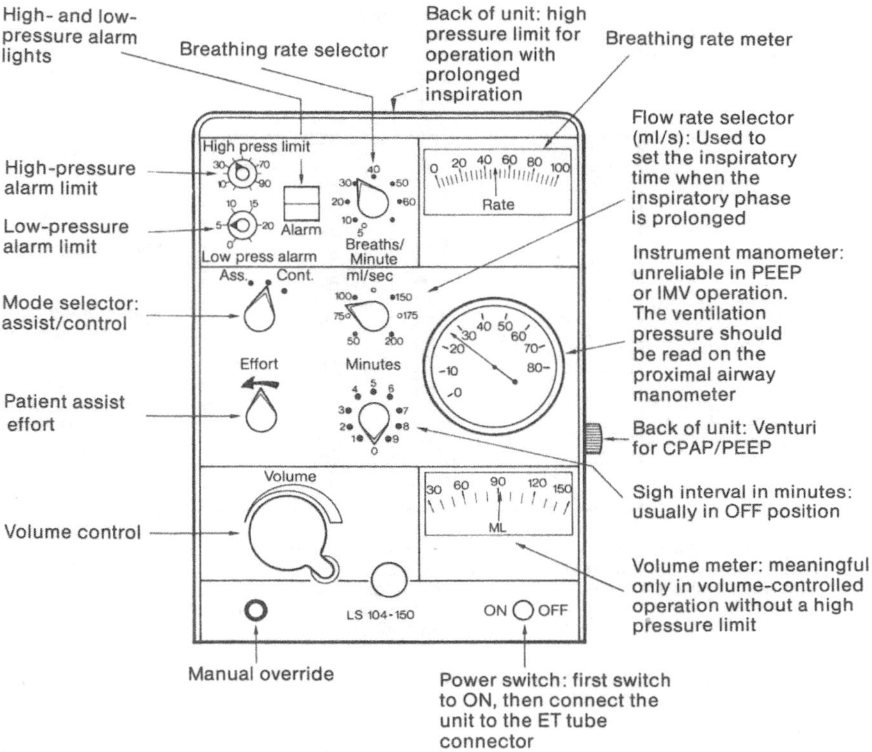

Fig. 17. Diagram of the Bourns LS 104–150 control panel

Disadvantage. The inspiratory phase is short and the peak pressure is high in volume-controlled operation; hence no inspiration plateau can be established. We usually operate the device in a modified pressure-limited mode with a prolonged inspiratory phase: A high tidal volume is set (100–120 ml), and the inspiratory pressure is limited to 20–25 cm H_2O with the knurled screw in back of the unit. The flow rate then regulates the inspiratory time. We use this ventilator in the volume-controlled mode for central respiratory disturbance and in postoperative states (e.g., after cardiac surgery).

7.4.4 Bourns BP 200

Time-controlled, pressure-limited ventilator for infants and neonates (Fig. 18). The unit produces a constant flow via a system of valves, and an electronic control system allows the largely independent control of all ventilation parameters. A highly versatile unit with capabilities for CPAP, PEEP, and IMV [7]. This unit allows control of ventilation with a prolonged inspiratory phase, owing to the very broad range of I : E

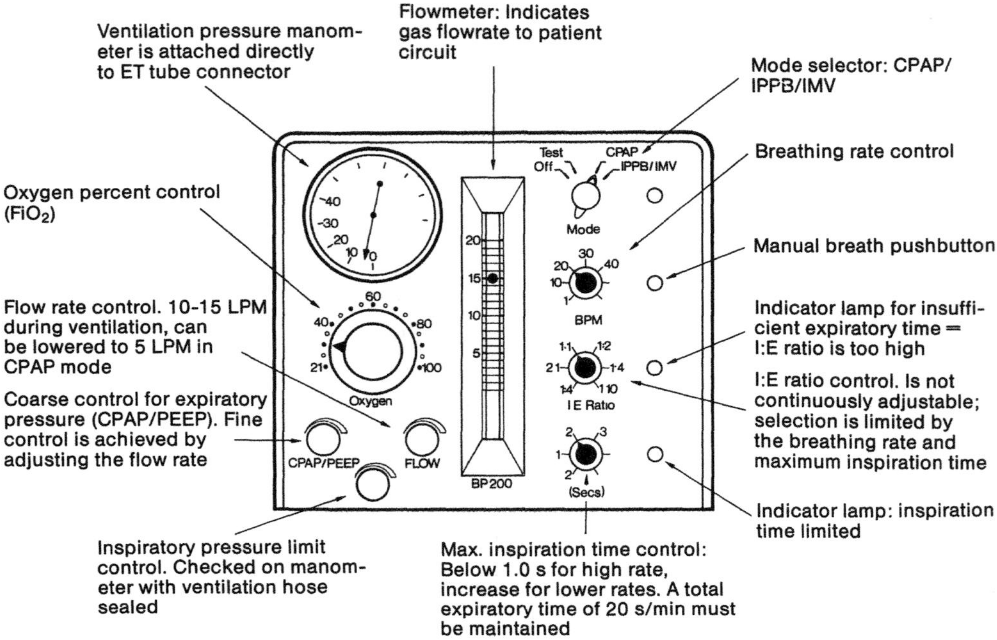

Fig. 18. Diagram of the Bourns BP 200 control panel

ratios and the fact that the inspiratory time can be directly limited and thus preselected [9].

Advantages. Built-in oxygen blender; IMV can be administered without accessory equipment.

Disadvantage. Has no low-pressure alarm, must always be used with a ventilation monitor. We prefer this clevice for ventilating infants with RDS.

7.4.5 Cavitron PV 10, Biomed MVP 10

Time-controlled, pressure-limited ventilator for infants and neonates (Fig. 19). The unit produces a constant gas flow via two flow regulators and a system of valves. Control is effected by pneumatic elements. Has precision controls for inspiratory time and expiratory pause; IMV operation is possible.

Advantages. Is independent of electric current owing to pneumatic control; has a very low gas consumption (practically identical to the patient flow).

Disadvantage. The rate and FiO_2 cannot be directly selected, but must be calculated. The respirator can be equipped with a supplementary oxygen blender if desired. It operates silently and has no low-pressure alarm; a ventilation monitor is required for continuous operation. We use the Cavitron for the transport of high-risk neonates, especially over great distances, and for ventilatory resuscitation in outlying hospitals.

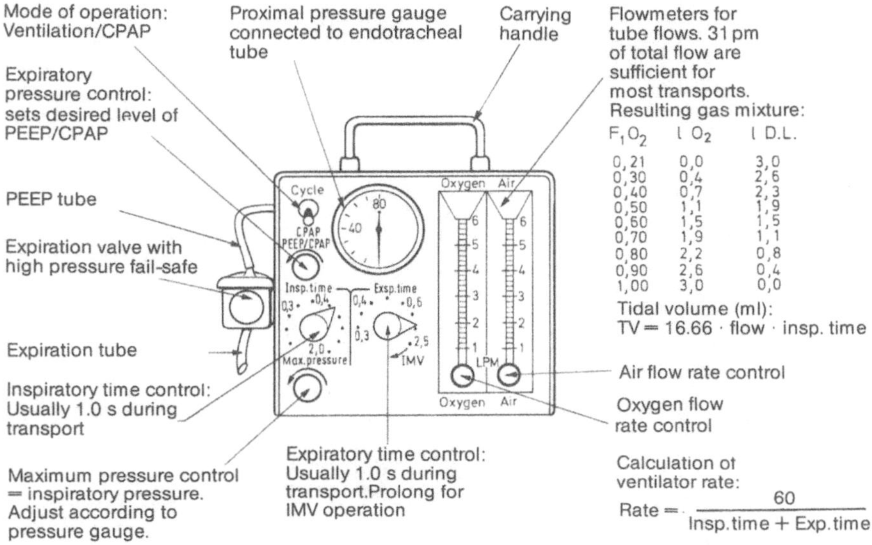

Fig. 19. Diagram of the Cavitron PV 10 and Biomed MVP 10 control panel

7.4.6 Ventilator Test Run

When

- At least once a week
- On assembly
- Before unit is put into operation.

How

Preferably with a model lung with a volume of 10–20 ml (rubber finger cots packed with swabs). Check the following:

- Wall connections
- Tubing system complete?
- When last disinfected?
- Supplementary valves in working order?
- PEEP or IMV system correctly assembled? Test-run ventilator for a period of 5 min
- Monitoring and alarm functions: Ventilation monitor? Oxygen blender working accurately? Manometer calibrated?

7.4.7 Basic Settings of a Neonatal Ventilator Ready for Use

- Respiratory rate 30/min
- Pressure 22/4 cm H_2O
- Inspiratory time 1.0 s
- I : E ratio 1 : 1
- FiO_2 0.6.

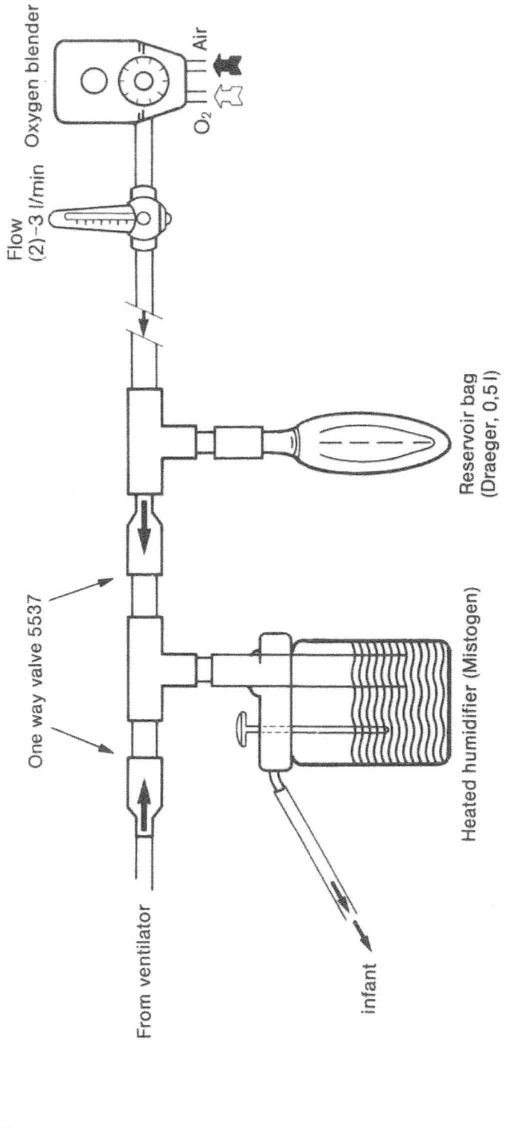

Fig. 20. System for administering IMV, can be installed on virtually any ventilator

7.4.8 Intermittent Mandatory Ventilation (IMV)

A form of ventilation specially adapted to the newborn infant: ventilation at a low rate, allowing the infant to breathe spontaneously between individual ventilator cycles. The technique can be combined with CPAP or PEEP. Spontaneous respiration can be progressively increased, so that the infant can be more easily weaned from the ventilator [7]. Fig. 20 shows a universal valve system with a reservoir bag; this system can be connected to any ventilator for administering IMV.

7.5 Continuous Positive Airway Pressure (CPAP)

7.5.1 Definitions (Fig. 21)

7.5.2 Principle

Increases the functional residual capacity; expands and maintains expansion of atelectatic areas of lung [13]. Surfactant release can occur only if the alveoli are adequately ventilated [39]. As collapsed lung areas are expanded, diffusion is improved and the PaO_2 is increased and $PaCO_2$ decreased.

7.5.3 CPAP System

Indication in respiratory distress syndrome: see hyperoxia test [5], p 64; nasal CPAP with a tube length of 3–4 cm is employed [33].

Apneic Attacks. Nasal CPAP with 2–cm tube length and a level of 2 cm H_2O (stimulates the respiratory receptors in the nose). Nasal CPAP reduces frequency of apnea by 69% [17].

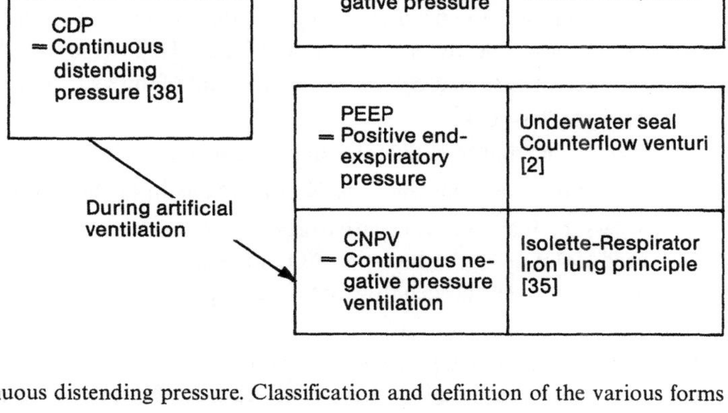

Fig. 21. Continuous distending pressure. Classification and definition of the various forms

Weaning. After severe respiratory distress syndrome or other long-term ventilatory support.

Technique. Minimal flow = 3X respiratory minute volume. Respiratory minute volume = 6–8 ml/kg X respiratory rate.

Procedure. CPAP flow of 3–5 LPM.
Initial CPAP level = 4–5 cm H_2O; increase in 2-cm increments to a maximum of 10 cm H_2O [10]. The blood gases must be monitored following each pressure change. The nasal tube is fixed [14] by means of a silicone flange which fits over the nose and is secured by a loose band about the head – similar to the method for nasotracheal tube fixation [3]. A simple CPAP system consists of an oxygen blender, heated humidifier, manometer, and underwater seal and is shown in Fig. 22.

7.5.4 CNP System (Pulmarca)

Opposite of CPAP: The chest is enclosed in a negative-pressure chamber; alveolar expansion is maintained by a continuous negative transthoracic pressure.

Indication. RDS, only relatively large infants (over 1500–2000 g) with good spontaneous respiratory activity whose respiratory failure is due mainly to impaired diffusion. Can be done only in infants with an umbilical artery catheter or, preferably, a transcutaneous electrode [26].

Technique

a) Place chamber into incubator, with inlet and outlet lines leading out of incubator (to avoid chilling), and connect.
b) Close chamber, set end expiratory pressure to −6 cm H_2O on upper dial.
c) Place infant into chamber. Pass monitor cable and umbilical catheter out through the seal, support the head with a pillow; do not overtighten the neck seal since an airleak is desirable and is compensated for by the flow, so that the desired negative pressure is maintained. Subaxillary placement of the seal is effective and lessens the risk of necrosis [41].
d) Close the incubator, adjust desired O_2 concentration in the incubator air.
e) Monitor by blood gas analysis, X-ray, etc., as in artificial ventilation.
f) If necessary, increase the negative pressure up to −10 cm H_2O [12]. When the PaO_2 exceeds 90 mm Hg, reduce the FiO_2 in stages. As soon as the FiO_2 reaches 0.4, gradually reduce the negative pressure in increments of 2 cm H_2O.

Risks. Pneumothorax (as in CPAP), necrosis at the neck, chilling (especially if the chamber is not preheated), danger of shock from fall of central venous pressure.

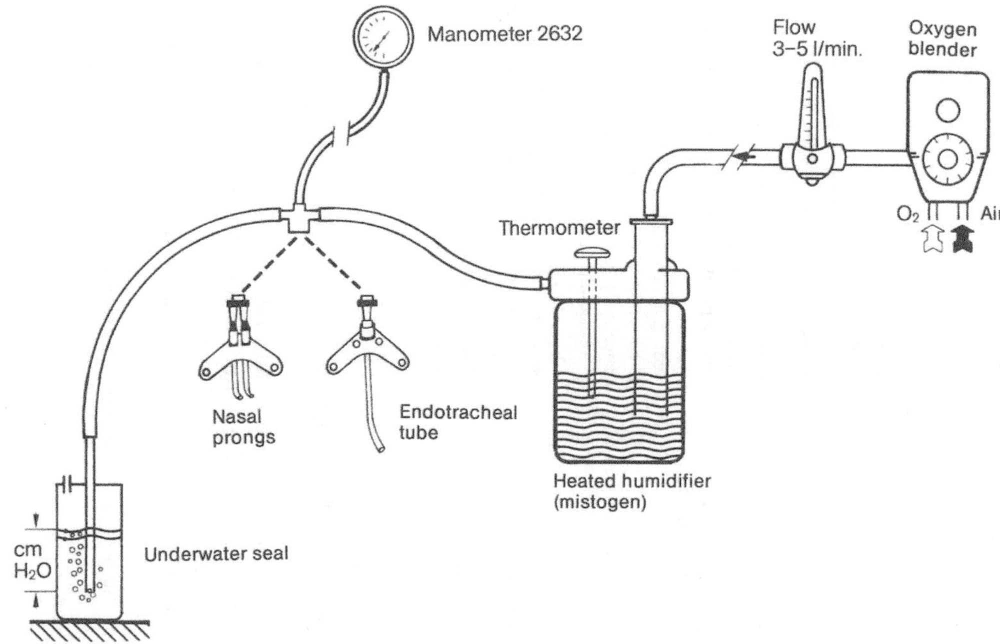

Fig. 22. Tubing system for continuous positive airway pressure (CPAP). The system can be fitted with adapters for a nasal or endotracheal tube

7.5.5 Comparison of CNP and CPAP (Table 31)

Table 31

CNP Pulmarca	CPAP Nasal prongs
No endotracheal tube needed	No endotracheal tube is needed
Mouth is free	Mouth is free
Access to infant restricted	Access to infant is unrestricted
Venous return ↑	Venous return ↓
Arterial puncture not possible; an umbilical artery catheter or transoxode is required	Monitoring by arterial puncture is possible
Feeding is possible	Feeding is problematic; risk of gastric distention and aspiration
Preheating is necessary, with possible loss of time	Preheating is unnecessary; system is ready for immediate use
No assembly is needed	Tubing system must be disinfected and connected to the oxygen blender and humidifier
Constant pressure is ensured	Unintentional pressure swings can occur if the tubing becomes kinked
Danger of necrosis at the neck	Danger of necrosis in the nose

7.5.6 Complications and Side Effects of CPAP

CPAP toxicity = CO_2 accumulation due to diminished expiration, especially with CPAP > 8–10 or PEEP > 6 cm H_2O. Respiratory acidosis, decreased minute volume, decreased venous return, cardiac failure.
Extra-alveolar collection of air (pneumomediastinum, pneumothorax, pneumopericardium, see p 118).
Danger of necrosis at the neck if a head box or Pulmarca is used [19].

7.6 Control of Ventilation

7.6.1 Control Scheme (Table 32)

Table 32. For simplicity, the acid-base derangements which usually accompany ventilatory changes in practice are disregarded here

Blood gas change	Means of correction
1. Hypercapnia: PCO_2 too high	Flow rate ↑ Respiratory rate ↑ Tidal or minute volume ↑ Dead space ↓
2. Hypocapnia: PCO_2 too low	Flow rate ↓ Respiratory rate ↓ Inspiratory pressure ↓ Tidal or minute volume ↓ Dead space ↑
3. Hyperoxemia: PaO_2 too high	FiO_2 ↓ PEEP ↓
4. Hypoxemia: PaO_2 too low	FiO_2 ↑ PEEP ↑ Inspiratory pressure ↑
5. Total ventilatory failure: PCO_2 too high and PaO_2 too low	I : E ratio ↑ Inspiratory pressure ↑ Inspiratory time ↑ Tidal or minute volume ↑
6. "CPAP toxicity": PCO_2 too high and PaO_2 normal or high	PEEP ↓

7.6.2 Changing the Ventilator Settings

Principle. Every change is documented and monitored by blood gas analysis. Only *one* parameter is changed at a time.

a) *When using pressure-controlled ventilators,* increase or decrease inspiratory pressure in increments of 2–5 cm H_2O; PEEP is usually 3–5 cm H_2O initially, is changed initially in stages of 5/min; in IMV and at rates below 15, increase or decrease in increments of 2/min.

b) *With volume-controlled ventilators* we use the following rule of thumb: Tidal volume including tube leak = 10–15 ml/kg body wt. The tidal volume is changed in increments of 5 ml; the respiratory rate and PEEP are changed as under a).

c) *Long expiratory times and low I : E ratios* were once preferred for newborns [28], but since the advent of PEEP and especially since the investigations of Reynolds [16, 30, 31], the inspiratory phase has become increasingly prolonged and the inspiratory flow reduced (plateau respiration). This makes it necessary to measure the inspiratory time; the Bourns LS 160 ventilation monitor can do this with precision, but a stopwatch can also be used. The optimal range for the inspiratory time is 1.0–2.0 s. It must be adjusted such that a total expiratory time of at least 20 s per minute is obtained. For preterm infants <1500 g, the inspiratory time should not exceed 1.5 s.

7.7 Examples of Ventilation

Some typical examples of ventilation including blood gas analyses and ventilator settings are given in this section. The arrows indicate the change made in the ventilator setting after a particular blood gas analysis.
Arterial PO_2 values are underlined, and warmed capillary PO_2 values are enclosed in parentheses.

7.7.1 Immature Preterm Infant with Apneic Attacks and Central Respiratory Disturbance (Table 33)

Table 33. Ventilation: volume-controlled/pressure-limited, brief attempt at spontaneous respiration. Bourns LS 104–150 ventilator; body weight 990 g, 29th week of gestation, 2nd day of life

Time:	3 : 00, etc.	4.00	5.00	6.00	8.00
pH	7,53	7,57	7,28	7,48	7,44
PCO_2	26	20	56	24	45
StB	24,5	23	22,5	21,5	28
BE	+1	−1	−2	−3	+5
PO_2	53	62	48	60	56
FiO_2	30%			→ 35%	→ 30%
Rate	25	→ 20	→ Spontane-	→ 15	→ 10
Pressure	15/3		ous after	15/3	
Vol.	20		20 min	20	
Insp. time	1,0			1,0	

7.7.2 **Preterm Infant, Stage-II RDS, Stabilization by Prolonged Inspiration** (Table 34)

Table 34. Ventilation: time-controlled/pressure-limited with IMV. Bourns BP 200 ventilator. Body weight 2170 g, 34th week of gestation, 2nd day of life

Time:	15:00, etc.	16.00	17.00	18.00	20.00	21.00	22.00	23.00
pH	7,30	7,40	7,47	7,42	7,55	7,48	7,49	7,44
PCO_2	95	47	40	49	31	33	44	42
StB	35	26,5	28	29	29	25,5	31	27
BE	+12	+3	+5	+6	+6	+2	+8	+4
PO_2	(36)	(63)	<u>50</u>	<u>42</u>	70	94	73	80
FiO_2	100%	100%	→ 60%	→ 65%	→ 70%		→ 65%	→ 60%
Rate	30		→ 25		25	→ 20	→ 18	→ 12
Pressure	20/3			→ 20/5	20/5		20/5	
Vol.								
Insp. time	1,0		→ 1,2		→ 1,5		→ 2,0	2,0

7.7.3 Preterm Infant, Stage-III RDS, Weaning by Use of IMV (Table 35)

Table 35. Ventilation: time-controlled/pressure-limited, IMV at decreasing rate, Bourns BP 200 ventilator. Body weight 1980 g, 33rd week of gestation, 4th day of life

Time:	1 : 00, etc.	4.00	7.00	9.00	13.00	18.00	21.00	0.00
pH	7,30	7,30	7,31	7,36	7,40	7,46	7,38	7,36
PCO_2	68	65	57	51	44	37	49	52
StB	26,5	25,2	24	25,5	25,5	17	26,5	25,5
BE	+3	+2	±0	+2	+2	+4	+3	+2
PO_2	75	72	96	80	76	91	84	72
FiO_2	70%	→ 65%	→ 60%	→ 55%	→ 45%		→ 40%	40%
Rate	28	→ 25		→ 20	→ 12	→ 8	→ 2	→ CPAP
Pressure	20/4	→ 18/3		18/3			18/3+4	L
Vol.								
Insp. time	1,3			→ 1,6	→ 2,0	2,0		

7.7.4 **Child of Diabetic Mother, Stage-IV RDS, Stabilization by High Inspiratory Pressure** (Table 36)

Table 36. Ventilation: pressure-controlled, high rate and high pressure. Bird Mark 8 ventilator. Body weight 3710 g, 36th week of gestation, 2nd day of life

Time:	3 : 00, etc.	5.00	6.00	10.00	16.00	16.30	17.00	17.30	18.00
pH	7,27	7,29	7,36	7,31	7,40	7,42	7,45	7,47	7,43
PCO_2	110	95	74	89	64	63	49	61,7	68
StB	38,5	35,5	35	34	34	34	31	39,5	39
BE	+16	+13	+12	+11	+11	+11	+8	+17	+15
PO_2	63	61	107	80	121	96	99	103	79
FiO_2	75%				75	→ 65	→ 60	→ 55	→ 50
Rate	40			→ 44	44	44	→ 40	→ 34	
Pressure	28/5	→ 30/7			→ 32/4	32/4		→ 30/5	
Insp. time	1,0				→ 0,8	→ 1,0	→ 1,2		→ 1,5

7.7.5 Heart Defect with Iatrogenic Hyperventilation (Table 37)

Table 37. Ventilation: volume-controlled, gradual reduction of rate to avoid hypoxia. Bourns LS 104–150 ventilator. Body weight 3470 g, 40th week of gestation, 7th day of life

Time:	3 : 00. etc.	4.00	5.00	6.00	8.00	11.00
pH	7,53	7,58	7,54	7,60	7,51	7,48
PCO_2	24	21	26	30	46	48
StB	23	23	24	32	35	33
BE	±0	±0	±2	+8	+12	+10
PO_2	(40)	(41)	(44)	58	(47)	(45)
FiO_2	60%				60%	
Rate	40	→ 35	→ 30	→ 25	→ 20	
Pressure	25/5				→ 20/5	→ 20/3
Vol.	(110)					
Insp. time	0,8		→ 1,0			
Alloferin	0,5 ml				0,5 ml	

7.7.6 Meconium Aspiration with Severe Respiratory Failure (Table 38)

Table 38. Ventilation: pressure-controlled, maximum rate and high pressure after relaxation. Bird Mark 8 ventilator. Body weight 4050 g, 40th week of gestation, 1st day of life

Time:	9 : 00, etc.	11.00	15.00	16.00	18.00	19.00	20.00
pH	7,12	7,17	7,36	7,38	7,50	7,56	7,46
PCO_2	>200	162	112	115	70	62	54
StB			>43	>43	>43	35	34
BE			> +20	> +20	> +20	+12	+11
PO_2	61	68	91	71	69	59	59
FiO_2	100%		100%→	90%→	85%		
Rate	50		50	→	40	→	30
Pressure	28/8→	30/8		30/8		30/8	
Vol.							
Insp. time	0,6			→	0,9	→	1,0
Na bicarb.	10 ml						
Lysine HCl					10 ml		
Alloferin	1 ml			1 ml			0,5 ml

7.8 Recognition of Equipment Malfunctions

7.8.1 Principle

Never try to repair a malfunctioning ventilator while a child is being ventilated with it! Replace it with a new ventilator, stabilize the child, and then check the defective unit.

7.8.2 Pressure-Controlled Ventilation

A prolonged inspiratory phase or failure to reach the preset inspiratory pressure despite adequate flow indicates a leak. The leak is often localized in the region of the humidifier, sealing rings, or water collector. Diminished breath sounds and low flow: Ceramic valve is dirty. Sudden high pressure which does not fall on expiration: Exhalation valve is dirty or jammed.

7.8.3 Volume-Controlled Ventilation with Prolonged Inspiration, High Volume, and Pressure Limit

Fall of respiratory rate is an indication that flow is below critical limit. Failure to reach inspiratory pressure or fall of rate: Gas supply to ventilator is too low.

7.8.4 CPAP and PEEP

The expiratory pressure displayed on the manometer deviates greatly from the level of the water column in the underwater seal: Flow is too low or too high.

References

1. Boros, S. J., Reynolds, J. W.: Hyaline membrane disease treated with early nasal endexpiratory pressure: one year's experience. Pediatrics *56*, 218 (1975)
2. Chernick, V., Vidyasagar, D.: Continuous negative chest wall pressure in hyaline membrane disease: one year experience. Pediatrics *49*, 753 (1972)
3. Cumarasamy, N., Nüssli, R., Vischer, D., Dangel, P. H., Duc, P. V.: Artifical ventilation in hyaline membrane disease. The use of positive endexpiratory pressure and continuous positive airway pressure. Pediatrics *51*, 629 (1973)
4. Dangel, P.: Organisation und Taktik der Intensivbehandlung von pädiatrischen und kinderchirurgischen Patienten. Klin. Päd. *186*, 120 (1974)
5. Davies, P. A., Robinson, R. J., Scopes, J. W., Tizard, J. P. M., Wigglesworth, J. S.: Medical care of newborn babies. Clinics in Developmental Medicine *44*, 55 (1972)
6. Doershuk, C. F., Fisher, B. J., Matthews, L. W.: Pulmonary physiology of the young child. In: Pulmonary Physiology of the Fetus, Newborn, and Child. Scarpelli, E. M. (ed.). Philadelphia: Lea & Febiger 1975
7. Downs, J. B., et al.: Intermittent mandatory ventilation: a new approach to weaning patients from mechanical ventilators. Chest *64*, 331 (1973)
8. Epstein, R. A.: The sensitivities and response times of ventilatory assistors. Anaesthesiology *34*, 321 (1971)
9. Mannino, F. L., Feldman, B. H., Heldt, G. P., DeLue, N. A., Wimmer, J. E., Fletcher, M. A., Gluck, L.: Early mechanical ventilation in RDS with a prolonged inspiration. Pediatr. Res. *10*, 464 (1976)
10. Fox, W. W., Berman, L. S., Downes, J. J., Peckham, G. J.: The therapeutic application of end-expiratory pressure in the meconium aspiration syndrome. Pediatrics *56*, 214 (1975)

11. GERARD, P., FOX, W. W., OUTERBRIDGE, E. W., BEAUDRY, P. H., STERN, L.: Early versus late introduction of continuous negative pressure in the management of the idiopathic respiratory distress syndrome. J. of Pediatrics *87*, 591 (1975)
12. GOMEZ, P. C. W., NOAKES, M., BARRIE, H.: A prognostic score for use in the Respiratory-Distress Syndrome. Lancet I, 808 (1969)
13. GREGORY, G. A., KITTERMAN, J. A., PHIBBS, R. H., TOOLEY, W. H., HAMILTON, W. K.: Treatment of the idiopathic respiratory distress syndrome with continuous positive airway pressure. New Eng. J. Med. *284*, 1334 (1971)
14. HARRIS, H., WILSON, S., BRANS, Y., WIRTSCHAFTER, D., CASSADY, G.: Nasal continuous positive airway pressure. Improvement in hyaline membrane disease. Biol. Neonat. *29*, 231 (1976)
15. HELLER, K.: Die Probleme der assistierten Beatmung bei Früh- und Neugeborenen. In: Pädiatrische Intensivmedizin (ed.) EMMRICH, P. Band 3, S. 30 Stuttgart: Thieme 1977
16. HERMAN, S., REYNOLDS, E. O. R.: Methods for improving oxygenation in infants mechanically ventilated for severe hyaline membrane disease. Arch. Dis. Child *48*, 612 (1973)
17. KATTWINKEL, J., NEARMAN, H. S., FANAROFF, A. A., KATONA, P. G., KLAUS, M. H.: Apnea of prematurity: Comparative stimulation and nasal CPAP. J. Pediatr. *86*, 588 (1975)
18. KEUSKAMP, D. H. G.: Charakteristik verschiedener Beatmungsgeräte. In: Anästhesie im Kindesalter, Bd. 2. München: J. F. LEHMANNS 1973
19. KRAUSS, D. R., MARSHALL, R. E.: Severe neck ulceration from CPAP head box. J. of Pediatrics *86*, 286 (1975)
20. KROUSKOP, R. W., BROWN, E. G., SWEET, A. Y.: The early use of continuous positive airway pressure in the treatment of idiopathic respiratory distress syndrome. J. of Pediatrics *87*, 263 (1975)
21. LEMBURG, P.: Erfahrungen mit neuen Respiratortypen für die Beatmung von Früh- und Neugeborenen. In: Pädiatrische Intensivmedizin. EMMRICH, P. (Ed.). Bd. 3, S. 16. Stuttgart: Thieme 1977
22. V. v. LOEWENICH: Positiver endexspiratorischer Druck beim Bird-Respirator. Diskussionsbemerkung. In: Pädiatrische Intensivpflege, 3. Symposion Stuttgart: Enke 1974
23. LLEWELLYN, M. A., SWYER, P. R.: Assisted and controlled ventilation in the newborn period: Effect on oxygenation. British J. of Anaestesia *43*, 926 (1971)
24. MOCKVIN, L. D., BANCALARI, E. H.: Early versus delayed initiation of continuous negative pressure in infants with hyaline membrane disease. J. of Pediatrics *87*, 596 (1975)
25. NELSON, N. M.: Neonatal pulmonary function. Pediat. Clin. North Amer. *13*, 769 (1966)
26. OBLADEN, M., WILLE, L.: Erfahrungen mit einer Unterdruckkammer zur Behandlung des Atemnotsyndroms. In: Perinatale Medizin. DUDENHAUSEN, J. W., SALING, E., SCHMIDT, E. (Ed.). Band 6, S. 319. Stuttgart: Thieme 1
27. O'BOYLE, M. P., FLETCHER, A. A., AVERY, G. B.: Objective early criteria for ventilatory assistance in ventilation of hyaline membrane disease. Pediatrics *51*, 748 (1973)
28. OWEN-THOMAS, J. B., ULAN, O. A., SWYER, P. R.: The effect of varying inspiratory gas flow rate on arterial oxygenation during IPPV in the respiratory distress syndrome. Brit. J. Anaesth. *40*, 493 (1968)
29. POWERS, W. F., SWYER, P. R.: The peripheral hemodynamic effects of continuous positive transpulmonary pressure breathing in neonates free from cardiorespiratory disease. Pediatrics *56*, 203 (1975)
30. REYNOLDS, E. O. R.: Effect of alteration in ventilation settings on pulmonary gas exchange in hyaline membrane disease. Arch. Dis. Child. *46*, 152 (1971)
31. REYNOLDS, E. O. R., Pressure waveform and ventilator settings for mechanical ventilation in severe hyaline membrane disease. Intern. Anaesthesiol. Clin. *12*, 259 (1974)
32. SCHACHINGER, H., FRANK, H. D.: Eine einfache Methode der exspiratorischen Druckerhöhung beim Bird Mark 8 mit Säuglingsventil. Z. prakt. Anästh. Wiederbel. *9*, 55 (1974)
33. SCHMID, F., DANGEL, P. H., DUC, G. V.: Nasale Anwendung von CPAP. In: Pädiatrische Intensivmedizin, EMMRICH, P. (Ed.). Bd. 3, S. 33. Stuttgart: Thieme 1977
34. SCHÖBER, J. G.: Maschinelle Beatmung von Neugeborenen und Frühgeborenen. Münch. med. Wschr. *115*, 581 (1973)

35. Stahlman, M. T., Malan, A. F., Shepard, F. M., Blankenship, W. J., Young, W. C., Gray, J.: Negative pressure assisted ventilation in infants with hyaline membrane disease. J. Pediatr. *76*, 174 (1970)
36. Suter, P. M., Fairley, H. B., Isenberg, M. D.: Optimum end-exspiratory airway pressure in patients with acute pulmonary failure. New Eng. J. Med. *292*, 284 (1975)
37. Uany, R., Shapiro, D. L., Smith, B., Warshaw, J. B.: Treatment of severe apnea in prematures with orally administered theophylline. Pediatrics *55*, 595 (1975)
38. Wung, J. T., Stark, R. I., Hegyi, T., Driscoll, J. M., James, L. S.: CDP: a major breakthrough. Pediatrics *58*, 783 (1976)
39. Wyszogrodski, I., Kyei-Aboagye, K., Taeusch, H. W., Avery, M. E.: Surfactant inactivation by hyperventilation; conservation by end-exspiratory pressure. J. Appl. Physiol. *38*, 461 (1975)
40. Boros, S. J., Orgill, A. A.: Mortality and Morbidity associated with pressure- and volume-limited infant ventilators. Am. J. Dis. Child. *132*, 865 (1978)
41. Keuth, U., Feldmann, E. M., Althaus, W., Fries, N., Zemke, M.: Erfolgreiche Behandlung neonataler Ateminsuffizienz mit kontinuierlich erhöhter transalveolärer Druckdifferenz. Paediatr. Prax. *16*, 445 (1976)

8 Long-Term Ventilation

M. Obladen

8.1 General Requirements

8.1.1 Prevention of Infection

Observe strict asepsis during suctioning! Touch the umbilical artery catheter only with sterile gloves. Disinfect hands before opening the incubator. Wipe all frequently used devices regularly with disinfectant and disinfect all tubing; see p 74.
Change the vaporizer jar, sterile water, and tubing sets daily [15].

Bacteriologic Screening of the Infant on Admission. Take smears twice a week to monitor bacterial growth.

Bacteriology of ET Tube. The growth of microorganisms in the ET tube alone is no indication for antibiotic therapy. Pseudomonas frequently grows in the trachea of infants receiving long-term ventilatory support. Routine bacteriologic smears are taken so that appropriate antibiotic therapy can be administered if a clinically manifest infection develops. No general prophylactic antibiotic therapy is given, but Polybactrin powder is used for umbilical care.
Infection can best be prevented by regular physio- und postural therapy.
Weak points are found and staff motivation is enhanced by thorough, unannounced bacteriologic inspections of the intensive care unit by the health authorities about twice a year (especially: wash basins, faucets, humidifiers, nebulizers, thermometers, incubator water, control knobs).

8.1.2 Suctioning

Hourly Tracheal Toilet. Aseptic technique [1]:
- Hyperventilate: five to ten breaths with Penlon bag (basic rule: thumb plus one finger per kg body wt).
- Instill 0.5–1 ml of 0.9% NaCl solution or 1 ml (0.2 mg) Chymotrypsin into the ET tube or suction catheter.
- Connect to ventilation system for 1 min.
- Turn the head to one side (to stretch the contralateral primary bronchus).

Table 39. Size of the suction catheter. The suction catheter must not seal the lumen of the ET tube: danger of atelectasis

ET tube Ø in mm Portex Blue Line or Rüsch nasal	Charrière Pharma-Plast suction catheter with rounded tip and two side holes
2.5	5
3	6
3.5	8
Oral suctioning	8

- With a sterile disposable glove, insert the suction catheter (with suction off) to about 1 cm beyond the end of the tube. Switch on suction for 5 s, withdraw the catheter with a rotary motion (to wipe out tube) (Table 39).
- Hyperventilate again as described above.
- Connect the ventilator again, then carefully suction the nose and throat (observe caution when suctioning the stomach and pharynx, especially in postasphyxic states: vagal stimulation, danger of cardiac arrest).
- Turn the head to the opposite side during the next suctioning.
- If the mucous is very viscous, instill the mucolytic agent *N*-acetyl cysteine diluted 1 : 1 with 0.9% sodium chloride, instead of alpha chymotrase.

8.1.3 Humidification and Nebulization

Routine nebulization is not necessary during long-term ventilation and even increases the risk of pulmonary infection. An ultrasonic nebulizer emits 100 000–200 000 *Pseudomonas* organisms per milliliter, and thus per minute after a few hours' use [17]. It is necessary only to compensate for the loss of nasal humidification due to the presence of the tube; otherwise, paralysis of the ciliary epithelia in the bronchial tree will result. The respiratory gas is best humidified by a heated vaporizer. The humidity of the respiratory gas should be at least 70% (vs 95% during nasal breathing). Excessive humidification or heating leads to a heavy condensation of water in the ventilator hose, especially if the tubing system is long. Regular checks are necessary due to the danger of overhydration, aspiration, or separations in the tubing system. We do not use an ultrasonic nebulizer in intubated neonates, but do use it for a brief period after extubation (see Sect. 8.4.2).

8.1.4 Heating

Respiratory gas should always be heated. This increases the water-vapor saturation of the gas and guards against paralysis of the bronchial ciliary epithelium. Newborns and infants undergo a considerable loss of water and calories during long-term ventilation:

- Specific respiratory water loss of the infant: 0.0286 g per respiratory time volume

- Specific respiratory caloric loss of the infant: 19.63 calories per respiratory time volume [3].

The losses that occur are fully compensated for if an inspiratory gas with a temperature of 32°–33° C and relative humidity of 85% is administered. We have obtained good results with the following gas temperatures: in the incubator, 34°; in the vaporizer jar with a 1-m hose length, 50° C. This gives a temperature of 30°–32° C at the ET connector. This temperature must be checked regularly due to the danger of overheating in case of a defect.
If the vaporizer is unheated, the water-vapor saturation is low, and there is a considerable risk of ET tube obstruction.

8.1.5 Physiotherapy

Physiotherapy is a radical measure which, in experienced hands, provides an effective means of removing bronchial secretions [33]. Its value in artificially ventilated neonates is disputed, and both positive [34] and negative effects [35] on oxygenation are reported. *After* ventilation is concluded, routine physio- and postural therapy can prevent the occurrence of a "wandering" atelectasis. We always perform physiotherapy in the following cases:
- Pneumonia
- Atelectasis
- Extubation after long-term ventilation.

Technique
a) Inhalation: 10 min with ultrasonic nebulizer: 1 ml *N*-acetyl cysteine plus 5 ml distilled water.
b) Vibration: Apply electric massager or toothbrush for 1 min, using 4-cm sponge attachment. Vibrate the chest bilaterally, using a rotary motion from the lung periphery toward the hilus while exerting a slight pressure during expirations. Vibration may be replaced with digital percussion if desired [5], but this must be done with extreme care to avoid rib fracture [24].
c) Compress the thorax by exerting a gentle pressure with the palm of the hand.
d) Apply oropharyngeal suction after coughing is initiated.

8.1.6 Postural Therapy

a) Reposition the infant every hour during long-term ventilation:
   - On back with small shoulder roll
   - On right side
   - Flat on stomach
   - On left side.
b) Give postural therapy for atelectasis, depending on localization (see Table 40).

Table 40. Postural therapy for atelectasis

Localization of atelectasis	Position
Superior lobe	
Apical segment	Upright, almost sitting
Anterior segment	Flat on back
Posterior segment, right	On stomach, right shoulder raised
Posterior segment, left	Sitting, left shoulder raised
Middle lobe, right	On left side with head low
Lingula, left	On right side with head low
Inferior lobe	
Anterior segment	On back with head low
Lateral segment, right	On left side with head low
Lateral segment, left	On right side with head low
Posterior segment	On stomach with head low
Superior segment	Flat on stomach

If the atelectasis does not respond to postural therapy, intratracheal suctioning should be applied after 48 h, and bronchial lavage should be attempted [7].

8.1.7 Feeding

Prolonged ventilation of the intubated neonate is *not* a contraindication for oral feeding with normal formula and volumes. We use either intermittent gastric tube feeding or continuous nasojejunal infusion (see p 44). The only contraindications for feeding which are associated with ventilation are:
- Drug-induced paralysis or
- extubation (6–h delay).

8.2 Supervision of the Neonate During Artificial Ventilation

The start of artificial ventilation almost never represents the solution to a clinical problem, but rather the beginning of a new series of problems [25]. Every artificially ventilated neonate must be constantly supervised and requires:
- A nurse, preferably providing care to the ventilated infants alone
- A vital function monitor for at least cardiac and respiratory activity
- A ventilation monitor for the technical functions of the ventilator
- A physicans' order sheet; each order is countersigned by the nurse providing care
- A 24-h flow-sheet with notes on all diagnostic and therapeutic data including changes in ventilator settings
- A progress chart in which all changes in clinical condition and examination findings are indicated.

8.2.1 Observation and Examination of the Artificially Ventilated Neonate [19]

Every Hour by the Nurse
Skin color
Peripheral blood flow
Body temperature
Heart rate (bracycardia during suctioning?)
Respiratory rate, retractions
Pulmonary auscultation (position of ET tube, flow rate, PEEP effectiveness, pneumothorax)
Observation of thoracic excursions: synchronous with respirator?

Every 4 h by the Nurse
Blood pressure
Activity
Spontaneous motor activity
Meconium or stool passage
Urine formation

General Examination Every 12 h by the Physician, Including at Least
Pulmonary auscultation
Cardiac auscultation (take briefly off ventilator or CPAP)
Gastric auscultation
Determination of liver size
Palpation of the abdomen
Femoral pulse
Fontanel.

According to Clinical Indication
Chest X-ray
ECG (especially during digitalization)
Phonocardiogram (especially if patent ductus is suspected)
Echocardiogram
Echoencephalogram (if hydrocephalus is suspected)
EEG (if cerebral hemorrhage is suspected).

8.2.2 Supervision by Monitor (see p 29)

8.2.3 Monitoring the Ventilator Settings

This must be done during each blood gas analysis, but at least once per hour. The following are checked:
FiO_2
Respiratory rate
Inspiratory pressure

Expiratory pressure
Inspiratory time (measure with stopwatch)
Tidal volume
Minute volume (measure with Wright respirometer)
Vaporizer temperature.
It is best to monitor the respirator function continuously, for instance with the Bourns LS 160 ventilation monitor, which not only monitors the upper and lower alarm limits for inspiratory pressure, PEEP, and rate, but also serves as an measuring instrument; the respiratory rate, inspiratory time, expiratory time, and I : E ratio are electronically measured and accurately displayed.

8.3 Relaxation

Goal. To coordinate the infant's breathing with the respirator. Muscle relaxation should be induced only if the infant is sedated. Often sedation alone is sufficient to interrupt "fighting" the ventilator.
0.5–1 mg/kg Dolantin alternating in 6–h intervals with
0.5–1 mg/kg Valium or 2–5 mg/kg Luminal.

8.3.1 Indication for Relaxation

Situations in which the infant is breathing strongly against the ventilator:
- Severe RDS in large newborns (usually children of diabetic mothers)
- Meconium aspiration, which requires high-pressure ventilation
- Interstitial emphysema with risk of pneumothorax
- Hyperexcitability (not to be confused with hyperventilation tetany)
- Convulsions [6].

Prerequisites for relaxation are:
No oral feeding
Change in position
Credé of bladder at regular intervals.

8.3.2 Dosage and Procedure

Alloferin. Initial dose 0.3 mg/kg, later reduced to 0.1 mg/kg. Duration of action about 30 min, but may last up to 12 h in small preterm infants.

Imbretil. Single dose 0.4 mg/kg; dosage must be adapted to individual, may be necessary to repeat in 2–h intervals (6).

Methylcurarin. Initial dose 0.7 mg/kg, later reduced to 0.3 mg/kg. Duration of action about 30 min (16).

8.4 Concluding Artificial Ventilation

8.4.1 Weaning from the Ventilator

Weaning from the ventilator should be considered if the infant
- Requires an FiO_2 of only 0.4
- "Fights" the ventilator, with good blood gas values
- Tolerates hourly suctioning with no deterioration of general condition
- Has RDS, is over 3 days old, and is maintained at PEEP of + 4 cm H_2O.

8.4.2 Procedure of Weaning

Wean the infant in stages. Change only one ventilator setting at a time, perform blood gas analysis after each change.

a) By IMV (intermittent mandatory ventilation; see p 82): Gradually reduce respiratory rate and prolong inspiratory time to increase spontaneous component of breathing (4).
b) By CPAP (see p 83): If spontaneous breathing is adequate, reduce expiratory pressure in increments of 2 cm H_2O. Try to remove from the ventilator at +2 cm H_2O. Analyze blood gases after 15 min (8).
c) By short periods off the ventilator: 5 min/h at first, then for longer periods.
d) In very immature preterm infants with a low respiratory drive, assist weaning by giving theophylline (see p 153) [30].

During the weaning phase ventilate the intubated patient briefly after each tracheal suctioning in order to shorten the recovery period.

8.4.3 Extubation

- Normally undertaken after 2–3 h of adequate spontaneous breathing through the tube.
- Should be done after 1 h of good spontaneous breathing in preterm infants <1500 g, in whom the tube may represent a significant dead space.
- Select a favorable time for extubation: preferably not at night or shortly before a change of shift.

8.4.4 Procedure of Extubation

Three to six h before the planned extubation, give 2 mg/kg Decortin IV.; 15 min before extubation premedicate with 0.01 mg/kg atropine. Aspirate gastric contents and suction airways.

Immediately Before Extubation. Repeat oral and nasopharyngeal suctioning. Hyperventilate carefully with Penlon bag, continue while the tube is withdrawn. Atelectasis is best avoided if the loosened tube is "blown out" with a sudden squezze on the Penlon bag. Immediately after extubation, lay infant on stomach, auscultate the lungs.
After 15 min: Blood gas analysis.
Give 2 mg/kg Decortin IV every 6 h for the next 24 h.
Wait 6 h before feeding.
Give physio- and postural therapy every hour [10]. Only in exceptional cases: one-half Tanderil suppository, 0.05% Nasivin nose drops or sedation.

8.5 Complications

8.5.1 Blockage of Endotracheal Tube

Symptoms. Acute deterioration, cyanosis, breathing against the ventilator, thoracic excursions out of synchrony with the ventilator, severe jugular and chest wall retractions, and absence of breath sounds on auscultation.
- Negative mirror test: A mirror held before the open tube shows no fogging during expiration.
- No secretions are obtained when suctioning is attempted.
- The suction catheter does not pass through the tube.

Treatment. Withdraw tube, ventilate with mask and oxygen until infant recovers, then reintubate.

Prophylaxis. When ventilation is done with properly warmed and humidified respiratory gas and regular tracheal toilet (see p 96), endotracheal tube obstructions are extremely rare.

8.5.2 Tube Dislocation

- Acute exacerbation of ventilatory status
- Thoracic excursions not synchronous with ventilator
- Faint breath sounds (this symptom is not reliable in very small preterms)

a) Dislocation into the hypopharynx: respiratory gas blows out the mouth during inspiration. Auscultation: squeaking, gurgling breath sound audible primarily over the throat.
b) Dislocation into the esophagus: abdominal distention, breath sounds audible over the stomach, negative mirror test.
c) Dislocation into a primary bronchus: Breath sounds not equally audible on both sides (not reliable).

Treatment. If dislocation is suspected, perform mirror test at once. If negative, examine by direct laryngoscopy; reintubate immediately if necessary.

Prophylaxis. Secure fixation of nasotracheal tube (see p 246); tube must be measured to correct size before intubation; check placement by X-ray after each intubation.

8.5.3 Accidental Disconnection

We have found that unintentional extubation almost never occurs when the Dangel fixation plate is used (see Fig. 22). However, the tube connector occasionally becomes detached in large, lively infants. If the ventilator has no leak alarm, a ventilation monitor should be used to indicate the interruption of ventilation before any deterioration of vital functions can occur.

8.5.4 Infection

This is one of the most serious complications of ventilation, especially in cases of prolonged intubation, faulty aseptic suction technique, and after aspiration. General antibiotic therapy of the ventilated infant or even general antibiotic prophylaxis increases the risk of pulmonary infection with Gram-negative pathogens.

8.5.5 Extra-Alveolar Collection of Air (see also pp 118 and 242)

Extra-alveolar air leakage can occur during practically any form of artificial ventilation. The smaller the child and the greater the impairment of his pulmonary compliance, the greater the risk. For pathogenesis, see p 118. Extra-alveolar air collection is especially common in the following situations:
- High ventilation rate with short inspiratory time
- High PEEP or CPAP [9]
- Acute resuscitation in situation with forced bag ventilation
- Insufficient sedation of a newborn who is breathing against the respirator

a) Interstitial emphysema
b) Mediastinal emphysema
c) Pneumothorax
d) Pneumopericardium (see p 144, 243)
e) Pneumoperitoneum.

Incidence
- RDS without ventilation: 3.5%
- RDS with CPAP: 11%
- RDS with PEEP: 24%–33% [20]

8.5.6 Disturbances of Venous Return

Pathogenesis. Prolonged inspiratory phase and high PEEP: "CPAP toxicity" (rise of PCO_2).
Decline in cardiac stroke volume
Cardiac failure
Hepatomegaly
Metabolic acidosis

Treatment. Reduce PEEP; if necessary replace CPAP with CNP.

8.5.7 Patent Ductus Arteriosus

This may be a complication of RDS in very small preterm infants below 1500 g [18, 26]. Ductal patency should be suspected with pulmonary exacerbation after the 3rd day of life, or in an atypical biphasic course of RDS in which weaning from the ventilator, cannot be accomplished after 5 days. Cardiomegaly (not mandatory), systolic or continuous murmur, pulmonary plethora, cardiac failure and hepatomegaly. For treatment, see p 140.

8.5.8 Inappropriate Secretion of ADH

Hyponatremia with normal potassium, possibly caused by a decrease in cardiac stroke volume [21] or hypoxia [28]. This is manifested by weight increase and edema.

8.6 Delayed Damage After Long-Term Ventilation

8.6.1 Pressure Lesions

The tracheal tube or its fixation can cause necrotic lesions, especially in the nose: enlargement of the nares, septal deviation, vestibular stenosis [12], or cleft nose. Intubation can also damage the larynx (laryngomalacia, vocal cord lesions, trachyphonia, subglottic stenosis [11]), the gums (grooving, splitting), and the occiput (occipital deformation, cerebellar hemorrhage [22]). The severity of the lesions is directly proportional to the duration of the intubation [11]. In general, these deformations tend to regress without profound residua and to heal amazingly well.

Prophylaxis

- Suspend the tubing system so that its weight can produce no lever action at the infant's nose.
- Change to the other nostril when reintubating.
- When ventilating for more than 8 days, rotate the tube placement from oral to right nostril to left nostril.

8.6.2 Bronchopulmonary Dysplasia

The lung undergoes considerable changes during long-term ventilation [29]. Bronchopulmonary dysplasia arises from a combination of oxygen toxicity, mechanical barotrauma [23], and the sensitivity of the very immature lung in its reactivity to these insults.

Opinion is divided as to whether bronchopulmonary dysplasia can be produced by oxygen and CPAP alone [2]. An FiO_2 of 0.6–0.8 for a duration of at least 44 h in respirator ventilation and 73 h in CPAP is necessary for the development of bronchopulmonary dysplasia [23]. For the pathogenesis of this disease. The radiologic findings and histology of the four stages of bronchopulmonary dysplasia are compared in Table 41. The treatment of bronchopulmonary dysplasia are compared in Table 41. The treatment of bronchopulmonary dysplasia is lengthy and unsatisfactory; steroids are ineffective. Treatment with vitamin E is currently under evaluation and shows some promise (31, 32, 36).

Table 41. Stages of bronchopulmonary dysplasia [14]

Stage	Radiologic findings	Histology
I	Increased density Air bronchogram	Loss of cilia Metaplasia and necrosis of the bronchial mucosa
II	Subtotal opacification Air bronchogram Cardiomegaly	Alveolar epithelial necrosis Thickening of capillary basal membrane
III	Diffuse honeycombed pattern	Extensive bronchial metaplasia Marked mucus secretion Focal alveolar emphysema Interstitial edema
IV	Striated pattern with radiolucent areas	Hypertrophy of peribronchial smooth musculature Exudation of macrophages, histiocytes, and foam cells Interstitial fibrosis Vascular changes consistent with pulmonary pressure

References

1. Ahnefeld, F. W., Halmágyi, M. (Hrsg.): Anaesthesie und Wiederbelebung bei Säuglingen und Kleinkindern. Anaesthesie und Wiederbelebung, Bd. 71. Berlin – Heidelberg – New York: Springer 1973
2. Berg, T. J., Pagtakhan, R. D., Reed, M. H., Langston, C., Chernick, V.: Bronchopulmonary dysplasia and lung rupture in HMD: Influence of continuous distending pressure. Pediatrics *55*, 51 (1975)
3. Dick, W.: Respiratorischer Flüssigkeits- und Wärmeverlust des Säuglings bei künstlicher Beatmung. In: Anaesthesiologie und Wiederbelebung, Bd. 62. Berlin – Heidelberg – New York: Springer 1972
4. Downs, J. B.: Intermittent mandatory ventilation: a new approach to weaning patients from mechanical ventilators. Chest *64*, 331–335 (1973)
5. Dunn, D., Lewis, A. T.: Some important aspects of neonatal nursing related to pulmonary disease and family involvement. Pediatr. Clin. North Am. *20*, 481 (1973)
6. Emmrich, P.: Erweiterte Anwendungsmöglichkeiten der vollständigen Relaxierung bei Neugeborenen und jungen Säuglingen. Mschr. Kinderheilk. *118*, 453 (1970)
7. Galvis, A. G., White, J. J., Oh, K. S.: A bedside washout technique for atelectasis in infants. Am. J. Dis. Child *127*, 824 (1974)
8. Gregory, G. A., Kitterman, J. A., Phibbs, R. H., Tooley, W. H., Hamilton, W. K.: Treatment of the idiopathic respiratory distress syndrome with continuous positive airway pressure. New Eng. J. Med. *284*, 1333 (1971)
9. Hall, R. T., Rhodes, P. G.: Pneumothorax and pneumomediastinum in infants with idiopathic respiratory distress syndrome receiving continuous positive pressure. Pediatrics *55*, 493 (1975)
10. Jordan, W. S.: New therapy for postintubation laryngeal edema and tracheitis in children. J. Am. Med. Ass. *212*, 585 (1970)
11. Joshi, V. V., Mandavia, S. G., Stern, L., Wigglesworth, F. W.: Acute lesions induced by endotracheal intubation. Occurrence in the upper respiratory tract of newborn infants with respiratory distress syndrome. Am. J. Dis. Child. *124*, 646 (1972)
12. Jung, A. L., Thomas, G. K.: Stricture of the nasal vestibule: A complication of nasotracheal intubation in newborn infants. J. Pediatr. *85*, 412 (1974)
13. Kuhns, L. R., Bednarek, F. J., Wyanan, M. L., Roloff, D. W., Borer, R. C.: Diagnosis of pneumothorax or pneumomediastinum in the neonate by transillumination. Pediatrics *56*, 355 (1975)
14. Laupus, W. E.: Bronchopulmonary dysplasia. In: Pulmonary disorders. Disorders of the respiratory tract in children. Vol. 1. Kendig, E. L. (Ed.). Philadelphia – London – Toronto: Saunders 1972
15. Lemburg, P., Sprock, I.: Bakteriologische Kontrollen in einer pädiatrischen Intensivpflegestation. Eine 3-Jahresübersicht. In: Pädiatrische Intensivpflege, 3. Symposion. Stuttgart: Enke 1973
16. v. Loewenich, V., Koch, H.: Pädiatrische Intensivbehandlung. Stuttgart: Thieme 1974
17. Marget, W., Adam, D., Daschner, F., Töpfl, C.: Bedeutung der mikrobiellen Disposition und Exposition bei der Neugeborenen-Intensivpflege. In: Pädiatrische Intensivpflege, 3. Symposion. Stuttgart: Enke 1973
18. Neal, W. A., Bessinger, F. B., Hunt, C. E., Lucas, R. V.: Patent ductus arteriosus complicating respiratory distress syndrome. J. Pediatr. *86*, 127 (1975)
19. Neidhardt, M., Emmrich, P.: Möglichkeiten der Beatmung in der pädiatrischen Intensivbehandlung. Mschr. Kinderheilk. *121*, 27 (1973)
20. Ogata, E. S., Gregory, G. A., Kitterman, J. A., Phibbs, R. H., Tooley, W. H.: Pneumothorax in the respiratory distress syndrome. Pediatrics *58*, 177 (1976)
21. Papageorgiou, A. N., Moffatt, M.: Bilateral pneumonia and inappropriate secretion of antidiuretic hormone in a premature infant. Canad. Med. J. *115*, 1119 (1976)

22. PAPE, K. E., ARMSTRONG, D. L., FITZHARDINGE, P. M.: Central nerve system pathology associated with mask ventilation. Pediatrics *58*, 473 (1976)
23. PHILIP, A. G. S.: Oxygen plus pressure plus time. Etiology of bronchopulmonary dysplasia. Pediatrics *55*, 44 (1975)
24. PUROHRT, D. M., CALDWELL, C., LEVKOFF, A.: Multiple rib fractures due to physiotherapy in a neonate with HMD. Am. J. Dis. Child. *129*, 110 (1975)
25. STEMMANN, E. A., LEMBURG, P.: Dauerbeatmung auf der pädiatrischen Intensivpflegestation. In: Pädiatrische Intensivpflege, 1. Symposion Suttgart: Enke 1971
26. THIBEAULT, D. W., EMMANOUILDES, G. C., NELSON, R. J., LACHMAN, R. S., ROSENGART, R. M., OH, W.: Patent ductus arteriosus complicating the respiratory distress syndrome in preterm infants. J. Pediatr. *86*, 120 (1975)
27. VERT, P., ANDRE, M., SIBOUT, M.: Continuous positive airway pressure and hydrocephalus. Lancet I, 319 (1973)
28. WEINBERG, J. A., WEITZMAN, R. E., ZAKAUDDIN, S., LEAKE, R. D.: Inappropriate secretion on antidiuretic hormone in a premature infant. J. Pediant *90*, 111 (1977)
29. WIEMERS, K., SCHOLLER, K. L.: Lungenveränderungen bei Langzeitbeatmung. Stuttgart: Thieme 1973
30. BARR, P. A.: Weaning very low birthweight infants from mechanical ventilation using intermittent mandatory ventilation and theophylline. Arch. Dis. Child *53*, 598 (1978)
31. BÖHLES, H.: Vitamin E in der Kinderheilkunde. Klin. Paediatr. *190*, 226 (1978)
32. EHRENKRANZ, R. A., BONTA, B. W., ABLOW, R. C., WARSHAW, J. B.: Amelioration of bronchopulmonary dysplasia after vitamin E administration: a preliminary report. N. Engl. J. Med. *229*, 564 (1978)
33. ETCHES, P. C., SCOTT, B.: Chest Physiotherapy in the Newborn: Effect on Secretions Removed. Pediatrics *62*, 713 (1978)
34. FINER, N. N., BOYD, J.: Chest Physiotherapy in the Neonate: A controlled Study. Pediatrics *61*, 282 (1978)
35. FOX, W. W., SCHWARTZ, J. G., SCHAFFER, Th.: Pulmonary physiotherapy in neonates: physiologic changes and respiratory management. J. Pediatr. *92*, 977 (1978)
36. NORTHWAY, W. H. u. J. R.: Bronchopulmonary dysplasia and vitamin E (Editorial). N. Engl. J. Med. *299*, 599 (1978)

9 Pulmonary Diseases

L. Wille and M. Obladen

9.1 Respiratory Distress Syndrome (Surfactant Deficiency)

Incidence. 1%–2% of all term infants, up to 14% of all preterm infants (particularly <1500 g, <32nd wk of gestation) [14, 43]. The incidence has not decreased during the last 10 years [49].

Pathogenesis. Pulmonary surfactant lowers the surface tension at the air-water interface of the alveoli, thus preventing alveolar collapse during expiration. Its absence causes decreased alveolar stability and is the crucial etiologic factor in RDS. Besides a quantitative decrease in the main component of surfactant, dipalmitoyl phosphatidylcholine (lecithin), the respiratory distress syndrome is characterized by a complete lack of the secondary component phosphatidylglycerol (Fig. 23) [22].

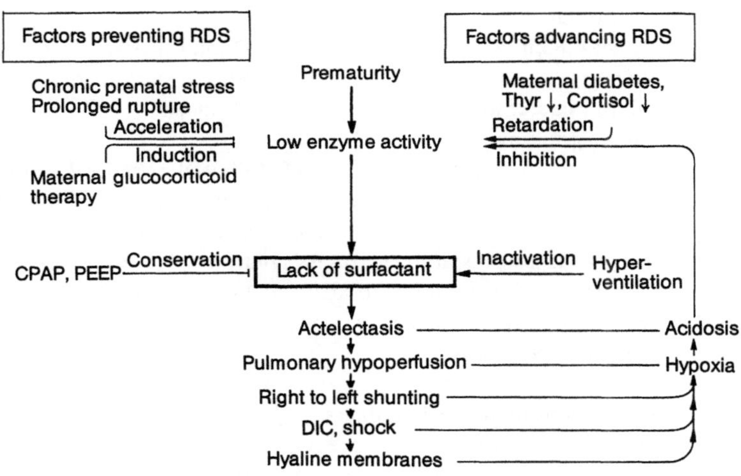

Fig. 23. Pathogenesis of respiratory distress syndrome and factors which can influence its course. (After Obladen, 1978 [33])

Pathophysiology
- Diminished lung compliance
- Reduced alveolar ventilation (microatelectases)
- Increased intrapulmonary shunt
- Cardiac right-to-left shunt (foramen ovale, ductus arteriosus)
- Reduced pulmonary capillary perfusion.

These changes cause a profound reduction in oxygen uptake and increase the alveolar-arterial gradient (A-aDO_2) for oxygen and carbon dioxide [25, 42]. Acidosis and hypoxia impede phospholipid synthesis de novo and create a pathogenic "vicious circle" [18]. Hyaline membranes develop as a consequence of pulmonary hypoperfusion and increased vascular permeability as is witnessed in shock lung. A severe from of respiratory distress syndrome can occur in the infants of diabetic, mothers [38, 41], even when at term, due to a developmental delay in lung maturation.

Prevention. Besides enzyme maturation, which is complete after the 35th week of gestation, there are prenatal factors which promote or inhibit the occurrence of the disease (see Fig. 23). Prophylaxis by administering dexa- or betamethasone to the gravida 24–72 h before delivery induces enzyme induction prematurely [10,28]. The risk of RDS can be assessed using amniocentesis to determine fetal lung maturity: a lecithin/sphingomyelin ratio > 2.0 and the presence of phosphatidylglycerol in the amniotic fluid indicate that RDS will not occur [17].

Clinical Features. The symptoms usually appear immediately postpartum or within the first 6 h of life:
- Tachypnea > 60/min
- Nasal flaring
- Sternal and intercostal retractions
- Expiratory grunting
- Diminished breath sounds
- Blue-gray skin color
- Cyanosis.

The disease peaks on the 2nd or 3rd day of life, followed by general improvement. The Fulham score [21], summarizes clinical, physical, blood-gas, and radiologic criteria of RDS and permits ongoing assessment of the disease (Fig. 24). A score > 15 in the 6th h of life strongly suggests respiratory distress syndrome. The diagnosis is confirmed by X-ray and a negative foam stability test [9, 12]: Aspirate from the pharynx or stomach is shaken with 95% ethanol; in the presence of mature surfactant, the foam layer which forms is stable after 15 min.

Radiologic Classification of RDS Stages [19]
I = fine granular densities
II = I + air bronchogram extending beyond heart contours
III = II + indistinct or partially obliterated heart and diaphragm contours
IV = "white lung."

Radiologic classification should be undertaken after the 6th h of life if possible: Prior to this time the fluid still present in the lung might create a false impression of RDS or increase the apparent degree of severity, or the RDS may not yet be visible due to a lack of hyaline membrane development and microatelectases. X-Ray findings can be improved by the use of increased transpulmonary pressures.

Differential Diagnosis

Group B streptococcal sepsis
Pulmonary hemorrhage
Pulmonary edema
Vitium cordis
PFC syndrome
Aspiration syndrome
Pneumonia
Extreme hemoconcentration variants (polycythemia, anemia)
Congenital diaphragmatic hernia
Transitory tachypnea
Malformation (airways, lung)
Congenital lobar emphysema
Acute metabolic disorders

- The chest X-ray is essential in all neonates with respiratory difficulty!
- The respiratory distress syndrome is extremely rare in the mature newborn and should be diagnosed by exclusion.
- Group B streptococcal sepsis may simulate the clinical and X-ray signs of RDS in term and preterm infants!

Therapy

1. Close observation of the high-risk neonate
2. Confirmation of diagnosis: Observation of progress (Fulham score), X-ray, foam stability test, hyperoxia test.
3. Special ventilatory support as indicated by the outcome of the hyperoxia test (see p 64).
   a) Mild RDS (X-ray stage I): Spontaneous respiration with elevated FiO_2, further PaO_2 checks, attempt nasal CPAP early if circumstances permit.
   b) Moderately severe RDS (X-ray stage II+III): Attempt nasal CPAP; proceed further according to hyperoxia test. Early CPAP conserves surfactant, may prevent use of mechanical ventilation as well as pulmonary complications, and improves the overall prognosis!
   c) Severe RDS (X-ray stage III+IV): Mechanical ventilation with prolonged inspiration [29]:

Ventilator setting	Initially	After stabilization
Breaths per minute	20–30	10–15
Insp. pressure (cm H_2O)	25–35	20–25
Insp. time (s)	1.0	1.5–2.0
PEEP (cm H_2O)	2– 4	2– 4

- Blood gas analysis after 15 min:
  Profound ventilatory failure ($= PCO_2 > 80$, $PaO_2 < 50$ mm Hg): Gradually increase peak inspiratory pressure until satisfactory ventilation of the lungs is achieved (stethoscope!). In RDS this is usually the case at inspiratory pressures of 25–30 cm H_2O
- Repeat blood gas analysis after 15 min:
  Isolated hypoxemia ($PaO_2 < 50$ mm Hg): Gradually prolong the inspiratory time up to a maximum of 2.0 s.
- Isolated hypercapnia ($PCO_2 > 80$ mm Hg): Briefly attempt a higher ventilation rate (up to 40–50/min) with a shortened inspiratory time.
- Only if the preceding scheme fails: Try ventilation by the method of Herman and Reynolds [37]. If the collapsed alveoli are successfully inflated, there will be a marked improvement of the PaO_2, which can generally be maintained even after the ventilator settings are carefully reduced. Reduction must be done gradually. Reduce the FiO_2 10% every hour if the PaO_2 exceeds 100 mm Hg. Rapid reduction in FiO_2 will cause a sudden fall of PaO_2 through an "oxygen flip-flop" (increased right-to-left shunt due to pulmonary vasoconstriction). We no longer favor high ventilation rates, especially with volume-controlled respirators, because:
- Satisfactory ventilation and a reduction of the O_2 demand can usually be achieved more easily with IMV than with controlled ventilation;
- High ventilation rates (hyperventilation) lead to the inactivation of surfactant through overdistension of the film and increased phospholipid turnover [6, 32] and
- The incidence of pneumothorax is lower at low ventilation rates with IMV.

With regard to the ventilator settings care must be taken that the expiratory time does not fall below 20 s/min! As a rule, only 5 days' ventilation is necessary in uncomplicated RDS. After this time increased secretion of phosphatidylinositol has usually produced enough surface-active material to maintain alveolar stability [32].

For discussion of weaning, see p 102.

4. Regular temperature checks: Maintain thermoneutral range (oxygen saving).
5. Frequent blood gas analyses: At least every 4 h after initial stabilization to assess:
   - Ventilator setting
   - Necessary FiO_2 (goal: PaO_2 of 60–70 mm Hg)
     With continuous monitoring by $tcPO_2$ (see p 67), an arterial blood gas analysis is generally necessary only every 14 h (arterial puncture)
   - Alkali therapy (goal: pH 7.30–7.50)
6. Buffers: No more than 10 mEq/kg body wt sodium bicarbonate in 4 h; monitor serum sodium levels thereafter. Infuse by continuous infusion over a 20–30 min period (beware of cerebral hemorrhage!). Correct ventilation; appropriate therapy for shock and early transfusion have made the use of buffer solution in RDS largely unnecessary [11].
7. Check blood pressure and hematocrit: Packed red cell transfusion if hematocrit is less than 45% or falls by more than 10% in shock or hypertension.
8. For details of long-term ventilation, see p 96.

9. Check FiO_2 and PaO_2, see p 67.
10. Check
   - Blood glucose 3 × daily
   - Hematocrit 1 × dialy
   - Electrolytes 1 × daily
   - Blood count 1 × daily (anemia, signs of infection)
   - Blood pressure every 4 h
   - Urine: fluid balance, pH, osmolarity.

Complications. See p 103.

Prognosis. The average mortality of RDS is as high as 30% [15], and as high as 16% under intensive care conditions [13]. The survival rate of preterm infants is today much better than previously considered [38, 44]; up to 50% for infants < 1000 g and up to 77% for infants of 1000–1500 g [42]. It is hoped that with the development of a suitable surfactant replacement therapy, the prognosis can be further improved [23].

9.2 Aspiration Syndrome

The incidence is 1%–3% of all newborns [3]. Small-for-date and postmature infants are the most susceptible. The history often shows:
- Fetus at risk (1-min Apgar < 6, fetal bradycardia, silent cardiotocography)
- Protracted, complicated delivery
- Presence of meconium in amniotic fluid.

Pathophysiology. Intrauterine hypoxia leads to mesenteric vasoconstriction and causes intestinal ischemia. It is followed by a transitory period of hyperperistalsis combined with atony of the anal sphincter which results in the passage of meconium. The hypoxia also triggers intrauterine breathing movements which cause the fetus to inhale amniotic fluid with meconium, vernix caseosa, and squamous epithelia [35]. The particles are inspired into the bronchioles with the first few breaths. This produces subsegmental atelectasis and areas of obstructive emphysema as well as a chemical pneumonitis [46]. These changes result in a reduced ventilation-perfusion ratio, an increased intrapulmonary shunt, a reduced diffusion capacity, and diminished lung compliance [4].
During the convalescent phase the aspirated material is absorbed and phagocytosed. Fibrosis, emphysema, and cystic changes may persist for weeks in serious cases.

Clinical Features. Immediately postpartum the skin is covered with meconium, and the skin, fingernails, and umbilical cord show a greenish-yellow discoloration. Severe respiratory depression, gasping, coarse rales, bradycardia, hypotension, shock symptoms, asphyxia livida or pallida.

Name:	Born:		Time:		Age:		Admission	6th h	12th h	24th h	48th h
Birth weight g.	> 1500	0	1001–1500	1	< 1000	2					
Temperature	stable	0	unstable (range ± 0.5°)	1	cold (< 35°)	2					
Heart rate (per min)	130–140	0	120–129 141–160	1	< 120 > 160	2					
Respiratory rate (per min)	< 50	0	51–70	2	> 70	3					
Cry	strong	0	fair	1	weak, absent	2					
Cyanosis	none	0	none in 100% O_2	2	present in 100% O_2	3					
Retractions	substernal	1	slight	2	moderate, severe	3					
Grunting	no	0	faint	1	loud	2					
Apnea	no	0	no	0	absent	3					
Air entry	faint	1	poor	2	very poor	3					
pH	7,3–7,4	0	7,2–7,29	2	< 7,2	4					
Base deficit	< 5	0	5–15	2	> 15	4					
pCO_2	< 45	0	45–60	1	> 60	2					
pO_2	normal	0	> 90 in 100% O_2	2 2	< 90 in 100% O_2	3 3					
X-ray	reticulo-granularity	1	air broncho-gram	2	air bron.+ atelectasis	3					
					Total:						

Fig. 24. Progress chart for neonates with respiratory difficulties. (After Gomez, 1969 (Fulham score) [21])

When spontaneous breathing is established: tachypnea, dyspnea, intercostal retractions, expiratory grunt, rhonchi, cyanosis.
Severe asphyxia can lead to the impairment of cardiovascular adaptation with a cardiopulmonary right-to-left shunt (persistent fetal circulation), cardiomegaly (cardiac failure: hypoxia , cor pulmonale) and peripheral hypoperfusion.
Cerebral alterations with increased intracranial pressure and convulsions are possible.

Radiologic Features. Symmetrically disturbed, somewhat dense, spotty, partially nodular lung infiltrates. Lungs hyperexpanded, diaphragm flattened, occasional pleural effusion. Interstitial emphysema, pneumomediastinum, pneumothorax may occur as complications [35].

Course. Full convalescence within 7–10 days; marked improvement is usually seen in 24–72 h.
In severe cases death can occur during the first minutes of life or the first 24 h. If the infant survives, a prolonged course of illness ensues.
Prophylaxis. Rapid termination of delivery in case of persistent intrauterine hypoxia.

Therapy

1. Do not ventilate before the airways are cleared!
2. Inspect the oropharynx under direct vision (laryngoscope), remove meconium-containing material with a large-bore suction catheter.
3. Immediate intubation and intratracheal suctioning.
4. Rapid aspiration of gastric contents.
5. Immediate ventilation if spontaneous breathing is poor: Several days of controlled ventilation are necessary for ventilatory failure (FiO_2 0.6: $PaO_2 < 50$ mm Hg, $PaCO_2 > 80$ mm Hg or recurrent apnea). Optimal ventilator settings: rate 20–30 BPM, volume 10 ml/kg, I:E ratio 1:2. Oxygenation can be improved by using a moderate PEEP of 4–7 cm H_2O [16] (reexpansion and continuous aeration of collapsed alveoli). In severe cases, muscular relaxation (see p 101) can aid in stabilizing the ventilation (improved thoracic compliance, no breathing against ventilator). Continued hypoxemia with a high A-aDO_2 gradient may indicate extensive atelectasis (persistent intrapulmonary shunt) or a persistent fetal circulation (intra- and extracardial right-to-left shunt). The latter can be diagnosed in some circumstances by a PaO_2 difference between the right radial artery and lower aorta. In these cases tolazoline may be given in an attempt to reduce pulmonary resistance (see p 142).
6. Intensive pulmonary physiotherapy (see p 98).
7. Buffering: Inject sodium bicarbonate (3 mEq/kg body wt) in 1:1 mixture with 5% glucose slowly through the umbilical vein (puncture, catheterization).
8. Bradycardia (<50/min): orciprenaline 0.1 mg/dose (=0.2 ml) VI
9. Shock: 5% human albumin infuse 10 ml/kg body wt.
10. Pneumothorax: Immediate thoracocentesis with chest tube placement with continuous drainage; see p 243.
11. Due to the possibility of cardiac failure (hypoxic cardiac injury, strain on right heart): early digitalization: digoxin 0.03 mg/kg/day, for loading dose, then 0.005–0.01 mg/kg/day.
12. We consider antibiotic therapy justified due to the secondary bacterial pneumonia which always develops.
13. Brain edema therapy for severe cerebral alteration: dexamethasone, 1.0 mg/kg/day in four doses. 20% mannitol, 2.0 ml/kg, with furosemide 1 mg/kg, several times daily; anticonvulsive therapy if needed (see p 150).

9.3 Pneumothorax

Incidence. Spontaneous, 1%–2% [2]; during CPAP or PEEP ventilation, 11%–33% [48, 50].

Predisposition
- Spontaneous pneumothorax with no discernible cause
- Respiratory distress syndrome
- Controlled ventilation
- Aspiration syndrome
- Improper resuscitation
- Staphylococcal pneumonia
- Congenital diaphragmatic hernia (contralateral)
- Pulmonary hypoplasia
- Renal dysplasia

Pathogenesis. Excessive intra-alveolar pressure readily leads to overexpansion and rupture of the alveoli. Air escapes along the perivascular sheaths into the interstitium (interstitial emphysema), and circumscribed air spaces (pseudocysts) may form within the lung parenchyma. If the alveolar leak persists, the air spreads along the peribronchial and vascular sheaths of the interstitium across the visceral pleura to the mediastinum (pneumomediastinum). The visceral and mediastinal pleurae being susceptible to rupture, air can penetrate into the pleural space and cause pneumothorax. Cervical emphysema can also develop. Unilateral or bilateral occurrence is possible, although the right side is usually affected [47]. If air escapes along the great vessels into the retroperitoneal space, pneumoperitoneum can occur (differentiate from gastrointestinal perforation). If air manages to cross the pericardial fold and enters the cavity of the pericardium, pneumopericardium results. Gas embolism may result from entrance of air into capillaries, pulmonary veins, or lymphatics [5, 36].

Clinical Features
Sudden respiratory distress (grunting)
Dyspnea
Tachypnea
Cyanosis
Development of shock symptoms
Intercostal retractions
Asymmetrical thoracic excursions
Cutaneous emphysema in some cases.
A life-threatening tension pneumothorax may be missed in small preterm infants!
The heart and respiratory rate are often reduced, as are the blood pressure and the amplitude of pulse pressure [24, 30]. When blood pressure is recorded via an umbilical artery catheter, the decrease in amplitude is useful for differentiating from tube obstruction [34]. Rapid development of respiratory acidosis, fall of the PaO_2. In the

continuous oxygen cardiorespirogram, abrupt changes in transthoracic impedance and a steady fall of the $tcPO_2$ may be early signs of impending pneumothorax [31].

Diagnosis

- If in doubt, rule out tube obstruction by immediate mirror test
- Auscultation: Absent or faint breath sounds, shift of heart sounds (left-sided pneumothorax)
- Thoracic transillumination: Illuminate over affected hemithorax [27] (oculus illuminator, 2.5 cm beam diameter)
- Test puncture: Perform immediately if shock symptoms are present! Puncture with 5-ml syringe with no. 14 cannula, filled with 0.9% NaCl. During aspiration: air bubble.

X-Ray. Taken only if the situation is not life threatening.

Radiologic Features. Mantle or tension pneumothorax. The lung is collapsed on the affected side and displaced from the lateral chest wall by a more or less broad area of lucency. As a rule the pneumothorax borders on the lateral edge of the lung, although air spaces may be present in various interlobular fissures and at the base. The ipsilateral diaphragm is flattened, the intercostal spaces are expanded, and the parietal pleura is arched. Serious cases show mediastinal herniation with displacement of the vascular pedicle and heart toward the contralateral side [35]. Differential diagnosis: lobar emphysema, large pulmonary cyst (pulmonary markings visible in radiolucent area!).

Therapy. Tension pneumothorax is a life-threatening emergency! Its successful treatment depends on immediate diagnosis, prompt surgical relief, and coordinated teamwork:

1. Interstitial emphysema/pneumomediastinum: No active intervention. During ventilation reduce CPAP, PEEP, peak inspiratory pressure, or prolonged inspiratory time if possible. Prevent breathing against ventilator.
2. Small pneumothorax with mild disturbance of respiration: sedation, immediate observation, close monitoring of blood gases. Avoid crying and any unnecessary manipulations (sedation). Absorption of the pneumothorax can be enhanced greatly by giving elevated levels of oxygen (FiO_2). However, this measure is not without its dangers due to possible hyperoxia and the risk of retrolental fibroplasia. It should be done only if means are available for continuous measurement of the PaO_2 (preferable with a transcutaneous electrode).
3. Large asymptomatic pneumothorax or tension pneumothorax: Immediate chest puncture with subsequent continuous drainage (for technique see p 243).

9.4 Acute Pulmonary Hemorrhage

Incidence. 1%–4%, occurring mainly in infants small for gestational age.

Pathology. The localization of the hemorrhage may be primarily interstitial (early stage) or alveolar (late stage).

Predisposition
- Severe perinatal asphyxia
- Hypothermia
- Rh erythroblastosis
- Congenital heart disease
- Hemorrhagic diathesis
- Respiratory distress syndrome
- Aspiration pneumonia
- Sepsis
- Immaturity

Pathophysiology. Investigations of tracheal secretions during acute pulmonary hemorrhage usually indicate pulmonary hemorrhagic edema [1, 8, 45]. It is assumed that an increased left-atrial pressure (left heart failure) and an increased pulmonary capillary pressure are the factors responsible. These also occur, however, in coagulopathy.

Clinical Features. Sudden, massive onset. The early form is manifested in the first 24 h of life, the late form between the 2nd and 4th day of life: sudden agitation, tachypnea, cyanosis, localized or generalized fine crackling rales, rapid progressive respiratory failure. A foamy, hemorrhagic secretion issues from the nose, mouth, and trachea. Differential diagnosis: the early form is difficult to distinguish from RDS. A high mortality accompanies pulmonary hemorrhage.

Radiologic Features. Fine reticulogranular lung markings during the first hours of life, often confused with RDS. Later mostly nodular or circumscribed, usually bilaterally distributed areas of clouding.
In massive hemorrhage, mostly bilateral, total to subtotal homogeneous opacification with sudden onset [35].

Prophylaxis. Avoidance or prompt treatment of perinatal asphyxia, hypothermia, or hypervolemia; prompt treatment of cardiac failure.

Therapy. The explanation of acute pulmonary hemorrhage as pulmonary hemorrhagic edema is suggestive of the appropriate therapy [26, 40, 44, 45]:
1. Immediate intubation and controlled ventilation with a moderate PEEP of 4–7 cm H_2O.

2. Digitalization with a loading dose (digoxin, 0.03 mg/kg, in three doses/day), maintenance dose 0.005–0.01 mg/kg/day.
3. Forced diuresis (furosemide 1 mg/kg, every 4–6 h).
4. Treatment of (mainly metabolic) acidosis: Buffering initially, then according to blood gas analyses.
5. Correct anemia and hypovolemia by packed red cell transfusion after prior diagnostic blood sample (blood count, coagulation status).
6. Correct coagulative disturbance: Fresh frozen plasma 10 ml/kg, taking into account the blood pressure or central venous pressure.
7. Fluid restriction: 60 ml/kg/day.

References

1. Adamson, T. M., Boyd, R. D. H., Norman, I. C. S., Reynolds, E. O. R., Shaw, J. L.: Haemorrhagic pulmonary oedema („massive pulmonary heamorrhage") in the newborn. Lancet *1*, 494 (1969)
2. Avery, E., Fletcher, B. D.: The lung and its disorders in the newborn infant p. 242. Philadelphia – London – Toronto: Saunders 1974
3. Bacsik, R. D.: Meconium aspiration syndrome. Pediatr. Clin. North Am. *24*, 463 (1977)
4. Bancalari, E., Berlin, J. H.: Meconium aspiration and other asphyxial disorders. Clin. Perinatol. *5* (2), 317 (1978)
5. Bauer, M., Otten, A., Briner, J.: Plötzlicher Tod durch massive Luftembolie bei Respirator-Beatmung im Neugeborenenalter. Helv. paediat. Acta *34*, 147 (1979)
6. Benzer, H.: Respiratorbeatmung und Oberflächenspannung in der Lunge. In: Anaesthesiologie und Wiederbelebung, Bd. 38, Berlin, Heidelberg, New York: Springer 1969
7. Chalmers, I., Dauncey, M. E., Verrier-Jones, E. R., Dodge, J. A., Gray, O. P.: Respiratory distress syndrome in infants of Cardiff residents during 1965–75. Brit. Med. J. *2*, 1119 (1978)
8. Cole, V. A., Normand, I. C. S., Reynolds, E. O. R., Rivers, R. P. A.: Pathogenesis of hemorrhagic pulmonary edema and massive pulmonary hemorrhage in the newborn. Pediatrics *51*, 175 (1973)
9. Cowett, R. M., Unsworth, E. J., Hakanson, D. O., Williams, J. R., OH, W.: Foam-Stability test on gastric aspirate and the diagnosis of respiratory-distress syndrome. N. Engl. J. Med. *293*, 413 (1975)
10. Dluholucky, S., Babic, J., Taufer, I.: Reduction of incidence and mortality of respiratory distress syndrome by administration of hydrocortisone to mother. Arch. Dis. Child. *51*, 420 (1976)
11. Eidelmann, A. I., Hobbs, J. F.: Bicarbonate Therapy Revisited. Am. J. Dis. Child. *123*, 847 (1978)
12. Evans, J. J.: Prediction of respiratory-distress syndrome by shake test on newborn gastric aspirate. N. Engl. J. Med. *292*, 1113 (1975)
13. Fanconi, A., Stoll, W., Duc, G., Bossi, E., Prodhom, S.: Das Atemnotsyndrom des Neugeborenen in der Schweiz. Schweiz. med. Wschr. *106*, 1426 (1976)
14. Farrell, P. M., Avery, M. E.: Hyaline membrane disease. Am. Rev. Respir. Dis. *111*, 657 (1975)
15. Farrell, P. M., Wood, R. E.: Epidemiology of hyaline membrane disease in the United States: Analysis of National Mortality Statistics. Pediatrics *58*, 167 (1976)
16. Fox, W. W., Berman, L. S., Downes, J. J., Peckham, G. J.: The therapeutic application of end-expiratory pressure in meconium aspiration syndrome. Pediatrics *56*, 214 (1975)

17. GLUCK, L., KULOVICH, M. V.: Lecithin/sphingomyelin ratios in amniotic fluid in normal and abnormal pregnancy. Am. J. Obstet. Gynecol. *115*, 593 (1973)
18. GLUCK, L. KULOVICH, M. V.: Fetal Lung Development – Current Concepts. Pediatr. Clin. North Am. *20*, 367 (1973)
19. GIEDION, A., HAEFLINGER, H., DANGEL, P.: Acute pulmonary x-ray changes in hyaline membrane disease treated with artificial ventilation and positive end-exspiratory pressure. Pediatr. Radiol. *1*, 145 (1973)
20. GOENEN, M., NINANE, J., DUCOFFRE, B., DECLERCK, Y., CLAUS, D., FERIERRE, G., VANMOERBEKE, R. M. T., MOULIN, D., DEMEYER, R., TREMOUROUX, J.: Hyaline Membrane Disease: Prognostic Factors and Medium-Term Follow-Up. Eur. J. Pediatr. *127*, 181 (1978)
21. GOMEZ, P. W. C., NOAKES, M., BARRIE, H.: A prognostic score for use in the respiratory-distress syndrome. Lancet *1*, 808 (1969)
22. HALLMAN, M., FELDMAN, B. H., KIRKPATRICK, E., GLUCK, L.: Absence of Phosphatidylglycerol in Respiratory-Distress syndrome in the Newborn. Pediatr. Res. *11*, 714 (1977)
23. IVEY, H. H., ROTH, St., KATTWINKEL, J.: Use of nebulized surfactants in treatment of the respiratory-distress syndrome (RDS) of infancy. Pediatr. Res. *10*, 462 (1976)
24. KITTERMAN, J. A., PHIBBS, R. H., TOOLEY, W. H.: Catheterization of umbilical vessels in newborn infants. Pediatr. Clin. N. Amer. *17*, 895 (1970)
25. KLAUS, M.: Respiratory problems. In: KLAUS, M., FANAROFF, A. H., Care of the high-risk neonate. p. 119, Philadelphia-London-Toronto: Saunders 1973
26. KOTAS, R. V., WELLS, TH. J., MIMS, L. C., TRAINOR, E. J., WILES, C. L.: A new model for neonatal pulmonary hemorrhage research. Pediatr. Res. *9*, 161 (1975)
27. KUHNS, L. R., BEDNAREK, F. J., WYMAN, M. L., ROLOFF, D. W., BORER, R. C.: Diagnosis of pneumothorax or pneumomediastinum in the neonate by transillumination. Pediatrics *56*, 355 (1975)
28. LIGGINS, G. C., HOWIE, R. N.: A controlled trial of antepartum glucocorticoid treatment for prevention of the respiratory distress syndrome in premature infants. Pediatrics *50*, 515 (1972)
29. MANNINO, F. L., FELDMAN, B. H., HELDT, G. P., DELUC, N. A., WIMMER, J. E., FLETCHER, M. A., GLUCK, L.: Early mechanical ventilation in RDS with a prolonged inspiration. Pediatr. Res. *10*, 464 (1976)
30. MERENSTEIN, G. B., DOUGHERTY, K., LEWIS, A.: Early detection of pneumothorax by oscilloscope in the newborn infant. J. Pediatr. *80*, 98 (1972)
31. MONIN, P., VERT, P.: Pneumothorax. Clin. Perinatol. *5* (2), 335 (1978)
32. OBLADEN, M., MERRITT, T. A., GLUCK, L.: Alterations in tracheal phospholipid composition during RDS. Pediatr. Res. *10*, 465 (1976)
33. OBLADEN, M.: Factors influencing surfactant composition in the newborn infant. Eur. J. Pediatr. *128*, 129 (1978)
34. OGATA, E. S., GREGORY, G. A., KITTERMAN, J. A.: Pneumothorax in the respiratory distress syndrome. Pediatrics *58*, 177 (1976)
35. OPPERMANN, H. C., WILLE, L.: Röntgenologie primär pulmonal bedingter Lungenveränderungen bei Früh- und Neugeborenen. Pediatr. Prax. *18*, 569 (1977)
36. OPPERMANN, H. C., WILLE, L., OBLADEN, M., RICHTER, E.: Systemic Air Embolism in the Respiratory Distress Syndrome of the Newborn. Pediat. Radiol., *8*, 139 (1979)
37. REYNOLDS, E. O. R.: Pressure waveform and ventilator settings for mechanical ventilation in severe hyaline membrane disease. Int. Anesthesiol. Clin. *12*, 259 (1974)
38. ROBERT, M. F., NEFF, R. K., HUBBELL, J. P., TAUSCH, H. W., AVERY, M. E.: Association between maternal diabetes and the respiratory-distress syndrom in the newborn. N. Engl. J. Med. *294*, 357 (1976)
39. SALING, E.: Oxygen-conserving adaption of the fetal circulation. In: Apley, J., Modern trends in Pediatrics 3. APLEY I. (ed.) Glasgow: Butterworth 1970
40. SAULE, H., ORTLIEB, R., LÖSCHER, T.: Mechanische Beatmung mit positiv endexspiratorischem Druck zur Behandlung der akuten Lungenhämorrhagie beim Neugeborenen. In: Pädiatrische Intensivmedizin, Emmrich, P. (Ed.), p. 26. Stuttgart: Thieme 1977

41. SMITH, B. T., GIROUD, C. J. P., ROBERT, M., AVERY, M. E.: Insulin antagonism of cortisol action on lecithin synthesis by cultured fetal lung cells. J. Pediatr. *87*, 953, (1975)
42. STEWART, A. L., TURCAN, D. M., RAWLINGS, G., REYNOLDS, E. O. R.: Prognosis for infants weighing 1000 g or less at birth. Arch. Dis. Childh. *52*, 97 (1977)
43. SWYER, P. R.: The intensive care of the newly born. p. 105. Basel–München: Karger 1975
44. THOMAS, D. B.: Survival after massive pulmonary hemorrhage in the neonatal period. Acta Peadiatr. Scand. *64*, 825 (1975)
45. TROMPETER, R., YA, V. Y. H., AYNSLEY-GREEN, A., ROBERTON, N. R. C.: Massive pulmonary hemorrhage in the newborn. Arch. Dis. Child. *50*, 123 (1975)
46. TYLER, D. C., MURPHY, J., CHENEY, F. W.: Mechanical and chemical damage to lung tissue caused by meconium aspiration. Pediatrics *62*, 454 (1978)
47. WILLE, L., OPPERMANN, H. C.: Das idiopathische Atemnotsyndrom: Pulmonale Veränderungen und Komplikationen unter Respiratortherapie bei Frühgeborenen. Röntgenbl. *29*, 278 (1976)
48. WUNG, J. T., STARK, R. I., HEGYI, T., DRISCOLL, L., ST., JAMES, L. ST.: CDP: A major breakthrough. Pediatrics *58*, 783, (1976)
49. WYSZOGRODSKI, I., KYEI-ABOAGYE, H. W., TAEUSCH, H. W., AVERY, M. E.: Surfactant inactivation by hyperventilation: conservation by end exspiratory pressure. J. Appl. Physiol. *38*, 461, (1975)
50. YU, V. Y. H., LIEW, S. W., ROBERTON, N. R. C.: Pneumothorax in the newborn – changing pattern. Arch. Dis. Child. *50*, 449 (1975)

10 Cardiological Problems in the Newborn

H. E. Ulmer

10.1 The Newborn with Congenital Heart Disease

According to extensive studies, the incidence of congenital heart disease is about 8.8 per 1000 livebirths [12]. Life-threatening cardiac symptoms develop in 2.3% of all liveborns during the neonatal period. The overall mortality associated with congenital heart disease in the first month of life is reported to be 1.2 per 1000 live births. Infants with congenital heart disease therefore still account for about 30% of all neonatal mortality [6]. The frequency of these cardiac disorders and the early, life-threatening symptoms explain why these infants represent a relatively high percentage (12%–15%) of cases in neonatal intensive care units. The most common congenital heart diseases with life-threatening symptoms, together with their relative diagnostic frequency, are listed in Table 42.

10.1.1 Differential Diagnosis of Congenital Heart Disease in the Newborn

The most revealing symptom of congenital heart disease in this age group, as opposed to older infants and children, is cyanosis, which is seen in two-thirds of these children. In one-half of cases, cyanosis is accompanied by congestive heart failure. Heart murmurs, arrhythmias, and heart failure without cyanosis occur as cardinal symptoms in only about one-third of these newborns.

Table 42. Relative diagnostic frequency of individual congenital heart disease with life-threatening symptoms in the newborn infant (in order of frequency [6])

Ventricular septal defect	15%
Transposition of the great arteries	11%
Tetralogy of Fallot and pseudotruncus	9%
Hypoplastic left heart syndrome	8%
Patent ductus arteriosus	7%
Coarctation of the aorta	7%
Endocardial cushion defects	5%
Malpositions	4%
Single ventricle	3%
Primary myocardial disease	2%
Other abnormalities	each < 1%

A guide to the differential diagnosis of the most important congenital heart defects in the neonatal period, as well as to therapeutic procedures, is given in Table 43 (Table 43, see p. 126/127).

It is equally important, however, to rule out diseases which are not of cardiac origin, but which often may be mistaken for heart disease in the newborn (see Table 44).

Table 44. Diseases which may be mistaken for congenital heart defects in the newborn

True diagnosis	Misinterpreted findings	Differential diagnosis by
Respiratory failure	Cyanosis and tachydyspnea	ECG and PCG are usually unremarkable; hyperoxia test: marked increase in arterial PO_2
Sepsis	ECG often resembles cardiomyopathy	Fall of platelet count, demonstration of organisms in blood culture
Severe anemia	Tachycardia, cardiac failure	Hb <10 g% Improvement after transfusion
Methemoglobinemia	Cyanosis and hypoxia	Arterial PO_2: normal Arterial saturation: low Detection of met-Hb
Hypoglycemia Hypocalcemia	Cardiomegaly	Serum-concentration Caution: Hypoglycemia may exist in severe cardiac failure
Congenital thyrotoxemia	Tachycardia, cardiomegaly, murmur	TSH, T3/T4, clinical picture
Extracardiac AV fistulae	Murmurs, cardiomegaly	Peripheral bruits, cranial auscultation!
Infant of a diabetic mother	Cardiomegaly, plethora	Maternal history, blood glucose determination
PFC-syndrome	Cyanosis	Tolazoline test in selected cases

10.1.2 General and Special Cardiological Diagnostic Tests in Suspected Neonatal Heart Disease

General cardiological diagnostic tests are noninvasive procedures used to investigate congenital heart disease before special diagnostic tests such as cardiac catheterization and angiocardiography are performed. In reference to the newborn period they include:

a) *History and Clinical Symptoms.* Difficulty in feeding, cyanosis (possibly dissociated), tachypnea, dyspnea, stridor, profuse sweating, thoracic thrill, absence of femoral pulses, blood pressure measurement on upper and lower extremities.

b) *Chest X-Rays.* The infant should preferably be in upright position if his condition permits. The heart size and configuration, superior mediastinal vascular roots, pulmonary vascularity, and visceral situs (location of stomach bubble) are assessed.

Table 43. Differential diagnosis of common congenital heart disease with severe symptoms in the neonatal period[a]

Defect	Symptoms	Heart size and shape in chest X-ray	Pulmonary vascularity
Simple D-transposition	Cyanosis, hypoxia, acidosis, usually on 3rd or 4th day of life	"Egg-on-side contour" with narrow superior mediastinum	Usually ++
Total anomalous pulmonary venous return to the heart	Cyanosis, cardiac failure	"Snowman silhouette" in 2/3 of cases	Usually ++
Ventricular septal defect	Cardiac failure, difficulty in feeding	Cardiomegaly	++
Patent ductus arteriosus	Cardiac failure, respiratory fail.	Cardiomegaly	++
Coarctation of the aorta	Cardiac failure, pulses: arm: + foot: −	Usually cardiomegaly	∅/+
Critical pulmonary stenosis	Cyanosis, shock	Usually cardiomegaly	∅/−
Tetralogy of Fallot	Cyanosis, no cardiac failure	Small with raised apex	−
Pseudotruncus	Cyanosis, no cardiac failure	Small with narrow superior mediastinum	−
Truncus arteriosus	Cardiac failure, possible cyanosis	Cardiomegaly	∅/++
Tricuspid atresia	Cyanosis, possible cardiac failure	Usually unremarkable	−/∅
Hypoplastic left-heart-syndrome	Shock, oliguria, most often seen on 1st or 2nd day	Cardiomegaly	−∅/+
Endocardial fibroelastosis	Progressive cardiac failure	Cardiomegaly	∅

[a] *NP*, neonatal period; *CC*, cardiac catheterization; *ACG*, angiocardiography; *BAS*, ballon atrioseptostomy; *LAD*, left-axis deviation in ECG; *LV*, left ventricle; ∅, normal; +, increased; −, decreased

In our opinion lateral or oblique projections rarely yield additional information during the neonatal period.

c) *Electrocardiogram.* Rhythm, rate, axis deviation, and signs of ventricular overload, hypertrophy or myocardial hypoxia are assessed using the six limb leads and the usual precordial leads.

ECG	PCG	Procedure during NP
Usually nonspecific	Often 	CC, ACG, BAS, artrioseptostomy
RVH	Usually 	CC, ACG, BAS, immediate surgery
RVH BVH	Usually 	CC and Pulmonary banding (as req.)
RVH BVH	Often nor more than 	Early ligature (as required)
RVH BVH	Often nor more than 	Preductal: resection
RVH	Usually 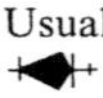	Commissurotomy
RVH	Often 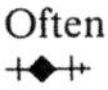	No digitalis, later CC
RVH	Often 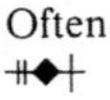	CC, ACG, anastomosis (as req.)
RVH BVH	Often 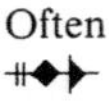	Banding (as req.), anastomosis (as req.)
LAD	Often 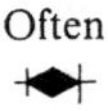	CC, ACG, BAS (as req.), anastomosis (as req.)
Often RVH; LV activity absent	Often 	Prognosis unfavorable
Hypervoltage	Usually 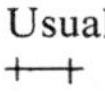	Attempt at conservative therapy; poor prognosis

d) *Auscultation and Phonocardiogram.* Because of the physiologic tachycardia of the newborn, phonocardiography is of particular value for the reliable differentiation and temporal correlation of heart sounds and murmurs. The absence of a murmur, e. g., in primary myocardial disease, is also of differential diagnostic significance.

e) *Echocardiogram.* Echocardiography, a noninvasive diagnostic procedure of increasing importance, is generally the province of the neonatal and pediatric cardiologist. It is increasingly used in the neonatal period to detect gross morphological anomalies (hypoplastic left-heart syndrome, transposition of the great vessels, valvular atresia, etc.) quickly and without discomfort in infants and newborns (8). Patent ductus arteriosus in preterm infants with respiratory distress syndrome (see p 140) can be diagnosed quite reliably by determining the relative diameters of the left atrium and aortic root ($LA/Ao > 1.3$) [30].

f) *Oximetry and Hyperoxia Test.* Though mostly performed invasively by the determination of arterial oxygen saturation (SaO_2) and arterial oxygen tension (PaO_2), this is included among the general diagnostic tests used by pediatric cardiologists. The degree of arterial hypoxemia provides information on the degree of physical impairment by congenital heart disease. Hyperoxia test (HOT): If the PaO_2 does not increase at all after 100% oxygen is administered for 10 min, or does not rise to approximately normal values, it must be assumed that a large intracardiac right-to-left shunt is present, due to an anatomic abnormality which prevents venous blood from passing through the lung for oxygenation. Although severe pulmonary diffusion barriers cannot be ruled out with absolute certainty in such cases, PaO_2 values below 35 mm Hg in the HOT are still a strong indication that complete transposition of the great arteries may be present [4].
The HOT should be performed whenever serious congenital heart disease is suspected. To avoid difficulties in performing subsequent cardiac catheterization from the right groin due to the formation of a hematoma, the right femoral artery should not be punctured.

Special cardiological diagnostic tests representing right and left heart cardiac catheterization and angiocardiography carry a reasonable risk during the neonatal period in relation to their diagnostic value. A mortality rate of 0.1% is assumed after the 1st month of life [6]. The mortality rate is considerably higher in the neonatal period, i. e., about 8.3% [33]. It must be noted, however, that this includes the natural mortality rate of these critically ill newborns; the fatal complication rate of the cardiac catheterization procedure itself is about 1%–2%, even in the first 4 weeks of life [6]. Nevertheless, cardiac catheterization of the newborn must always regarded as an emergency procedure whose indication strongly depends upon the severity of the individual case. In our opinion, the indications for cardiac catheterization in the neonatal period are present when, according to the presumptive diagnosis based on the general cardiologic diagnostic tests:

- A clinically urgent correction of a heart defect is necessary and possible in the 1st month of life or shortly therafter, or
- an incurable defect is suspected, or nonstructural heart disease cannot be excluded and the possibility of an operation must be ruled out by catheterization.

The latter indication in many cases facilitates the decision as to the extent of further intensive measures, such as long-term ventilation. The indication for cardiac catheterization in the neonatal period should not be a purely diagnostic one. The procedure is done under local anesthetic and usually via the right greater saphenous vein. The umbilical vein may be used in the first days of life as long as the ductus venosus is still patent, or when it is held open by an umbilical vein catheter passed into the right atrium.

10.1.3 Cardiac Surgery in the Newborn

Cardiac surgery is undertaken in the 1st month of life only in newborns who are in an imminent danger of death. The surgical procedures most frequently performed are:

a) Atrioseptectomy by the Blalock-Hanlon technique in transposition of the great arteries
b) Resection in the coarctation of the aorta of the pre- or juxtaductal type
c) Aortopulmonary shunt operations in pulmonary stenosis or pulmonary atresia with or without ventricular septal defect
d) Pulmonary valvulotomy by the Brock technique in critical pulmonary stenosis
e) Ligation of a persistent ductus arteriosus
f) Corrective operations for total anomalous drainage of the pulmonary veins.

The mortality rate for these operations is still generally high except for ductal ligation, even in centers with considerable experience in cardiac surgery during infancy [34]. Other operations for a variety of specific defects are described [1]. It has to be pointed out that the operative mortality decreases by about two-thirds past the 3rd month of life. Thus, it is the task of neonatal intensive care to minimize cardiorespiratory or other complications in those newborns, until a more favorable time of operation.

10.2 Urgent Cardiac Diagnosis in the Newborn

It is impossible to discuss in this text every kind of congenital heart disease that results in serious clinical symptoms during the neonatal period. The discussion here must be limited to abnormalities which are frequent or typical in terms of diagnostic and therapeutic procedures. More comprehensive descriptions are found in the literature [6, 1, 19, 16, 25, 27].

10.2.1 Transposition of the Great Arteries (TGA)

Definition. In the so-called simple transposition of the great arteries (TGA), the aorta arises from the right ventricle, and venous blood is pumped unsaturated back into circulation. In contrast the pulmonary artery arises from the left ventricle and returns saturated arterial blood back to the lungs. In the most common form, the d-TGA ("dextro-transposition"), the aorta is located to the right and in front of the pulmonary artery. In simple d-TGA there is no other concomitant cardiac malformation.
In "complex" TGA the transposition of the aorta and pulmonary artery is associated with any of various other cardiac malformations – often a ventricular septal defect or

subvalvular pulmonary stenosis (19). It is also possible for the atria and the two ventricles to be inverted in relationship to one another. Simple TGA is preponderant by a factor of about 2 : 1. Males seem to be preferentially affected.

Pathophysiology. In d-TGA, oxygenated blood can enter the systemic circulation only through a patent foramen ovale, a patent ductus arteriosus, or a ventricular septal defect. Venous blood can reach the pulmonary circulation only by the same route. If the foramen ovale and ductus arteriosus close after birth, as is usual, the blood flows cannot be adequately shunted, and life-threatening arterial hypoxemia will develop.

Clinical Picture. Simple d-TGA should be suspected in infants who appear normal at birth, but who in 3–4 days develop rapidly increasing cyanosis, tachypnea, and acidosis, initially without signs of cardiac failure. In cases of complex d-TGA, e. g., if a significant ventricular septal defect is also present, the symptoms usually take longer to develop, and 8–14 days may pass before marked signs of cardiac failure appear. Infants with TGA are often large for gestational age. Maternal diabetes is disproportionately frequent.

Diagnosis. In typical cases the X-ray shows a normal-size or slightly enlarged "egg-on-side" heart contour completed by a narrow superior mediastinum due to the dextroposition of the aorta (Fig. 25). The pulmonary vascularity is increased with an associated VSD, but tends to be decreased with an associated pulmonary stenosis. The ECG initially often shows only an age-related normal pattern. PCG in simple TGA demonstrates only a mild uncharacteristic systolic murmur and sometimes a split second heart sound. In complex TGA the phonocardiographic findings depend on the associated defects. In the hyperoxia test (see p 128) the PaO_2 hardly increases during 100% O_2 breathing, since the hypoxemia is not caused by pulmonary undersaturation; rather, the possibilities of the oxygen uptake are anatomically fixed and limited, e. g., by the foramen ovale. PaO_2 values below 35 mm Hg are strongly indicative of d-TGA; even with associated VSD they are seldom higher than 50 mm Hg [4].

Management. The suspected presence of d-TGA is an absolute indication for immediate cardiac catheterization. The diagnosis has to be confirmed by angiocardiography demonstrating the aorta arising from the venous ventricle, to the right and in front of the pulmonary artery. In the balloon atrioseptostomy technique of Rashkind [20], a balloon-tipped catheter filled with contrast medium is passed into the left atrium, inflated, and withdrawn back through the foramen ovale, thereby creating a defect in the atrial septum and providing arterial blood with an access to the systemic circulation. If this procedure is ineffective, it may be necessary in some cases to create an atrial septal defect operatively by the Blalock-Hanlon technique [10]. The nature and timing of further palliative measures beyond the neonatal period are determined by the associated defect. Total correction by the Mustard technique is usually performed around the 1st year of life.

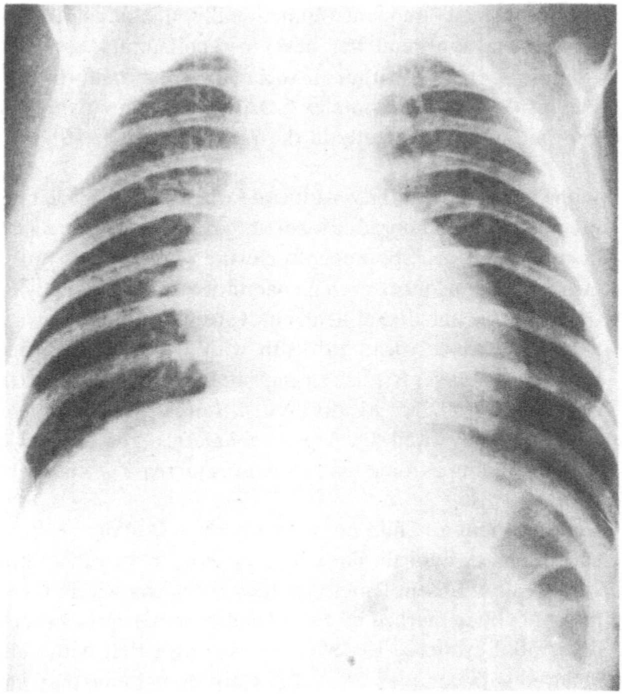

Fig. 25. X-Ray of infant with transposition of the great vessels: slightly enlarged "egg-on-side" heart with narrow superior mediastinum and moderate increase in pulmonary vascularity (M. M., ♂, 6th day of life, d-TGA with VSD)

10.2.2 Coarctation of the Aorta (COA)

Anatomy. The classification of COA depends on the anatomical site of the coarctation in relation to the ductus arteriosus [16]:

a) *Preductal* (*Preligamentous*) *COA* (formerly called "infantile" type). Coarctation proximal to the ductus arteriosus or obliterated ligamentum arteriosum. Associated cardiac malformations are obligatory, with a large patent ductus, often with hypoplasia of the aortic arch, with aortic stenosis, hypoplastic left ventricle, ventricular septal defect. Collaterals to the lower half of the body are poorly developed, mostly because this kind of coarctation has had little effect on the circulation in utero.

b) *Postductal* (*Postligamentous*) *COA* (formely called "adult" type). Coarctation distal to the ductus arteriosus or ligamentum arteriosum. Associated cardiac malformations are less frequent. Collaterals to the lower body half are usually well developed, since the coarctation has had intrauterine effects.

c) *Juxtaductal* (*Juxtaligamentous*) *COA*. Coarctation just opposite to the aortic orifice of the ductus arteriosus or ligementum arteriosum. Associated cardiac malformations are frequent. Functionally, juxtaductal COA usually parallels the preductal type, and well developed collateral vessels are rare.

"Simple" COA, i. e., without associated cardiac malformations, is almost exclusively of the postductal type. Complex COA with accompanying malformations is diagnosed ten times more frequently in the 1st month of life [6].

Pathophysiology. In the postductal form of COA, the left heart is subjected to both a pressure load and an additional volume load from the left-to-right shunt across the ductus arteriosus. Spontaneous closure of the ductus thus represents a relief for the heart in the long term, even if coarctation should actually increase slightly due to the traction from the ductal ligament. Closure of the ductus arteriosus in the preductal form of COA can lead to death within a few hours, because it produces a life-threatening left ventricular strain, and the blood supply to the lower body half via the right-to-left shunt is critically limited. Since this kind of coarctation has had little effect in utero, few well-developed collaterals to the lower body are available. Accompanying cardiac malformations increase the severity of the condition.

Clinical Picture. Children with simple COA of the postductal type are usually asymptomatic at birth. The main symptom in the other forms is severe cardiac failure with weak or absent femoral pulses, appearing within the 1st week of life. Preductal forms are often marked by an isolated cyanosis of the lower half of the body, so-called differential cyanosis. Experience has shown that with conservative measures, even children with complex COA of the postductal type may improve after a few days or weeks; preductal forms, on the other hand, generally show a short recovery period following conservative treatment and again exhibit the picture of severe cardiac failure after 1–2 days.

Diagnosis. Blood pressure measurements by sphygmomanometer or ultrasonic probe in the first days of life often yield normal or slightly elevated pressures (70–90 mm Hg) in the upper extremities, while the pressures in the lower extremities (popliteal artery, dorsalis pedis) rarely exceed 50 mm Hg. The X-ray generally shows considerable cardiac enlargement and signs of pulmonary congestion. The ECG shows evidence of a right ventricular or biventricular hypertrophy, which in the postductal form successively gives way in typical cases to a more or less pronounced left ventricular hypertrophy. The PCG shows a systolic murmur which extends beyond the second sound and which may be continuous.

Preductal coarctation is indicated in the differential hyperoxia test if, during simultaneous arterial blood sampling while 100% O_2 is administered, the PaO_2 of the left femoral artery (beware: hematoma formation on right groin) shows no increase relative to the right radial artery. It has been proven recently that transcutaneously measured arterial PO_2 values (tc-PaO_2) are as reliable as PaO_2 measurements by arterial samplings [4].

Management. If preductal COA is suspected, an urgent indication exists for cardiac catheterization and angiocardiography to localize the stricture and identify associated cardiac malformations before an operation is performed. The operative possibilities range from resection of the COA with ductal ligation to supplementary aortoplasty and pulmonary banding [1]. The mortality rate is between 35% and 60%, depending on the necessary extent of the operation. Later reoperations are necessary in about one-fourth of the patients [1, 34].

10.2.3 Hypoplastic Left Heart Syndrome (HLHS)

Anatomy. The hypoplastic left heart syndrome encompasses a group of cardiac malformations consisting of:

- Varying degrees of hypoplasia or atresia of the aortic and/or mitral valve, and
- hypoplasia of the left ventricle, the ascending aorta, and the aortic arch.

Various individual types can be distinguished according to the degree of hypoplasia of the two valves of the left heart [32]. The combination of aortic atresia and mitral hypoplasia with a hypoplastic left ventricle is the most common. The branching of the coronary arteries is normal as a rule. Males predominate by 3 : 1.

Pathophysiology. Common to all forms is an anatomically determined decrease in arterial blood supply to the peripheral circulation. Mixing of the venous and arterial blood takes place in the right atrium caused by a complete left-to-right shunt via the patent foramen ovale. The systemic circulation is usually supplied with the mixed blood shunted through the widely patent ductus arteriosus. The oxygen saturation in the right atrium, right ventricle, pulmonary artery, aorta and the retroperfused coronary arteries is identical.

Clinical Features. The infants are almost always admitted in the first days of life with signs of severe cardiac failure in a shock-like state with initially moderate cyanosis. The arterial pulses are weak in both the upper and lower extremities and may vary in intensity, depending on functional constriction of the ductus arteriosus. The further course almost always leads to oliguria and anuria caused by renal hypoperfusion.

Diagnosis. The chest X-ray usually shows marked cardiomegaly despite the hypoplasia of one ventricle. The pulmonary vasculature appears congested to the point of pulmonary edema. The ECG may be a valuable guide, with evidence of strain and hypertrophy of the right ventricle and, typically, the absence of left ventricular activity in the left-precordial leads. Ordinarily the second sound in the PCG is not split due to the aortic atresia. Gallop rhythm and nonspecific systolic murmurs are not uncommon. A valuable part of the noninvasive diagnosis is the echocardiogram [8], which demonstrates the hypoplastic left ventricle, and the absence of normal aortic or mitral valve movements. In the hyperoxia test, the PaO_2 may be over 50 mm Hg, with regularly no difference between the pre- and the postductal parts of the circulation.

Management. Even if the diagnosis appears established by general diagnostic tests, cardiac catheterization with angiocardiography should still be performed. The angiocardiogram is necessary for excluding malformations such as preductal coarctation of the aorta or isolated aortic arch atresia, for which at least palliative operative consequences are available (1). Even palliative operations for hypoplastic left heart syndrome have a mortality rate of 95%–100% [1] and are extremely problematic. The majority of children with HLHS die in the 1st month of life because of intractable cardiac failure and consecutive prerenal kidney failure.

10.2.4 Primary Myocardial Disease

Definition. Primary myocardial disease encompasses a group of nonstructural heart disease in which the myocardium is damaged at the cellular level, and there is no structural malformation in the form of congenital heart disease. The following etiologic distinctions are made:

Inflammatory Processes. Acute myocarditis (e. g., from Coxsackie-B infection).

Degenerative Processes. Primary and secondary cardiomyopathies of the congestive type (CCMP) or the hypertrophic type (HCMP).
- Primary CCMP, e. g., endocardial fibroelastosis (EFE)
- Secondary CCMP, e. g., in certain neuromuscular diseases
- Primary HCMP, e. g., idiopathic hypertrophic subaortic stenosis
- Secondary HCMP, e. g., in glycogenosis (Pompe's disease).

Posthypoxic States. e. g., due to severe perinatal asphyxia, special forms of the persistent fetal circulation syndrome [26], or as the result of severe and persistent hypoxemia of pulmonary origin.
Often this diagnosis has to be confirmed by later histologic studies of the myocardium. Even postmortem differentiation between connate myocarditis or endocardial fibroelastosis is of practical significance. It is noteworthy that some forms of the primary cardiomyopathies have a high risk of recurrence in a family.

Pathophysiology. Cardiac failure in acute myocarditis of the newborn is accompanied by dilatation of the ventricles with a small stroke volume and a low cardiac output despite a high ventricular preload due to increased end diastolic ventricular pressures and volumes. Atrial pressures and the pulmonary capillary pressure are elevated. The cause of these hemodynamic changes is the inflammatory rupture of myocardial fibers, as well as the edematous swelling of the cardiac muscle, which greatly impairs myocardial contractility and hinders the uptake of energy-rich substrates and oxygen. Isolated endocardial fibroelastosis (EFE) is now regarded mainly as the end stage of prior intrauterine myocarditis [17]. The functional state of the hypodynamic myocardium is morphologically based on increasing fibroid degeneration in the subendocardial region. This usually proceedes during recurrent episodes.

Clinical Picture. Infants with cardiomyopathies generally develop progressive cardiac failure, usually without marked cyanosis, as well as feeding problems and failure to thrive toward the end of the neonatal period or in early infancy. Clinical symptoms of Coxsackie myocarditis, however, usually appear in the 1st week of life; the course is more fulminant and is accompanied in one-third of cases by seizures or other central nervous symptoms. Primary myocardial disease caused by severe perinatal asphyxia usually presents the clinical picture of cardiogenic shock in the neonate.

Diagnosis. The X-ray in primary myocardial disease generally shows a bilaterally dilated heart which shows only weak contractions during fluoroscopy or echocardiography. Myocarditis, obstructive or congestive cardiomyopathy cannot be differentiated by plain film X-ray in this period of life. The ECG findings in endocardial fibroelastosis are marked by left ventricular hypertrophy and manifestations of the damage to the left heart in the form of ST – depressions or negative T waves, as well as an often grotesque hypervoltage which is seldom seen in structural congenital heart disease. Low voltage, conduction disturbances, and cardiac arrhythmias, on the other hand, are more indicative of inflammatory heart disease. Here, however, the ECG findings are highly uncharacteristic and only indicative in about 15%–20% of cases [17]. A heart murmur is usually absent. The heart sounds are remarkably faint, suggesting the term "large mute heart of infancy" to characterize the situation in primary myocardial disease. Ventricular performance and myocardial contractility can be quantitatively analyzed by echocardiographic estimation of the right and left ventricular systolic time intervals [11]. If primary myocardial disease is suspected, serologic tests should be done in the mother and child in an attempt to demonstrate or rule out infectious origin, e. g., Coxsackie-B, mumps, influenza, herpes, rubella, or cytomegalic viruses or toxoplasmosis, either acquired connately or during pregnancy.

Management. If the diagnosis of primary myocardial disease is clearly established by echocardiography or serologic investigations, cardiac catheterization may not be indicated in the neonatal period. As compared to connate myocarditis, endocardial fibroelastosis has a decidedly poor prognosis. Despite intensive anticongestive therapy, children with this kind of heart disease generally do not survive the 1st month of life [25]; with a later onset of symptoms, the course may be prolonged over a period of years [24]. The outcome of postasphyctic myocardial disease depends strongly on the effectiveness of the initial measures in the first hours of the cardiogenic shock. In many cases the prognosis is determined by the consecutive cerebral damage or renal failure.

10.3 Cardiological Emergencies in the Newborn

10.3.1 Congestive Heart Failure

Congestive heart failure in newborns and young infants is often manifested initially by a rapid weight gain of about 80–100 g/day despite difficulties in feeding. Profuse sweating, especially of the face during feeding, and tachypnea in excess of 60/min are

also seen. On examination the arterial pulses are soft, the heart rate is accelerated, the liver is enlarged, the eyelids are edematous, and the muscles are generally hypotonic; the end expiratory rales of the fluid-filled lungs are audible on auscultation. Tachydyspnea with bronchospasms, cold extremities, pretibial edema and anasarca, as well as oliguria or anuria, are additional, but late symptoms in advanced cardiac failure. The X-ray shows an enlarged heart. Ventricular performance cannot be assessed by ECG or PCG, but can be by echocardiography [11]. The differentiation between right- or left-sided heart failure is of little consequence in terms of treatment. In any event, right and left heart failure are usually combined in the newborn.
The therapeutic guidelines for treating congestive heart failure in the newborn are summarized in Table 45. The nature and extent of the measures chosen are dictated by the degree of cardiac failure. Thus, reduction of fluid intake combined with digitalization is sufficient in many newborns. The risk of relatively high digitalis concentrations must be taken into account temporarily in some infants.

Note on I (Table 45). Selection of the cardiac glycoside should always be decided on the basis of personal experience. Pure glycosides are preferable to mixed preparations. We have obtained good results with digoxin and β-acetyldigoxin in the dosages indicated in Table 45. In view of the uncertain absorption conditions in acute cardiac failure, the loading dose should be routinely administered parenterally! The information in Table 45 regarding glucagon therapy is based on experiences obtained elsewhere.

Note on II. Aldosterone antagonists have proved beneficial in newborns. However, they should always be used adjunctively in combination with other diuretics. Maximal effect is usually achieved in 2 or 3 days.

Note on III. A total fluid volume of one–tenth the body weight should not be exceeded as long as fluid restriction is necessary. The fluid balance is maintained best by weighing the infant once or twice daily (can also be done in the incubator). If a splint is applied or the infant is intubated, etc., the new baseline weight should be determined.

Note on IV. Maintenance of the acid-base balance is particularly important in cyanotic defects, for acidosis causes additional pulmonary vasoconstriction. Even catecholamine therapy is ineffective in an acidic milieu. A Hb value below 14 g% and an erythrocyte count below 4.0 million/mm^3 are indicative of anemia in the newborn. The transfusion of packed red blood cells (10 ml/kg body wt.) may produce marked improvement in such cases.
Cyanotic spells are caused by paroxysmal constriction of the infundibulum of the right ventricle in heart defects with right ventricular outflow tract obstruction. Consecutive hypoxia and acidosis further promote the constriction and lead to acute cardiac decompensation. Correction of the acidosis, 100% oxygen respiration, and the slow intravenous infusion of morphine preparations (morphine sulfate 0.1–0.2 mg/kg body wt.) usually interrupt the cyanotic spell. Maintenance therapy with propranolol (5 mg/kg body wt./day, orally in three doses) is continued until operation. Elevated hematocrit values over 70% can be temporarily lowered in larger infants by reduction

Table 45. Guidelines for the treatment of congestive heart failure in the newborn

Principles	Basic therapy for congestive heart failure	Adjunctive therapy for pulmonary edema and cardiogenic shock
I. Increase of myocardial contractility	– *Digoxin*, *β*-acetyldigoxin *Preterm infants:* LD: 0.03 mg/kg IV/IM[a] MD:0.005–0.01 mg/kg/day[b] *Mature infants:* LD: 0.03–0.04 mg/kg IV/IM MD: 0.005–0.01 mg/kg/day 0.005 mg/kg below the age of 14 days 0.010 mg/kg beyond the age of 14 days *Older infants:* LD: 0.04 mg/kg IV/IM MD: 0.01 mg/kg/day Loading dose always parenterally! If maintenance does is given orally, increase by 20% of the parenteral MD	– *Dopamine* infusion: 0.25–0.50 mg/kg/hr – *Glucagon* infusion: 0,05–0,1 mg/kg/hr
II. Promotion of diuresis	– *Furosemide* 1–5 mg/kg every 4–6 h	– *Sprionolactone* 4 mg/kg/day IV (init.) 2 mg/kg/day orally (maint.)
III. Nutritional and fluid support	– Total daily volume supp.: max. 1/10 of body weight 8–12 meals, tube feeding Fluid balance by weighing 1–2 times per day	– Parenteral nutrition 60–80 ml/kg/day, salt fraction = 1/10–1/5
IV. Maintenance of homeostasis	– Careful adjustment of: Acid-base balance Electrolyte balance Carbohydrate balance Transfusion of packed red Cells 10 ml/kg, as required	
V. Economizing measures	– Incline patient (30–45°) administer 40% O_2 – *Phenobarbital* 5 mg kg/day orally	– *Morphine sulfate* 0.1–0.2 mg/kg SC Increased admin. of O_2 Intubation and artificial ventilation PEEP of 4–6 cm H_2O

[a] *LD*, complete loading dose IV, intravenous IM, intramuscular
[b] *MD*, maintenance dose per day SC, subcutaneous

transfusion (10 mg/kg body wt.) and replacement with an equal volume of low-molecular dextran to avoid thromboembolic complications.

Note on V. By inclining the patient, the liver is placed lower and breathing is facilitated. O_2 concentrations over 40 vol.% are necessary and effective in cyanotic children only if pulmonary edema is also present and interfering with pulmonary diffusion. Sedation provides a useful means of conserving oxygen by reducing the increased work of respiration. Manifest pulmonary edema is improved by PEEP ventilation.

10.3.2 Cardiac Arrhythmias

The most frequent deviations from the sinus rhythm in the newborn are extrasystoles. These involve premature cardiac contractions that arise primarily in response to a heterotopic supraventricular impulse. P waves are visible, and the QRS complex is usually not deformed. As a rule, no treatment is necessary. Supraventricular extrasystoles combined with sinus tachycardia can often be early symptoms of heart disease and disappear after digitalis therapy is begun.

First- and second-degree AV blocks are frequently the result of digitalis toxicity. On withdrawal of digitalis, the heart rate quickly returns to normal. Delays of AV conduction in the newborn are not a pressing reason for decreasing the dosage, if the positive inotropic action of this dosage is required clinically, and no higher degrees of blockage are observed during monitoring.

In complete heart block (third-degree AV block) the ventricular rate in newborns is usually about 60–80/min, while the artrial rate generally exceeds 100/min. If this disorder of the AV-conduction occurs congenitally in combination with cardiac failure, it is associated with structural heart disease in about 50% of cases [6]. Complete heart block occurring suddenly in the newborn is indicative of severe hypoxia, toxic or inflammatory myocardial damage with a poor prognosis. If the ventricular rate falls below 50/min, treatment with orciprenaline (0.05–0.1 mg) subcutaneously or, in less dramatic cases, two drops of the 2% solution on the tongue, is indicated. This may be repeated up to eight times in 24 h. Little experience is available to date with pacemaker therapy in newborns.

In cardiac arrest by asystole (see Table 46), 0.1–0.25 mg orciprenaline and 5 ml sodium bicarbonate are injected into a central venous infusion catheter or directly into the heart and then are distributed by cardiac massage. It has to be pointed out that catecholamines are virtually ineffective in a strongly acidic milieu.

Cardiac massage without artificial ventilation is useless! Emergency treatment is followed if necessary by a continuous drip infusion of dopamine, 0.25 mg/kg/h.

In circulatory arrest from ventricular fibrillation or ventricular flutter, a completely irregular ECG trace is obtained. Individual QRS complexes are no longer discernible. External cardiac massage and artificial ventilation must be instituted immediately. Transthoracic electrical defibrillation in the newborn is performed using 10–25 W s. In many cases defibrillation must be repeated several times within a short period. If a defibrillator is not available, pharmacologic defibrillation can be attempted by the intracardiac or central venous injection of lidocaine, 5 mg/kg body wt. In extreme situations it may be necessary to arrest the heart by the intracardiac injection of KCl solution, (2 mEq/kg), and then immediately afterward to restimulate the heart beat with intracardial orciprenaline. For the first 8 h following defibrillation, a prophylactic infusion of lidocaine (0.1–0.2 mg/kg/min). It must be borne in mind that lidocaine has a markedly negative inotropic and chronotropic side effect.

Table 46. Treatment of life-threatening cardiac arrhythmias in the newborn

General immediate measures:		
	– External cardiac massage – Ventilation with 100% O_2 – Correction of acidosis (sodium bicarbonate, 2.5–5 mEq/kg) – ECG monitoring	
Cardiac arrhythmia	**Acute therapy**	**Follow-up treatment**
Asystole	– *Orciprenaline* 0.1–0.25 mg, intracardially – and/or *calcium gluconate* 10% solution (1–2 ml/kg) intracardially	– *Dopamine* by continuous drip infusion (0.25 mg/kg/h)
Supraventricular paroxysmal tachycardia	– *Bilateral ocular compression* – *Rapid digitalization* (2 × 50% LD within 1 h) – *Verapamil IV* (0.3 mg/kg as maximal single dose) dissolved in 5 ml 5% glucose, give 1 ml/min of the solution until heart rate *begins* to fall)	
Atrial flutter or fibrillation with a high ventricular rate	– *Rapid digitalization* – *Verapamil* (as above) – *Electrical defibrillation* (10–25 Ws)	– Digitalis maintenance
Ventricular flutter Ventricular fibrillation	– *Electrical defibrillation* – *Lidocaine* (5 mg/kg) intracardially	– *Lidocaine* by continuous drip infusion (0.1–0.2 mg/kg/min)

Supraventricular paroxysmal tachycardia may be also life threatening if prolonged. In some cases it can be diagnosed and treated prenatally. Initial treatment in the newborn consists of a forceful bilateral ocular compression of about 5-s duration. Regardless of the success of this or additional measures, rapid parenteral digitalization is warranted. If a sinus rhythm is not established by the first digitalis injection, it is usually achieved on injection of verapamil (0.3 mg/kg). However, this may be done only under ECG supervision. In our nursery the calculated individual dose is diluted with 5% glucose solution to a total of 5 ml. This solution is then injected at a rate of 1 ml/min under ECG supervision until the tachycardic rate tends to fall by about 10%. The change to a sinus rhythm then occurs spontaneously several seconds later. Residual solution still present in the infusion system must be aspirated. Deaths have been reported from excessive injection rates and dosages. Follow-up care consists mainly of digitalis maintenance for at least the 1st year of life. For details on the prevention and treatment of recurrences of cardiac arrhythmias see special references [7].

Atrial flutter and atrial fibrillation are rare cardiac arrhythmias in newborns, but they are dangerous and resistant to therapy. In atrial flutter the atrial rate may reach

350/min, usually with some degree of atrioventricular block mostly of 4 : 1 or 2 : 1. In atrial fibrillation, on the other hand, the atrial rate is usually indeterminate, and conduction to the ventricles is irregular (tachyarrhythmia absoluta). At these higher degrees of atrioventricular block, immediate digitalization and, if required, later cardioversion are necessary. Atrial flutter with 1 : 1 conduction is a life-threatening situation. By increasing the degree of atrioventricular blockade with verapamil IV (0.3 mg/kg), the ventricular rate usually can be lowered. Immediate cardioversion is performed in emergencies [36].
The danger of atrial fibrillation lies in an inadequate blood supply to the peripheral circulation. The formation of atrial thrombi in prolonged atrial fibrillation is another danger. Paroxysmal atrial fibrillation usually responds well to digitalis therapy. In persistent forms verapamil can be given adjunctively by a short infusion over a 1–h period (0.3 mg/kg/h). If this fails, cardioversion is performed. The prognosis of atrial flutter and fibrillation is serious in the newborn, but better than in older children.

10.3.3 Patent Ductus Arteriosus in Premature Infants with Respiratory Distress Syndrome

Pathophysiology. After the 20th week of gestation, fetal ductus tissue shows a vasoconstriction in response to an increase in the O_2 concentration of the perfusing blood [27]. The vasodilating action of local E-type prostaglandins is no longer fully operative. However, in about 70% of all premature infants with a birth weight below 1750 g, the ductus arteriosus remains patent for a time after birth. If a respiratory distress syndrome (RDS) is also present, this incidence is still higher [18]. In a third of these cases the ductus closes spontaneously within a few days. In another third it persists without remarkable complications for a longer period but finally also closes spontaneously [27]. However, in another third of these preterm infants with RDS the ductus arteriosus remains patent, possibly caused by an increased local prostaglandin E activity. The hemodynamic consequence is a considerable left-to-right shunt through the ductus with pulmonary hypercirculation, hypertension, and congestion.

Clinical Features. The clinical manifestations are a combination of persistent respiratory failure and increasing cardiac failure in a preterm infant with X-ray evidence of RDS, but no signs of any other congenital heart defect. The recurrence of respiratory failure after initial improvement and the occurrence of apneic spells around the 5th day of life are typical. In most of the cases it is impossible to wean the infants from the ventilator.

Diagnosis. On physical examination there is liver enlargement. So-called bounding pulses are corresponding to a large amplitude of the arterial blood pressure with low diastolic values. Auscultation and phonocardiography disclose at least a systolic murmur, which in about three out of four cases is accompanied by diastolic components. The ECG is usually not specific and shows few changes not exceeding the physiologic right ventricular strain associated with age. The chest X-ray shows cardiomegaly and increased pulmonary vascularity only in certain cases, but always reveals a clouding of the lung fields which is difficult to distinguish from the changes in uncomplicated RDS. Echocardiography contributes significantly to the diagnosis, based on the ratio of the diameter of the left atrium (LA) to that of the aortic root (AO). If the LA:AO ratio is over 1,3, the diagnosis of patent ductus arteriosus in this situation is considered established [5]. Demonstration of the left-to-right shunt through the patent ductus by cardiac catheterization or angiocardiography is necessary only in exceptional cases [27, 5].

Management. Corrective therapy in this life-threatening disorder of the premature infant consists in surgical closure of the patent ductus. On the other hand, indomethacin, an inhibitor of prostaglandin synthesis, has been successfully used for pharmacologic ductus closure for several years [27, 5, 15].

The indication for pharmacologic or surgical closure of the ductus with RDS is present when intractable cardiac failure is still present 24 h after the start of conservative medical therapy (see p 137) or if artificial ventilation is required further on. If artificial ventilation is not needed to maintain adequate oxygenation and a satisfactory acid-base balance, and there is no decompensated congestive heart failure, the pharmacologic or surgical closure of the ductus is not indicated in the preterm infant with RDS. The mortality rates for primary surgical and pharmacologic closure at large neonatal or cardiological centers are the same: about 10%–15% [24, 15]. Inasmuch as the failure rate for pharmacologic closure is also about 10%, primary pharmacologic treatment appears justified as a rule. Contraindications for the use of indomethacin are hemorrhage, thrombopenia with thrombocyte counts below 100 000/mm^3, hyperbilirubinemia with more than 10 mg% indirect bilirubin, and an elevated serum creatinine of more than 1.2 mg% [15].

Indomethacin is administered orally by a gastric tube in a single dose of 0.2 mg/kg body wt. as a suspension in 5% glucose solution (0.2 mg/ml). This may be repeated twice at 12–h intervals. If no significant effect is observed 24 h after the third dose, *immediate* surgical ligature of the ductus is necessary. This surgical intervention is also indicated if a deterioration of cardiac or respiratory function occurs during pharmacologic therapy. If the pharmacologically closed ductus becomes reopened and the above clinical picture reappears, the course of medicinal therapy may be repeated, but no sooner than 3 days after the last dose of indomethacin. In most infants, more than one dose of indomethacin, but not more than one course, is required to effect closure of the patent ductus. Successful closure of the ductus is evidenced by an immediate improvement of respiratory function to the extent that artificial ventilation is usually no longer necessary within 24 h after the last dose of indomethacin. The heart murmur generally disappears in a few hours, the liver and heart return to normal size, and the echocardiographic LA : AO ratio decreases below 1, 0. A constant side effect of indomethacin therapy is a transitory impairment of renal function, indicated by a rise in blood urea nitrogen and fluid retention which lasts no more than a few days. Fluid restriction, the use of diuretics, or the infusion of dopamine in low doses may be temporarily indicated. Follow-up examinations of children 1 year after pharmacologic ductus closure have as yet shown no lasting changes in the heart, lungs, central nervous system, or kidneys [15].

The use of indomethacin for ductus closure in preterm infants still represents an unconventional therapy with possible unknown long-term effects. It should therefore be used only in pediatric cardiology centers and with the informed consent of the parents. Different legal regulations in different countries have to be regarded.

10.3.4 Persistent Fetal Circulation Syndrome

Pathophysiology. Persistent fetal circulation (PFC) exists when the pulmonary vascular resistance does not decrease normally during postnatal physiologic adaptation, but remains high, and the fetal circulatory pathways temporarily persist (Fig. 26). The consequences are pulmonary hypertension as well as decreased pulmonary blood flow due to a large right-to-left shunt through the patent ductus arteriosus and the foramen ovale [14, 29]. A distinction is made between a primary or idiopathic form of PFC, a morphological abnormality of the pulmonary vascular musculature [14], and a secondary form of PFC, in which vasoconstriction of the arterial pulmonary circulation is usually reactive to a persistent hypoxia and/or acidosis associated with an underlying disease, such as perinatal asphyxia, meconium aspiration, polycythemia, as well as severe bacterial or viral infections [14, 26]. Accessory myocardial ischemia can complicate the course considerably; this condition is sometimes called

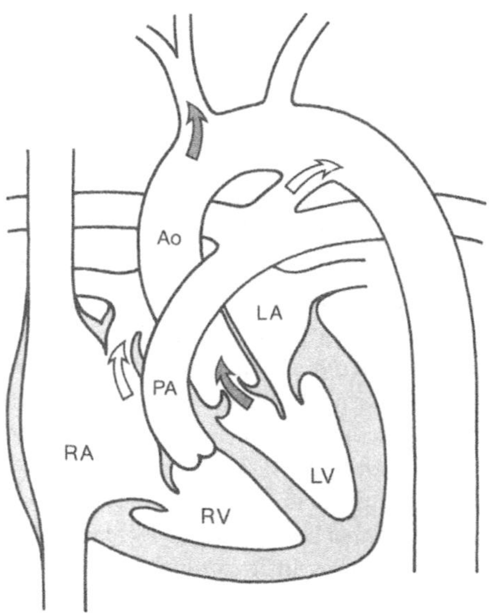

Fig. 26. Graphic representation of the central hemodynamics in the PFC syndrome. The high pulmonary vascular resistance causes a right-to-left shunt through a patent farance ovale as well as through the patent ductus arteriosus to the descending aorta (*light arrows*). In contrast, the ascending aorta is supplied with oxygenated blood deriving from the left ventricle (*dark arrows*)

complex PFC to distinguish it from simple PFC, which is more favorable prognostically [14, 26]. The consequences of persistent fetal circulatory pathways are serious arterial hypoxemia and severe cyanosis from the large right-to-left shunt into the systemic circulation.

Clinical Features. The patients are usually mature term infants with considerably generalized cyanosis which is always present at birth or occurring in the first hours of life, tachydyspnea, and frequently a late systolic heart murmur. In the typical case of primary PFC of the simple type, no signs of cardiac failure are evident. The arterial blood pressures and palpable pulses are unremarkable. On the whole, the clinical picture is like that seen in the presence of severe congenital heart disease with cyanosis. This impression is strengthened in the complex form with signs of cardiac failure. Despite intensive therapeutic measures such as high oxygen administration, ventilation, correction of acidosis and digitalization, about 10%–20% of the children do not survive this condition and die mostly within 1 day from the fatal consequences of prolonged hypoxemia [26].

Diagnosis. The first step in diagnosis is to effectively rule out cardiogenic, respiratory, hematogenic, or central nervous causes of the cyanosis. The chest X-ray in the typical primary PFC syndrome shows a normal heart size and configuration as well as some decrease in pulmonary vascularity. There is no clouding or opacification of the lung fields. The ECG usually shows no specific changes in the simple form of PFC. Late systolic heart murmurs from a transitory tricuspidal or mitral valve insufficiency can frequently be demonstrated by phonocardiography [14, 31]. Echocardiography in simple PFC shows impairment of the right ventricular performance. In the complex form there is left ventricular impairment as well [26, 23]. Polycythemia can be ruled out by determination of the hematocrit or hemoglobin and methemoglobinemia by determination of the Met-Hb level. The majority of cases show an increase of right-to-left shunt in the differential hyperoxia test (see p 132) during 100% O_2 respiration. Arterial blood from the lower regions of the body supplied by the descending (postductal) aorta (e. g., the left femoral artery) shows no increase in PaO_2, because this blood is shunted past the lung through the patent ductus arteriosus. On the other hand, the PaO_2 values from regions supplied by the ascending (preductal) aorta (e. g., the right brachial artery) increase markedly during 100% O_2 respiration in primary PFC [14]. Simultaneous transcutaneous oxygen measurements ($tcPO_2$) have proved to be sufficiently reliable and offer a means of continuous PaO_2 monitoring [2, 4].

Management. If cyanotic congenital heart disease cannot be ruled out with suffcient certainty, cardiac catheterization with angiocardiography is indicated. Aortography is also necessary in some cases, because right ventricular angiocardiograms may give the erroneous impression of an interrupted aortic arch or a preductal coarctation of the aorta [31]. If the presence of congenital heart disease is unlikely and there is no adequate basis for a respiratory, hematologic or neurologic cause of the central syanosis, a single test injection of tolazoline in an attempt to decrease the pulmonary vascular resistance should be considered. Tolazoline is a vasodilating agent of the α-

receptor blocking type, which dilates not only the pulmonary vessels, but also the arteries of the systemic circulation [9]. Contraindications for the tolazoline test are PaO_2 values over 60 mm Hg in the hyperoxia test, congestive heart failure, or concurrent treatment with sympathomimetics [22, 9]. Arterial blood pressures below 60 mm Hg systolic in the mature term infant are another contraindication for tolazoline administration. In such cases the peripheral vasodilatation caused by tolazoline can cause serious arterial hypotension [14, 22]. Initially a single test dose of 1 mg/kg tolazoline is injected undiluted intravenously within a 30–s period [14]. An increase in the postductal arterial blood PaO_2 by more than 15 mm Hg is interpreted as a positive response [9]. If the improvement is not lasting, tolazoline can be administered by continuous infusion in a dosage of 1–2 mg/kg/min.

The infusion should be gradually decreased if the oxygen concentration of the inspired air can be reduced to 60% and the inspiratory pressure to 30 cm H_2O [9]. Continuous tolazoline infusion is usually necessary for only a few hours, but may be necessary and proven effective for up to several days [9]. During the infusion the arterial blood gases and arterial blood pressure have to be checked at regular intervals. A fall of blood pressure should be treated by volume replacement, e. g., human albumin, but not with sympathomimetics [14]. Other possible complications requiring withdrawal of tolazoline are oliguria from a transitory impairment of renal function and gastrointestinal bleeding due to the histamine – like action of tolazoline [9]. A mortality rate of 10% is reported for tolazoline therapy in the PFC syndrome [14, 22]. The prognosis of the complex form with myocardial involvement is poorer still and depends largely on the underlying disease [26].

The treatment of persistent fetal circulation with tolazoline represents an unconventional therapy which is not yet generally accepted. It should therefore be used only in pediatric cardiology centers and with the informed consent of the parents. Different legal regulations in different countries have to be regarded.

10.3.5 Pneumopericardium

Pathophysiology. Pneumopericardium occurs when air enters the pericardial sac, usually from the mediastinum. Spontaneous pneumopericardium is a rare disease. In the overwhelming majority of cases this life-threatening condition occurs as a complication of ventilation with IPPV or PEEP. As a rule, interstitial pulmonary emphysema, pneumomediastinum or pneumothorax are simultaneously observed [3]. The invasion of air into the pericardial sac leads to cardiac compression, especially in the region of the atria and the large veins, and thus causes upper inflow obstruction. If the intrapericardial pressure increases further, cardiac tamponade may result.

Diagnosis. The clinical picture of cardiac tamponade is marked by acute onset of cyanosis, an extensive drop in blood pressure, and bradycardia. The heart sounds are faint, and a low-voltage ECG is obtained. The X-ray shows microcardia, and a pericardial air gap can be demonstrated in typical cases (Fig. 27). The small heart is usually encircled by a more or less broad, sharply defined area of lucency. In about

30%, however, the pneumopericardium was not diagnosed clinically until postmortem examination [21].

Management. The prognosis is poor; there is a mortality rate of about 75% [21]. If no cardiac tamponade is present, a reduction of inspiratory pressure and PEEP is recommended during ventilation [35].

In microcardia with shock symptoms, immediate pericardial puncture and catheter drainage is the only life-saving approach (for technique see p 242). Recurrent tamponade has occurred in about 50% of cases in which the drainage was withdrawn too soon [21]. The catheter should therefore be left in place as long as positive pressure ventilation is continued.

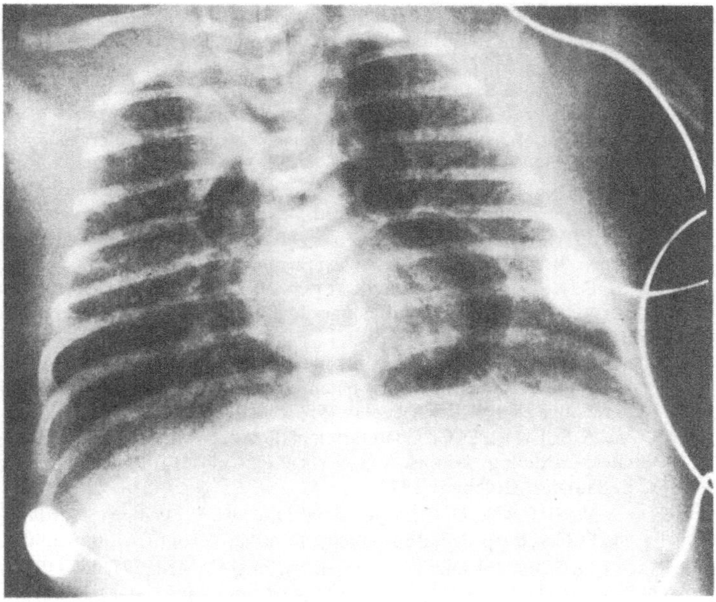

Fig. 27. Pneumopericardium in a newborn infant. The broad intrapericardial air gap, which leads to microcardia by compression, is clearly visible. Pneumomediastinum is also present. The condition was successfully treated by transthoracic catheter drainage (S. N., ♀, 3rd day of life, RDS III-IV, PEEP ventilation)

References

1. Billig, D. M., Kreidberg, M. B.: The Management of Neonates and Infants with Congenital Heart Disease. New York. London: Grune & Stratton 1973
2. Boyle, R. J., Oh, W.: Transcutaneous pO_2 monitoring in infants with persistent fetal circulation who are receiving tolazoline therapy. Pediatrics *62*, 605 (1978)

3. Brans, Y. W., Pitts, M., Cassady, G.: Neonatal Pneumopericardium. Am. J. Dis. Child. *130*, 393 (1976)
4. Bucher, H. U., Arbenz, U., Bucher, A.: $tcPO_2$ in Pediatric Cardiology: Application During Ballon Septostomy, Tolazoline Administration, and in Children With Right-to-Left Shunt Birth Defects *15*, 355 (1979)
5. Friedmann, W. F., Hirschklau, M. J., Printz, M. P., Pitlick, P. T., Kirkpatrick, St. E.: Pharmacologic Closure of Patent Ductus Arteriosus in the Premature Infant. N. Engl. J. Med. *295*, 526 (1976)
6. Fyler, D. C., Rosenthal, A.: Neonatal Heart Disease in: Neonatalogy, Pathophysiology and Management of the Newborn, p. 295. Philadelphia-Toronto: J. B. Lippincott Company 1976
7. Gelband, H., and Rosen, M. R.: Pharmacologic Basis for the Treatment of Cardiac Arrhythmias Pediatrics *55*, 59 (1975)
8. Godman, M. J., Tham, P., Kidd, B. S. C.: Echocardiography in the evaluation of the cyanotic newborn infant. Brit. Heart J. *36*, 154 (1974)
9. Goetzmann, B. W., Sunshine, P., Johnson, J. D., Wennberg, R. P., Hakkel, A., Merten, D. F., Bartoletti, A. L., and Silverman, N. H.: Neonatal hypoxia and pulmonary vasospasm: Response to tolaziline. J. Pediatr. *89*, 617 (1977)
10. Hallmann, G. L., Cooley, D. A.: Surgical Treatment of Congenital Heart Disease. Philadelphia: Lea & Febiger 1975
11. Hirschfeld, S., Meyer, R., Schwartz, D. C., Korfhagen, J., and Kaplan, S.: Measurement of Right and Left Ventricular Systolic Time Intervals by Echocardiography Circulation 51, 304 (1975)
12. Hoffman, S. I. E., Christianson, R.: Congenital heart disease in a cohort of 19, 502 births with long term follow up. Am. J. Cardiol. *42*, 941 (1978)
13. Keck, E. W.: Pädiatrische Kardiologie, Herzkrankheiten im Säuglings- und Kindesalter. München, Berlin, Wien: Urban Schwarzenberg 1972
14. Levin, D. L., Heymann, M. A., Kittermann, J. A., Gregory, G. A., Phibbs, R. H., and Rudolph, A. M.: Persistant pulmonary hypertension of the newborn infants. J. Pediatr. *89*, 626 (1976)
15. Merritt, T. A., Disessa, T. G., Feldman, B. H., Kirckpatrick, St. E., Gluck, L., and Friedmann, W. F.: Closure of the patent ductus arteriosus with ligation and indomethacin: A consecutive experience. J. Pediatr. *93*, 639 (1978)
16. Nadas, A. S., Fyler, D. C.: Coarctation of the Aorta with Congestive Failure in Infancy. In: Pediatric Cardiology Nadas, A. S., Fyler, D. C., p. 461. Philadelphia, London, Toronto: W. B. Saunders Company 1972
17. Nadas, A. S., Fyler, D. C.: Myocardial Diseases. In: Pediatric Cardiology Nadas, A. S., Fyler, D. C. (Ed.). p. 217. Philadelphia, London, Toronto: W. B. Saunders Company 1972
18. Nadas, A. S.: Patent Ductus Revisited. N. Engl. J. Med. *295*, 563 (1976)
19. Paul, M. H.: D-Transposition of the Great Arteries. In: Heart Disease in Infants; Children and Adolescents Moss, A. J., Adams, F. H., Emmanonilides, G. C. (eds.) The Williams & Wilkins Co., Baltimore 1978, p. 301
20. Rashkind, W. G., Miller, W. W.: Creation of an Atrial Septal Defect without Thoracotomy. JAMA *196*, 991 (1966)
21. Reppert, S. M., Ment, L. R., Todres, I. D.: The treatment of pneumopericardium in the newborn infant. J. Pediatr. *90*, 115 (1977)
22. Riemenschneider, Th. A., Nielson, H. C., Ruttenberg, H. D., Jaffe, R. B.: Disturbances of the transitional circulation: Spectrum of pulmonary hypertension and myocardial dysfunction. J. Pediatr. *89*, 622 (1977)
23. Riggs, T., Hirschfeld, S., Fanaroff, A., Liebmann, J., Fletcher, B., and Meyer, R., with the technical assistance of C. Bormuth: Persistance of fetal circulation syndrome: An echocardiographic study. J. Pediatr. *91*, 626 (1977)
24. Rittenhouse, E. A., Doty, D. B., Lauer, R. M., Ehrenhaft, J. L.: Patent ductus arteriosus in premature infants, indications for surgery. J. Thorac. Cardiovasc. Surg. *71*, 187 (1976)

25. Rowe, R. D., Mehrizi, A.: Endocardial Fibroelastosis, In: The Neonate with Congenital Heart Disease. p. 260. Philadelphia, London, Toronto: W. B. Saunders Company 1968
26. Rowe, R.: Abnormal pulmonary vasoconstriction in the newborn. Pediatrics *59*, 318 (1977)
27. Rudolph, A. M.: The Ductus Arteriosus and Persistent Patency of the Ductus Arteriosus. In: Congenital Diseases of the Heart. p. 168. Chicago: Year Book Medical Publishers 1974
28. S. 233 in 17
29. Schöber, J. G., Mocellin, R., Bühlmeyer, K.: Persistierender fetaler Kreislauf bei reifen Neugeborenen. Monatschr. Kinderheilkd. *124*, 430 (1976)
30. Silverman, N. H., Lewis, A. B., Heymann, M. A., Rudolph, A. M.: Echocardiographic Assessment of Ductus Arteriosus Shunt in Premature Infants. Circulation *50*, 821 (1974)
31. Silverstein, E. F., Ellis, K., Casarella, W. J., Steeg, C. N., and Gersony, W. N.: Persistance of the fetal circulation: Radiologic considerations. Am. J. of Roentgenol. *128*, 781 (1977)
32. Sinha, S. N., Rusnak, S. L., Sommers, H. M., Coll, R. B., Muster, A. J., Paul, M. H.: Hypoplastic left ventricle syndrome: Analysis of thirty autopsy cases in infants with surgical considerations. Am. J. Cardiol. *21*, 166 (1968)
33. Stanger, P., Heymann, M. A., Tarnoff, H., Hoffmann, J. I. E., Rudolph, A. M.: Complications of Cardiac Catheterization of Neonates, Infants, and Children. A three year study. Circulation *50*, 595 (1974)
34. Stark, J., Hucin, B., Aberdien, E., Waterston, D. J.: Cardiac surgery in the first year of life: Experience with 1.049 operations. Surgery *69*, 483 (1971)
35. Wille, L., Oppermann, H. C.: Das idiopathische Atemnotsyndrom: Pulmonale Veränderungen und Komplikationen unter Respiratortherapie bei Frühgeborenen. Röntgen-Bl. *29*, 278 (1976)
36. Wolf, D.: Vorhofflattern, Vorhofflimmern. In: Pharmakotherapie im Kindesalter. Schweier, P. und Wolf, H. G. (Ed.) S. 580. München: Hans Marseille Verlag, 1975

11 Neurologic Diseases

L. Wille

11.1 Postasphyxia Syndrome

This consists of pulmonary, cardiovascular, metabolic, and/or cerebral complications following perinatal asphyxia. Evaluation, observation of clinical course, and treatment are required. Certain neurologic symptoms are of long-term prognostic significance in these neonates [7, 13, 20, 32].

Pulmonary Complications
Transitory tachypnea
Respiratory distress syndrome
Aspiration syndrome.

Cardiovascular Complications
Persistent fetal circulation [21]
Bradycardia
Transient cardiomegaly/cardiac failure [21]
Pallor (peripheral hypoperfusion)
Systolic or continuous murmur (tricuspidal insufficiency).

Metabolic Complications
Metabolic acidosis
Hypoglycemia
Hypocalcemia
Hyperbilirubinemia
Disturbance of thermoregulation
Increased oxygen consumption
Increased ADH production.

Cerebral Complications
Apathy/hyperexcitability
Irregular breathing/apnea
Wide fluctuations of body temperature
Difficulties in swallowing (poor feeding)
Abnormalities of eye movement

Facial grimacing/fixed gaze
Poor crying
Symptoms of increased intracranial pressure (tense fontanel, mydriasis, nonreactive pupils)
Convulsions/cyanotic spells
Disturbances of primitive reflexes
Pathologic reflexes
Neurovegetative symptoms.

Renal Complications
Acute tubular necrosis
Acute medullary necrosis
Acute renal failure.

Diagnosis
Chest X-ray
ECG, PCG
Blood gas analysis
EEG
Lumbar puncture/computerized tomography (as required)
Coagulation analysis, blood glucose, calcium, bilirubin.

Therapy
- Incubator care, monitoring
- Maintenance of neutral thermal environment
- Early feeding and/or parenteral infusion
- Correction of metabolic disturbances (acidosis, hypoglycemia, hypocalcemia)
- F_IO_2 corresponding to PaO_2
  Meconium aspiration; see p 115
  Respiratory distress syndrome; see p 111
- Cardiomegaly/heart failure: digitalization (see p 137)
- Persistence of fetal circulation: mechanical ventilation if necessary; attempt to lower pulmonary hypertension (see p 142)
- Patent ductus arteriosus: pharmacologic or surgical closure of the ductus as required (see p 140) [11, 16].
- Cerebral symptoms (brain edema, convulsions): brain edema therapy:
  dexamethasone, 1 mg/kg body wt./day in four doses. Fluid restriction (60 ml/kg/day).
  mannitol, 20%, 2 ml/kg/6 h combined with furosemide 1 mg/kg.
- Anticonvulsive therapy (see p 152)
- For treatment of acute renal failure, see p 163.

Neurologic symptoms which are highly unfavorable prognostically [2, 32] are:
Initial apnea > 10 min
Nonreactive pupils
Absence or disappearance of all primitive reflexes
Asymmetrical neurologic findings and asymmetrical transillumination
Asymmetrical neurologic findings and feeding difficulties
Asymmetrical neurologic findings and apneic spells
Apathy with subsequent hyperexcitability and hypertonia of extensors

11.2 Neonatal Seizures

Incidence. 0.2–0.8%. Convulsions during the first 3 days of life and after the 8th day of life are usually the result of cerebral damage. Convulsions between the 5th and 8th day of life are often caused by metabolic disturbances [5]. Seizures are the expression of a central nervous disorder which can have local or general causes. Convulsions can lead to irreversible cerebral injury. The prognosis depends on recognition of etiology and prompt treatment!

Clinical Features. Range from intermittent focal, multifocal, or generalized muscular twitching with no significant impairment of consciousness to unilateral or generalized grand mal seizures with eye deviation and coma.
The classic, tonic-clonic, generalized grand mal seizure is rare. Tonic seizures are common, characterized by extension of the limbs, or by flexion of the upper limbs and extension of the lower limbs. Also common are transient hypotonia, clonic movements of individual limbs, rolling of the eyes, irregular breathing, apneic spells, tremor, twitching of the eyebrows, nystagmus, smacking movements, and cyanotic episodes [14].

Etiology. Occasionally the history (course of pregnancy, mode of and nature of the delivery) or clinical picture (sepsis, meningitis) makes the etiology clear (Table 47).

Diagnosis

1. Mandatory tests:
   Blood glucose
   Calcium
   Magnesium
   Phosphorus
   Blood count with thrombocytes
   Prothrombin time (Quick test)
   Blood gas analysis
   ECG (prolonged Q-T interval).

Table 47. Causes of neonatal seizures [4, 8]

I. Metabolic
1. Hypoglycemia
2. Hypocalcemia
3. Hypomagnesemia
4. Pyridoxine (B_6)
   a) Dependency
   b) Deficiency
5. Hypo- (<130 mEq/l) and hypernatremia (>150 mEq/l)
6. Aminoacidemia (see p 174)
7. Bilirubin
   a) Kernicterus
8. Drug withdrawal
   a) Heroin
   b) Barbiturates
   c) Alcohol
9. Polycythemia

II. Infection
1. Sepsis
2. Meningitis
3. Encephalitis

III. Hemorrhage
1. Trauma
   a) Subarachnoid
   b) Subdural
   c) periventricular, intracerebral
2. Maternal anticonvulsive therapy

IV. Thrombosis

V. Hypoxia (perinatal complications)
1. Without secondary cerebral hemorrhage
2. With periventricular hemorrhage
3. With periventricular and intraventricular hemorrhage

VI. Developmental anomalies
1. Cerebral dysgeneses
2. Incontinentia pigmenti
3. Degenerative cerebral disorders

2. The following tests may be done, depending on the clinical situation and other findings:
   a) Blood culture, lumbar puncture (exclusion of meningitis; if cerebral hemorrhage is presumed, delay puncture until 7th day of life), funduscopy
   b) Suspected cerebral cause: cranial X-ray (fracture), echoencephalogram (dysgenesis, hematoma, hygroma), transillumination, EEG, computerized axial tomography
   c) Dehydration/edema: sodium, chlorine, potassium
   d) Suspected metabolic diseases, see p 174.

Therapy. Frequent or continuous seizures require immediate treatment, because they can result in brain injury! [28]

1. General measures:
   - Manage in incubator
   - Maintain patent airways by placing head on side (vomiting!)
   - Cardiac and respiratory monitoring
   - Persistent apneic spells: mask ventilation; intubation and controlled ventilation if required.
2. Before receipt of biochemical analyses
   Treat according to the principal etiologies, with frequent periods of observation:
   a) 20% glucose, 2 ml/kg IV
   b) 10% calcium gluconate, 1–2 ml/kg slowly IV
   c) 40% magnesium sulfate, 0.1 ml/kg IM
   d) Pyridoxine (benadon), 50 mg/dose IV, under EEG control if possible.
   e) Cerebral hemorrhage: Fresh frozen plasma at 8–h intervals, 10 ml/kg IV; transfusion with packed red cells if necessary.
3. Symptomatic therapy
   Persistent seizures
   a) Clonazepam 0.1 mg/kg/dose slowly IV, repeat hourly as needed.
   b) Uncontrollable seizures:
   Phenobarbital initial dose 15 mg/kg/day, maintenance dose 3–4 mg/kg/day; Chloral hydrate, 30 mg/kg/day (clysma) as needed.
4. Specific treatment
   In accordance with biochemical analyses.

11.3 Recurrent Apneic Spells

Definitions

1. Periodic breathing
   Breathing for 10–15 s at a rate of 50–60 BPM. The breathing becomes increasingly shallow and terminates in a brief apnea of 5–10 s duration with no change in heart rate or skin color.
2. Apneic spells
   Respiratory arest > 20 s

Types of Apnea

1. Apnea after hypoventilation
2. Apnea after hyperventilation or hyperactivity
3. Apnea with manifest CNS symptoms [3].

Predisposition

Hypoxia	Hypoglycemia	Increased intracranial pressure
Acidosis	Hyperglycemia	Convulsions
Hypothermia	Electrolyte disturbances	Respiratory failure
Extreme immaturity	Dehydration	
Malnutrition	Hyperbilirubinemia	
Anemia	Cerebral hemorrhage	
Sepsis/meningitis		

Incidence. Twenty-five to 50% of all extremely premature infants (<30 weeks gestation). Occurs between 3rd day and 4th week of life. May persist for several weeks.

Clinical Features. Respiratory arrest accompanied by bradycardia, hypoxia, acidosis, flaccidity, apathy, and hypertension which appear immediately or within 5–30 s after the pause in breathing.

Etiology. Uncomplicated apneic spells are an expression of neuronal immaturity. They tend to occur in the preterm infant during REM sleep and are caused by the inhibition of sensory input (afferents) and motor output (efferents) of the central nervous system [9, 13, 22].

Therapy

1. General measures
   Avoid unnecessary handling
   Manage in incubator
   Maintain neutral thermal environment
   Correct metabolic disturbances
   Correct acidosis
   Screen for infection
   Treat for anemia.

If apnea recurs on feeding, change to nasojejunal tube or parenteral nutrition.

2. Tactile and proprioceptive stimuli: Strike gently, use water mattress.
3. Increase F_IO_2 to 0.25–0.30: Apneic spells can sometimes be prevented or reduced in this way. PaO_2 is best monitored by continuous recording with a transcutaneous electrode.
4. Pharmacologic therapy. [1, 2, 10, 23, 27]:

   Theophylline
   Initial dose: 6 mg/kg orally
   Maintenance dose: 2 mg/kg orally every 12 h.

   The therapeutic plasma level is between 6 and 13 μg/ml. Xanthine therapy leads to an improvement of the oxygen cardiorespirogram [17]. Side effects: Tachycardia >180/min, diuresis, hyperglycemia, glucosuria and blood pressure fluctuations [15]. If the infant does not respond, convulsive apnea is excluded (EEG).
5. Mask ventilation: First with ambient air (F_IO_2 0.21), then with increased oxygen concentration of circumstances warrant (beware of retrolental fibroplasia!).

6. Nasal CPAP [18, 24].
   Mode of action: Probably stimulation via inflation reflex and prestretching of intercostal muscles (increased impulse rate of muscle spindle afferents). Give CPAP of 2–3 cm H_2O by nasal prongs.
7. Ventilate for recurrent apneic spells of long duration.

Evaluation. Impedance pneumography, plethysmography combined with oxygen-cardiorespirography for optimal monitoring of the severity of apneic spells, fall of heart rate, duration of bradycardia and depth of hypoxemia [18]. The apnea mattress is an acceptable but less recommended alternative.

11.4 Intracranial Hemorrhage [29]

11.4.1 Subdural Hemorrhage

Causes

a) Tentorial laceration with rupture of the sagittal sinus, vein of Galen, or lateral sinus
b) Falx laceration with rupture of the inferior sagittal sinus
c) Rupture of superficial cerebral veins (cerebral convexity).

Etiology. Almost exclusively traumatic.

Clinical Features. Massive hemorrhage results in symptoms characterized by stupor or coma, asymmetrical eye deviation, unequal pupils (may indicate affected side), tachypnea, nuchal rigidity, retrocollis, opisthotonos. The final stage is marked by fixed, dilated pupils followed by respiratory arrest. Surviving infants may be left with hydrocephalus from obstruction to flow of cerebrospinal fluid.
Hemorrhage over the hemispheres may show no clinical signs, or convulsions with focal symptoms. Subdural hemorrhage may develop into a chronic subdural hygroma.

Diagnosis. Echoencephalography, electroencephalography, computerized axial tomography. Lumbar puncture: Fluid is usually colorless. In laceration of the arachnoid the fluid is burgundy red, later becoming xanthochromic with an elevated protein content. The bilirubin formed may diffuse through the arachnoid and also lead to xanthochromia. If subdural hygroma is suspected: Transillumination, fontanel puncture, computerized axial tomography, possibly carotid angiography.

Therapy. In chronic subdural hygroma, rapid drainage of the effusion:

a) Repeated fontanel punctures
b) Surgical inspection: If the hygroma has not been drained in 2–3 weeks, continuous drainage for several days through subdural drains is necessary. In some cases the hygroma must be surgically exposed and cleared [30].

11.4.2 Primary Subarachnoid Hemorrhage

Generally the hemorrhage covers the hemispheres or it may be localized.

Cause. Trauma or hypoxia.
Small hemorrhages produce no clinical symptoms and have a good prognosis. Even extensive hemorrhages may be clinically silent.

Symptoms. The main symptoms are convulsions, which usually have their onset on the 2nd day of life. These infants often appear well between seizures. The prognosis in such cases is good. In massive subarachnoid hemorrhage the course is rapid and fatal. Neurologic residua are rare in survivors. The most frequent sequela is hydrocephalus caused by the impaired flow of cerebrospinal fluid.

Therapy. No effective intervention is possible; hydrocephalus is treated later if necessary.

11.4.3 Periventricular Intracerebral (Intraventricular) Hemorrhage

Etiology. Unclear; hypoxia [25], hyperosmolarity and hypernatremia [12, 16, 31], and disorders of the perinatal circulation with an increase in cerebral capillary and venous pressure [6, 30] have been postulated.

Clinical Features. Intraventricular hemorrhage is seen in preterm infants. The onset of symptoms depends on the timing of the insult causing the hemorrhage. Symptoms usually appear 24–48 h after birth: Severe respiratory difficulties, bulging fontanel, falling hematocrit, unequal pupils, flaccid quadriparesis, tonic extension of the limbs, coma, and terminal apnea. Occasionally the symptoms take several days to appear: sudden stupor, pallor, and fall of hematocrit.
In many infants the deterioration is saltatory with intermittent periods of stabilization followed by further deterioration.

Therapy. The outcome depends mostly on the extent of the hemorrhage. Survivors are treated for hydrocephalus.

References

1. Aranda, J. V., Sitar, D. S., Parsons, W. D., Loughnan, P. M., Neims, A. H.: Pharmacokinetic aspects of theophylline in premature newborns. N. Eng. J. Med. *295*, 413 (1976)
2. Bednarek, F. J., Roloff, D. W.: Treatment of apnea of prematurity with aminophylline. Pediatrics *58*, 335 (1976)
3. Belgaumkar, T. K., Scott, K. E.: Apnea in premature infants: Recording by arterial catheter. Eur. J. Pediatr. *123*, 301 (1976) .
4. Brown, J. K.: Convulsions in the newborn period. Dev. Med. Child. Neurol. *15*, 823 (1973)
5. Brown, J. K., Cockburn, F., Forfar, J. O.: Clinical and chemical correlates in convulsions of the newborn. Lancet *1*, 135 (1972)

6. Cole, V. A., Durbin, G. M., Olafson, A., Reynolds, E. O. R., Rivers, R. P. A., Smith, J. F.: Pathogenesis of intraventricular haemorrhage in newborn infants. Arch. Dis. Child. *49*, 722 (1974)
7. DeSouza, S. W., Richards, B.: Neurological sequelae in newborn babies after perinatal asphyxia. Arch. Dis. Child. *53*, 564 (1978)
8. Freeman, J. M.: Neonatal seizures – diagnosis and management. J. Pediatr. *77*, 701 (1970)
9. Gabriel, M.: Zur Apnoe-Genese gesunder Neugeborener. Monatsschr. Kinderheilk. *125*, 181 (1977)
10. Giacoia, G., Jusko, W. J., Menke, J., Koup, J. R.: Theophylline pharmacokinetics in premature infants with apnea. J. Pediatr. *89*, 829 (1976)
11. Goetzman, B. W., Sunshine, P., Johnson, J. D., Wennberg, R. P., Hackel, A., Merten, D. F., Bartoletti, A. L., Silverman, N. H.: Neonatal hypoxia and pulmonary vasospasm: Response to tolazoline. J. Pedriatr. *89*, 617 (1976)
12. Hambleton, G., Wiggelsworth, J. S.: Origin of intraventricular haemorrhage in the preterm infant. Arch. Dis. Child. *51*, 651 (1976)
13. Kattwinkel, J., Nearman, H. S., Fanaroff, A. A., Katona, P. G., Klaus, M. H.: Apnea of prematurity. J. Pediatr. *86*, 588 (1975)
14. Kruse, R.: Epilepsien des Kindesalters. In: Neuropädiatrie Matthes, A., Kruse, R. (ed.) S. 353. Stuttgart: Thieme 1973
15. Larcher, V. F., Gamsu, H. R., Sanderson, M. C., Drayton, M., Sandhu, B.: Theophylline toxicity in a neonate. Arch. Dis. Child. *53*, 757 (1978)
16. Levin, D. L., Heymann, M. A., Kitterman, J. A., Gregory, G. A., Phibbs, R. H., Rudolph, A. M.: Persistent pulmonary hypertension of the newborn infant. J. Pedriatr. *89*, 626 (1976)
17. Peabody, J. L., Neese, A. L., Philip, A. G. S., Lucey, J. F., Soyka, L. F.: Transcutaneous Oxygen monitoring in aminophylline-treated apnoic infants. Pediatrics *62*, 698 (1978)
18. Pörksen, Chr., Ehlers, H., Bensan, I., Hürter, P.: CPAP als Therapie bei Apnoeanfällen Frühgeborener. Mschr. Kinderheilk. *124*, 432 (1976)
19. Prod'hom, L. S.: Die Erkrankungen des Fetus und des Neugeborenen. In: Lehrbuch der Pädiatrie. Fanconi, G., Wallgren, A. (Ed.). S. 281. Basel-Stuttgart: Schwabe 1972
20. Prod'hom, L. S.: Prognose von intensiv behandelten Neugeborenen. Pädiatr. FortbildK. *41*, 347 (1975)
21. Riemenschneider, Th. A., Nielsen, H. C., Ruttenberg, H. D., Jaffe, R. B.: Disturbances of the transitional circulation: Spectrum of pulmonary hypertension and myocardial dysfunction. J. Pediatr. *89*, 622 (1976)
22. Schulte, F. J.: Apnea. Clin. Perinatol. *4* (1), 65 (1977)
23. Shannon, D. C., Gotay, F., Stein, I. M., Rogers, M. C., Todres, I. D., Moylan, F. M. B.: Prevention of apnea and bradycardia in low-birth-weight infants. Pediatrics *55*, 589 (1975)
24. Speidel, B. D., Dunn, P. M.: Effect of continuous positive air-way-pressure on breathing pattern of infants with respiratory-distress syndrome. Lancet *1*, 302 (1975)
25. Thomas, D. B.: Hyperosmolality and intraventricular haemorrhage in premature babies. Acta Paediatr. Scand. *65*, 429 (1976)
26. Turbeville, D. F., Bowen, F. W., Killam, A. P.: Intracranial hemorrhages in kittens: Hypernatremia versus hypoxia. J. Pediatr. *89*, 294 (1976)
27. Uauy, R., Shapiro, D. L., Smith, B., Warshaw, J. B.: Treatment of severe apnea in prematures with orally administered theophylline. Pediatrics *55*, 595 (1975)
28. Volpe, J. J.: Neonatal seizures. Clin. Perinatol. *4* (1), 43 (1977)
29. Volpe, J. J.: Neonatal intracranial hemorrhage. Clin. Perinatol. *4* (1), 77 (1977)
30. Weinmann, H. M.: Subdurales Hämatom in: Neuropädiatrie. Matthes, A., Kruse, R., (ed.) p. 291. Stuttgart: Thieme 1973
31. Wigglesworth, J. S., Keith, I. H., Girling, D. J., Slade, S. A.: Hyaline membrane disease, alkali, and intraventricular haemorrhage. Arch. Dis. Child. *51*, 755 (1976)
32. Ziegler, A. L., Calame, A., Marchand, C., Passera, M., Reympod-Goni, Prod'hom, L. S.: Cerebral distress in full-term newborns and its prognostic value. A follow-up study of 90 infants. Helvetica Paediatr. Acta *31*, 299 (1976)

12 Acute Abdominal Diseases

L. Wille

12.1 Acute Gastrointestinal Diseases

Most acute gastrointestinal diseases requiring urgent surgical intervention can be identified preoperatively by following a systematic procedure [2, 9, 11, 15, 23]:

Family History. Familial diseases (e.g., cystic fibrosis, Hirschsprung's disease), hydramnios.

Patient History

Main symptoms:
1. Vomiting
2. Abdominal distention
3. Failure to pass meconium

The appearance of the symptoms and the sequence of their onset provide a clue as to the level of the stenosis or atresia. Watch for initial passage of meconium, feeding behavior, and passage of stool.

Clinical Features

1. Vomiting (bile-stained) without abdominal distention (high intestinal obstruction).
2. Vomiting with general abdominal distension indicates low intestinal obstruction).

Also Watch for. Tense, shiny abdominal skin, engorged veins, muscular defense, ascites, resistances.

Diagnosis (Tables 48–50)
Abdominal transillumination
Abdominal radiographs (upright)
Sonography
Urography with lower cavography (or tomography)
Cystourethrography
Barium enema/gastrointestinal passage
Genitography
Cholegraphy
Scintigraphy
Aortography (transumbilical)
Computerized tomography.

The extent to which, and sequence in which, these diagnostic procedures are performed depend upon the individual case.
Essential for the optimal care of the newborn are modern, efficient diagnostic facilities and close cooperation with a pediatric surgical department.

Table 48. Differential diagnosis of abdominal diseases with acute respiratory symptoms (23)

Esophageal atresia
Isolated tracheoesophageal fistula
Diaphragmatic hernia (congenital)
Diaphragmatic paralysis
Secondary respiratory difficulties due to aspiration or thoracic displacement (ileus, abdominal mass)

Table 49. Differential diagnosis of ileus (modified from [23])

Peritonitis
Duodenal obstruction (extrinsic, intrinsic)
Small bowel atresia or stenosis
Necrotizing enterocolitis
Meconium ileus
Mesenteric cysts, congenital adhesions
Colonic atresia or stenosis
Anorectal agenesis
Hirschsprung's disease
Meconium plug syndrome
Functional intestinal obstruction
Internal hernia
Small left colon syndrome

Differential Diagnosis

The differential diagnosis is based on the classic symptoms: recurrent vomiting, abdominal distension, abdominal mass, failure to pass meconium or stools, sometimes combined with respiratory difficulties (Tables 48–51).

Table 50. Differential diagnosis of duodenal obstruction and peritonitis [23]

Duodenal obstruction	
Duodenal atresia, stenosis (membranous form, etc.)	
Annular pancreas	
Volvulus (various forms of malrotation)	
Congenital adhesions, preduodenal portal vein	
Peritonitis	
Fetal (aseptic)	Meconium peritonitis Urinary ascites Bile ascites
Postnatal (septic)	With intestinal perforation (with or without discernible cause) Without intestinal perforation (omphalitis, vascular, enteral)

Table 51. Differential diagnosis of abdominal masses [2, 15]

Extraperitoneal masses
Hydronephrosis, hydroureter, full bladder
Infantile cystic kidney
Renal vein thrombosis
Neoplasms (Wilms' tumor, neuroblastoma, teratoma)
Hydrometrocolpos
Ovarian cyst, tumor
Anterior meningocele
Intraperitoneal masses
Neoplasms (hemangioma, lymphangioma, hepatoblastoma)
Subcapsular hepatic hematoma
Malformations (duplicature)
Hepatosplenomegaly
Meconium ileus
Meconium pseudocyst
Mesenteral cyst
Choledochal cyst
Splenic tumor

Table 52. Acute abdominal diseases [7, 16, 17, 20]

Disease	Clinical symptoms
Esophageal atresia	Maternal hydramnios; regurgitation immediately postpartum, frothy salivation, paroxysmal or permanent respiratory distress, acute deterioration during feeding
Isolated tracheoesophageal fistula	Cough, respiratory distress on feeding, recurrent atelectasis and aspiration pneumonia, abdominal distension
Diaphragmatic hernia (congenital)	Life-threatening respiratory distress may occur immediately postpartum, symptoms of shock/ileus. Faint breath or bowel sounds over affected hemithorax. Shift of cardiac dullness and apex beat, "paradoxical" respiration when viewed from side, scaphoid abdomen
High intestinal obstruction: extrinsic duodenal stenosis, intrinsic duodenal atresia, annular pancreas, malrotation, jejunal atresia, multiple atresias	1st–2nd day of life: (bilestained) vomiting, upper abdominal distension; possibly intermittent symptoms and peristaltic waves, melena
Low intestinal obstruction: ileal atresia, meconium ileus, Hirschsprung's disease, colonic atresia, microcolon, meconium plug syndrome, anorectal atresia	2nd–4th day of life: meconium-stained vomitus, general distension, at times visible peristalsis, failure to pass meconium
Gastrointestinal perforation (peritonitis): meconium ileus, sepsis, exchange transfusion, Hirschsprung's disease, malrotation with volvulus	1st week of life: Refusal of feeds, vomiting, abdominal distension, possibly with dyspnea, cyanosis and shock
Necrotizing enterocolitis	1st week of life: vomiting, fever, bloody dyspeptic stools, abdominal distension; later shock with sepsis and peritonitis

Radiographic diagnosis	Preoperative therapy
Chest and abdominal films; level of blind pouch is demonstrated with radiopaque catheter	Prompt recognition is vital! Pass suction catheter into blind upper pouch, transport with upper body raised (20°), immediate operation
Filling of esophagus (balloon catheter), demonstration of fistula in semilateral and prone position	Physical and antibiotic therapy until operation. Nasojejunal tube feeding is possible
Abdominal film, lateral and AP chest films. If in doubt, administer contrast medium	Administer oxygen, decompress the stomach with a nasogastric tube to continuous drainage. Immediate operation
Upright abdominal film. Air insufflation and/or contrast examination of gastrointestinal tract if necessary	Gastric evaluation, nasogastric decompression, intermittent suctioning, fluid and electrolyte replacement, total parenteral nutrition, consultation with pediatric surgeon
Upright abdominal film (e. g., Wangensteen film), retrograde contrast examination of colon if necessary	Fluid and electrolyte replacement, abdominal decompression by nasogastric drainage, consultation with pediatric surgeon
Upright and/or lateral supine abdominal film	Adequate oxygenation, shock therapy, correction of electrolyte and acid-base derangements. Nasogastric drainage. Immediate operation!
Upright abdominal film	Gastric drainage, antibiotic therapy, electrolyte and fluid replacement. Operate if perforation is present or clinical deterioration

12.2 Necrotizing Enterocolitis [6, 18, 19, 21]

Predisposition. Preterm infants between 1200 and 2000 g with perinatal distress and hypoxemia (RDS, sepsis, congenital defect, hypothermia) are most prone to develop necrotizing enterocolitis. Other risk factors have been implicated: umbilical vessel catheterization, blood exchange transfusion, hyperosmolar feedings, pathologic intestinal flora, and patent ductus arteriosus.

Clinical Features

Early Signs
Temperature instability
Apathy
Irritability
Abdominal distension
Demonstration of occult blood in the stool

Typical Symptoms
Delayed gastric emptying
Bile-stained vomiting
Abdominal tenderness
Faint or absent bowel sounds
Gray-blue skin color
Shock symptoms
Acidosis
Consumption coagulopathy
Vasomotor collapse.

Radiographic findings
Intestinal distension (small bowel)
Fluid levels
Pneumatosis intestinalis
Accumulation of gas in portal venous system
Pneumoperitoneum
Persistent dilated intestinal loop

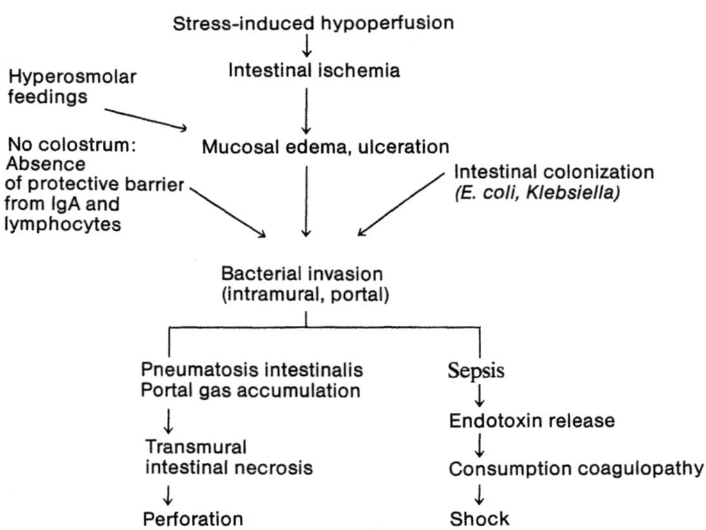

Fig. 28. Pathogenesis of necrotizing enterocolitis [6]

Laboratory findings
Leukopenia or leukocytosis
Signs of disseminated intravascular coagulation (thrombocytes < 50 000, PTT and PT prolonged)
Blood and cerebrospinal fluid cultures are sterile initially, but often become positive.

Therapy. After the diagnosis is established, good interdisciplinary cooperation between neonatal intensive medicine and pediatric surgery is essential!

– Close evaluation	Blood gases
Clinical symptoms	Blood count
Blood pressure	Electrolytes
Respiration	Coagulative status
Heart rate	Plain X-ray films: Frequency according to clinical course.

- Withdrawal of oral feedings for 10 days to 3 weeks, depending on the severity of the condition.
- Nasogastric residual drainage
- Maintenance of fluid and electrolyte balance (replacement).

Note. Fluid and electrolytes bog down in the third space (gastrointestinal tract) and require intensive hydration therapy.

- Shock therapy: Fresh blood transfusion (10 ml/kg) to maintain the systolic blood pressure
- Adequate intravenous caloric nutrition (without fat)
- Antibiotic therapy
  Cefoxitin, 100 mg/kg/day in three doses
  Tobramycin, 4 mg/kg/day in 2 doses, possibly 2 mg/kg orally q. 4 hr [5]. We prefer this combination due to the possibility of anaerobic infection.

Indication for Surgical Intervention
Pneumoperitoneum
Persistent dilated intestinal loop
Persistent peritonitis.
The proper timing for surgical intervention can be determined only by continuous supervision and frequent X-rays. The multiple perforations, chiefly in the region of the ileum and colon, confront the pediatric surgeon with a problematic situation and require great expertise in operative methods and techniques.

12.3 Acute Renal Failure

Preliminary Remarks. Immediately after birth the kidneys, along with other organ systems, are given the task of maintaining and controlling homeostasis of the organism (Table 53). The immature renal function of newborn infants results from a

Table 53. Renal function in the neonate [4]

Glomerular filtration rate	26 ± 1.7 ml/min
Renal plasma flow	88 ± 4.2 ml/min
Urine osmolarity	450–700 mosmol/l
Bicarbonate threshold	21–22 mosmol/l
Urine volume	30–300 ml/day

structural immaturity which causes a low glomerular filtration rate, poor concentrating capacity, incomplete reabsorption of bicarbonate, glucose and amino acids, as well as an ineffective secretion of organic acids in the proximal tubule and limited ammonia production in the distal tubule [10, 12, 14].

Although these functional restrictions are age-related, biologically reasonable, and entirely adequate for healthy neonates, they limit the ability of the kidneys to adapt to nonphysiologic stresses (hypoxia, shock) [8]. (Fig 29).

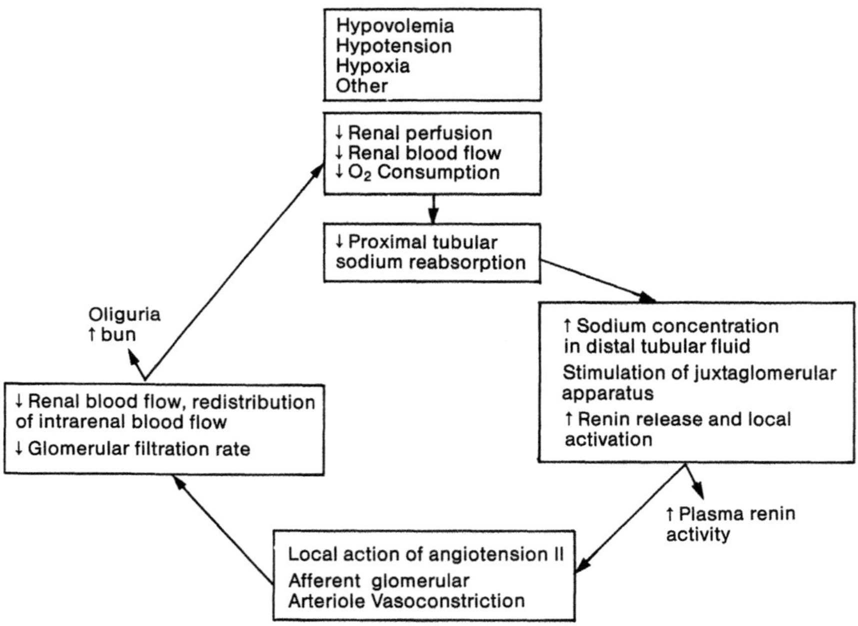

Fig. 29. Pathophysiology of acute renal failure [10]

Definition. Acute renal failure refers to a sudden impairment of renal function characterized by oliguria or anuria, water and electrolyte imbalance, acid-base disturbances, and an elevated concentration of renal products in the serum (urea, creatinine) [3, 4, 13].

Urinary output	<15 ml/kg body wt./day
Serum creatinine	>1.8 mg/100 ml
Serum urea	>40 mg/100 ml

Etiology. The causes of acute renal failure in the neonate are listed in Table 54. The prerenal form of acute renal failure represents a purely functional restriction of excretory renal output as a result of diminished perfusion pressure. It can be relieved by prompt volume substitution and/or normalization of the systolic blood pressure. If treatment is delayed or irreversible damage is present, an organically fixed acute renal failure will develop. The renal form of acute renal failure results from congenital malformations or an impairment of renal function occurring as part of a complex syndrome. The latter is the most frequent cause in the neonatal period.
The postrenal form of acute renal failure is most commonly caused by congenital obstructions to urinary outflow but is rarely seen in the neonatal period.

Table 54. Causes of acute renal failure in the neonate [3, 4, 10]

Prerenal	
Hypovolemia	Perinatal hemorrhage, dehydration, diarrhea, consequence of surgery
Heart failure	Congenital defects
Hypotension	Sepsis, coagulation defect, hemorrhage, hypothermia
Hypoxemia	Asphyxia, respiratory distress syndrome, pneumonia, cardiac surgery
Renal	
Congenital	Agenesis, hypoplasia, multi- or polycystic degeneration, nephrotic syndrome, nephritis
Acquired	Renal vein or renal artery thrombosis, renal cortical necrosis, nephrotoxins, disseminated intravascular coagulation, trauma, untreated prerenal causes
Postrenal	
Obstructive uropathy	Urethral stricture, urethral valve, meatal stenosis, ureteral stenosis, renal tumors, etc.

Clinical Features
History. Maternal diabetes, oligo- or polyhydramnios, perinatal hemorrhagic shock.

Nonspecific Symptoms. Reluctance to feed, vomiting, pallor, weak pulse.

Cardinal Symptoms. Oligo- or anuria, overhydration (edema, weight gain); this leads to hypertension, cardiac failure, pulmonary edema, cerebral edema, and convulsions.
Findings. Palpable enlargement of kidneys, ascites, among others.

Singular umbilical artery, typical facies (Potter), low-set ears, meningomyelocele, and polydactyly may be signs of a severe renal malformation.

Laboratory Findings

Serum

Urea, creatinine, potassium, calcium, phosphate, magnesium

Urinary Status. Hematuria, proteinuria, cylindruria. Specific weight < 1.010, pH > 6.0, electrolytes, creatinine (Table 55).

ECG. The ECG in hyperkalemia shows a flat P wave, widened QRS complex, prolonged T-R interval, ST depression and spiked T wave.

Table 55. Differentiation between the prerenal and renal forms of renal failure [10, 13]

		Prerenal	Renal
Urine/plasma	Osmolarity	2.0	1.0
	Creatinine	20:1	5:1
	Urea	10:1	5:1

Diagnosis. Acute renal failure is diagnosed if no urine has been passed by 48 h postpartum or if oligo- or anuria occurs during the course of the neonatal period. Ultrasonography, retrograde urography, and cystoscopy are performed, depending on the individual case.

Infusion urography is of no diagnostic value in the anuric stage and leads to an unnecessary osmolar load!

Therapy. The treatment of acute renal failure requires a systematic procedure. We have found the following scheme to be of value (Fig. 30) [22]:

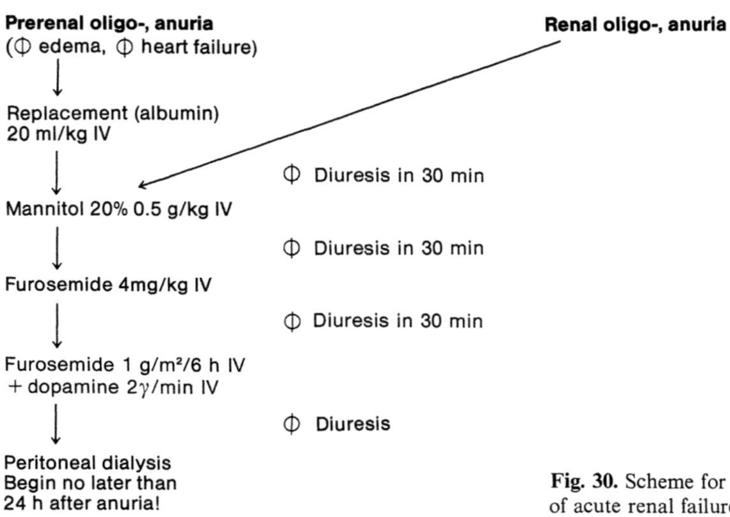

Fig. 30. Scheme for the treatment of acute renal failure

When combined, furosemide and dopamine exert a synergistic diuretic action. Conservative treatment may be sufficient in oliguric renal failure. Mannitol is contraindicated in this stage of acute renal failure due to its osmotic properties, but further attempts with furosemide are permissible.

Maintenance of fluid and electrolyte balance:

- Fluid restriction: 20 ml/kg/day (insensible losses)
- Sodium administration: Corresponds to urine output of previous day (sodium bicarbonate!)
- Potassium restriction
- Hyperkalemia (> 6.0 mEq/l): 0.5–1.0 ml 10% calcium gluconate/kg body wt. over 2–4 min (under ECG control)
  Correction of acisdosis (2–3 mEq sodium bicarbonate/kg body wt.)
  4 ml 20% glucose IV with 0.2 IU insulin/kg in 30 min
  Resonium A: 1.1 g/kg reduces hyperkalemia by 1 mEq/l
  Dosage: 0.5–1.5 g/kg in three to four doses (clysma, orally)
- Hypocalcemia: 5 ml 10% calcium gluconate/kg/day
- Blood pressure check every 2–6 h

Weight checks: every 6 h; physiologic weight loss is 1%–2%/day.

Nutrition: High-caloric feeding by central venous catheter; 50% glucose, L-amino acids, Intralipid if required.

Treatment for hypertension.

Overhydration is often unavoidable in anuric patients, even with strict adherence to the therapeutic plan, and peritoneal dialysis should be performed. Even in newborn infants, this is a technically simple procedure.

Table 56. Pharmacologic treatment of neonatal hypertension [1]

Dihydralazine	1–9 mg/kg/day IV, p.o.
Methyldopa	5–50 mg/kg/day IV, p.o.
Propranolol	0.5–2.0 mg/kg/day IV, p.o.
Diazoxide	5 mg/kg/dose IV
Na-nitroprusside	2.5–5 μg/kg/min IV

Indications for peritoneal dialysis:
Intractable anuria after 24 h!
Hyperkalemia > 6.5 mEq/l
Serum urea > 100 mg/100 ml
Overhydration, hypertension, heart failure
Uncorrectable acidosis
For technique of peritoneal dialysis see p. 247.

References

1. ADELMAN, R. D.: Neonatal hypertension. Pediatr. Clin. North Am. *25*, 99 (1978)
2. ALLEN, R. G.: Tumor masses of the neonate, Clin. Perinatol. *5* (1), 115 (1978)
3. ANAND, S. K., NORTHRAY, J. D., CRUSSI, F. G.: Acute renal failure in newborn infants. J. Pediatr. *92*, 985 (1978)
4. ASHINGBERG, L. C., ZEIS, P. M., HAGEMAN, J. R., VIDYASAGAR, M. J.: Acute renal failure in the newborn. Crit. Care Med. *5*, 36 (1977)
5. BELL, M. J., SHACKELFORD, P. G., FEIGIN, R. D., TERNBERG, J. L., BROTHERTON, TH.: Alteration in gastrointestinal microflora during antimicrobial therapy for necrotizing enterocolitis. Pediatrics *63*, 425 (1979)
6. BURRINGTON, J. D.: Necrotizing enterocolitis in the newborn infant. Clin. Perinatol. *5* (1), 29 (1978)
7. CREMIN, B. J., CYWES, S., LOUW, J. H.: Radiological Diagnosis of digestive tract disorders in the newborn. London: Butterworth 1973
8. DRAGO, J. R., ROHNER, RH. J., SANFORD, E. J., MAESELS, M. J.: Perinatal asphyxia and renal failure in neonatal patients. J. Urol. *118*, 80 (1977)
9. HANDERSON, K. C., TURCH, E. M.: Differential diagnosis of abdominal masses in the neonate. Pediatr. Clin. North Am. *24*, 557 (1977)
10. JAIN, R.: Acute renal failure in the neonate. Pediatr. Clin. North Am. *24*, 605 (1977)
11. KAISER, G.: Chirurg. Eingriffe in den ersten 3 Lebenstagen. Pädiat. Fortbk. Praxis *41*, 134 (1975)
12. LEAKE, R. D.: Perinatal nephrobiology: A developmental prospective. Clin. Perinatol. *4*, 321 (1977)
13. MEHLS, O., GILLI, G.: Akute Niereninsuffizienz S. 9.21. in: Pädiatrie in Praxis und Klinik. BACHMANN, K. D., EWERBECK, H., JOPPICH, G., KLEIHAUER, E., ROSSI, E., STALDER, G. (Hrsg.). Stuttgart: Thieme 1978
14. NASH, M. A., EDELMANN, C. M.: The developing kidney. Nephron *11*, 71 (1973)
15. OPPERMANN, H. C., GREINACHER, I., WILLE, L., WILLICH, E.: Präoperative radiologische Diagnostik bei abdominalen Raumforderungen im Neugeborenen- und frühen Säuglingsalter. Abstracta Congressus Paediatrico-Chirurgicus Bohemoslovacus *103* (1978)
16. POZNANSKI, A.: Radiologic examinations in the neonatal intensive care unit, in: Practical approaches to Pediatric Radiology, p. 61. Chicago: Year Book Medical Publishers 1976
17. RAFFENSPERGER, J. G., SEELER, R. A., MONCACLA, R.: The acute abdomen in infancy and childhood. Abdominal masses in infancy. p. 21. Philadelphia-Toronto: Lippincott 1970
18. REID, W. D., SHANNON, M. P.: Necrotizing enterocolitis – a medical approach to treatment. C. M. A. J. *108*, 573 (1973)
19. ROSEGGER, H.: Die nekrotisierende Enterocolitis. Pädiatrie and Pathologie *12*, 349 (1977)
20. SILVERMAN, A., ROY, C. C., COZZETO, F. J.: Pediatric Clinical Gastroenterology, p. 47: Gastrointestinal emergencies of the neonate. St. Louis: Mosby 1971
21. WERNER, J. P., PRINGSHEIM, W., HELWIG, H., SCHÄFER, G.: Entstehung und Verlauf der nekrotisierenden Enterokolitis bei Frühgeborenen. In: Pädiatrische Intensivmedizin. Bd. 3, S. 209. EMMRICH P. (Hrsg.). Stuttgart: Thieme 1977
22. WILLE, L., MEHLS, O., GILLI, G.: Akute Niereninsuffizienz beim Neugeborenen. Ther. Umschau 29, 8590 (1979)
23. WOLF, H. G.: Präoperative Notfalldiagnostik beim Neugeborenen und Säugling. Praxis *53*, 1254 (1964)

13 Disorders of Metabolism

L. Wille

13.1 Hypoglycemia

Definition [8]

Term infants:	<30 mg% during the first 72 h
	<40 mg% after the 72–h limit
Preterm infants:	<20 mg% in the first week of life
	<40 mg% thereafter.

Blood glucose is determined by glucose oxidase method.

Incidence [8, 16]. Two to 4.4 per 1000 term births, 15.6 per 1000 preterm births; 20% in infants small for gestational age, 17.8% in severe erythroblastosis.

Etiology [6]. Hypoglycemia is currently classified as follows according to clinical course, onset of symptoms, duration, response to therapy, and underlying primary disease [8, 14, 16]:

Early transient adaptive hypoglycemia
Secondary hypoglycemia
Classic transient neonatal hypoglycemia
Severe recurrent hypoglycemia.

However, we believe that the classification given in Table 57 is better from a didactic and therapeutic standpoint.

Clinical Features. Often asymptomatic; in symptomatic hypoglycemia the symptoms are usually nonspecific:

Apathy	Apneic spells
Hypotonia	Cyanosis
Hyperexcitability	Hypothermia
Convulsions	Bradycardia
Reluctance to feed	Tachycardia

Radiography. Cardiomegaly in some cases [24].

Diagnosis. Screening with Dextrostix (Ames) or, preferably, with Reflotest hypoglycemia test strips (Boehringer/Mannheim Co.). If predisposing risk factors are

Table 57. Classification of hypoglycemia (modified from [6])

Pathophysiologic mechanism	Common states	Differential diagnosis Uncommon states, partly theoretical at present	Infants at risk
Deficient intake		Delayed feeding	
Inadequate liver glycogen stores	Prematurity, intrauterine malnutrition, dysmaturity, perinatal hypoxia	Glycogen synthetase deficiency	Preterm infants, SGA infants, perinatal asphyxia, discordant twin
Defect in metabolic pathways which lead to glucose		Type I glycogenosis, glyconeogenesis defects, galactosemia, fructose intolerance, fructose 1,6-diphosphatase deficiency, epinephrine ↓ (*Zetterström*), cortisol ↓, glucagon ↓, growth hormone ↓	
Increased peripheral consumption Hyperinsulinism	Maternal diabetes, macrosomia, Rh erythroblastosis	Islet cell adenoma, nesidioblastosis, β-cell hypoplasia, Wiedemann-Beckwith-Combs, leucine-induced hypoglycemia	Infants of diabetic mothers, macrosomia, Rh eryhtroblastosis after exchange transfusion
Anaerobic energy production, heat production	Hypoxia, severe cardiac failure, hypothermia		Hypoxia, respiratory distress, congenital defects, hypothermia, sepsis
Congenital defects of amino acid metabolism		Maple syrup disease, proprionic acidemia, methylmalonic adidemia, tyrosinosis	
Pathogenesis unclear	Polycythemia	Cardiomegaly which is correctible by glucose administration	Polycythemia

present, blood glucose should be checked in the 2nd, 4th, 6th, 12th, 24th, and 48th hours of life.
In the presence of symptoms or Dextrostix values ≤25 mg% (color scale), the glucose level is determined by the glucose oxidase method. Once hypoglycemia has been demonstrated, frequent determinations are made at least every 2–4 h, depending on the clinical situation.

Prophylaxis. Screening of high-risk infants, early feeding, systemic buffer therapy for birth asphyxia, adequate oxygenation, maintenance of neutral thermal environment, hematocrit determination (polycythemia).

Therapy. Most investigators agree that even asymptomatic hypoglycemia represents a potential hazard and should be treated.

Immediate Measures. If clinical symptoms are present or if a blood glucose ≤25 mg% has been indicated by Dextrostix, take a blood sample for enzymatic glucose determination. Then give the infant 20% glucose, 3 ml/kg IV (=0.6 g/kg) immediately followed by the infusion of 10% glucose, 60–115 ml/kg/24 h (=4–8 mg/kg/min). Do not await the results of the enzymatic determination!

Recurrent Hypoglycemia (hypoglycemia uncontrolled after 4–6 h). Infuse 15% glucose, 100–115 ml/kg/day (=10–12 mg/kg/min); if this fails to maintain the blood glucose within normal limits, give prednisolone, 1 mg/kg IV q. 6 h; change to oral route later (prednisone, 1 mg/kg/day) if possible.

Intractable hypoglycemia. Glucagon, 0.03–0.1 mg/kg q. 4–6 h (exception: SGA infants). If glucagon is ineffective, try diazoxide, 15–20 mg/kg/day orally in three doses; start with low dosage.
Persistent hypoglycemia requires thorough diagnostic clarification!

13.2 Infants of Diabetic Mothers

Etiology and Pathophysiology. Maternal diabetes mellitus (White classification). Functional fetal hyperinsulinism, diminished response to glucagon and epinephrine, and decreased basal STH level are held responsible for impaired basal glucose homeostasis; the hepatic production of glucose by glycogenolysis and glyconeogenesis is diminished [1, 8, 13, 18].

Clinical Features. The severity of the clinical picture depends partly on the severity of the maternal diabetes mellitus as well as the quality of prenatal dietary and medical care.
The infants are usually large for gestational age (White A, B, C); they are rarely small for date (White D, E, F).

Hypoglycemic symptoms are present (see p 169). Cardiomegaly and cardiac failure may be present [23, 30].
Complications [10, 13, 20, 21, 25]:

Stillbirth	Hyperbilirubinemia
Prematurity	Respiratory distress syndrome
Congenital malformations (e. g., heart, caudal regression syndrome)	Renal vein thrombosis
	Hydrops fetalis
Metabolic or electrolyte imbalance (hypoglycemia, hypocalcemia, hypomagnesemia)	Polycythemia
	Cardiomyopathy

Diagnosis. Screening with Dextrostix (or Reflotest strips) immediately after birth and again after 1, 2, 4, 6, 12, 24, 36, 48, 72, and 96 h of life.
In the presence of clinical symptoms or Dextrostix values ≤25 mg% (color scale), check glucose by glucose oxidase method. If hypoglycemia is established, recheck at least every 4 h depending on clinical situation. Also: blood gas analysis, calcium and magnesium determination.

Prophylaxis. Close supervision of the pregnancy and good medical management of the diabetic gravida. Give newborn 10% glucose, 100 ml/kg/day by intravenous infusion. Start of feeding depends on clinical situation in the 4th-6th h of life.

Therapy

- If clinical symptoms are present, take blood sample for enzymatic glucose determination; immediately give 20% glucose, 3 ml/kg IV (=0.6 g/kg), followed by infusion of 10% glucose, 60–115 ml/kg/day (=4–8 mg/kg/min).
- Recurrent hypoglycemia (uncontrolled after 4–6 h): Infuse 15% glucose, 100–115 ml/kg/day (= 10–12 mg/kg/min; increase to 14–18 mg/kg/min if necessary). If this fails to keep the blood glucose within normal limits, give glucagon, 0.3 mg/kg IM in intervals of 4–6 h.
- If there is no response to glucagon, try prednisolone, 1 mg/kg IV q. 6 h; later change to oral route if possible (prednisone, 2 mg/kg/day).
- As the oral feeding regime is increased, reduce the intravenous glucose accordingly (feeding volume + drip infusion = 100 ml/kg/day). Recheck blood glucose due to possible reactive hypoglycemia.

13.3 **Hyperglycemia** (see Table 58)

Table 58

Etiology	Pathogenesis	Clinical features	Prognosis and Therapy
1. Cerebral injury (perinatal asphyxia, intracranial hemorrhage) [28]	Disturbance of glucostatic control mechanisms	See under Postasphyxia Syndrome and Cerebral Hemorrhage	See under Postasphyxia Syndrome and Cerebral Hemorrhage
2. Intravenous hyperalimentation [28]	Excessive glucose infusion per unit time during parenteral nutrition	Often dehydration, increased serum osmolality, glucosuria	Risk of Candida sepsis with fatal course. Reduction of glucose infusion. Careful, gradual reduction of serum osmolality (beware: convulsions, intracranial hemorrhage)
3. Transient diabetes mellitus [5, 8, 22, 27, 29]	Unknown, numerous pathogenetic hypotheses have been advanced	Weight loss, dehydration, polydipsia, polyuria, hyperglycemia (up to 2300 mg%), in rare cases ketonuria, high-grade emaciation, whiteness. SGA infants are usually affected; onset occurs between the 1st week and 44th day of life.	Duration of illness varies. Insulin therapy is required: 1–3 units/kg/-day. Always start with only 0.2 units insulin/kg, followed by continuous insulin infusion. Careful rehydration with 1/4–1/3 saline solution over 48–72 h. Give sodium as chloride and bicarbonate. If urine output is adequate, give potassium chloride (20–40 mEq/l) and calcium gluconate, 0.5 g/12 h.
4. Persistent neonatal diabetes mellitus [11, 27, 29]	Diminished response of β-cells to various attempts at stimulation	Clinical and biochemical symptomatology as under 3; this clinical picture is rare	Differentiation from 3: Infant is small for gestational age; ketosis is absent, the insulin demand is increased. Failure to recover spontaneously. Treat as under 3

Table 59. Classification of congenital aminoacidopathies with severe neonatal disease [26]

Amino acid classification	*Disorder*	*Clinical findings*	*Laboratory findings*	*Enzymatic defect*
Branched chain	Branched chain ketoaciduria (maple syrup urine disease)	Feeding difficulty, lethargy, coma, maple syrup-like odor	Metabolic acidosis; hypoglycemia; elevated blood and urine leucine, isoleucine and valine; branched-chain ketoaciduria	Branched chain ketoacid decarboxylase
	Valinemia	Feeding difficulty, vomiting, lethargy	Elevated blood and urine valine	Valine: α-ketoglutarate transaminase
	Isovalericacidemia	Progressive neurologic dysfunction, odor of "sweaty feet"	Metabolic acidosis; elevated blood and urine isovaleric acid	Isovaleryl-CoA dehydrogenase
	β-Hydroxyisovaleric aciduria	Feeding difficulty, acrid urine odor	Urinary excretion of β-hydroxyisovaleric acid and β-methylcrotonylglycine	β-Methylcrotonyl-CoA carboxylase (?)
	Propionicacidemia (ketotic hyperglycinemia)	Feeding difficulty, vomiting, lethargy, seizures	Metabolic ketoacidosis; hypoglycemia; hyperammonemia; hyperglycinemia and -uria; long-chain ketonuria; elevated blood and urine propionate	Propionyl-CoA carboxylase
	Methylmalonic aciduria (B_{12}-unresponsive)	Feeding difficulty, vomiting, lethargy	Metabolic ketoacidosis; hypoglycemia; hyperammonemia; hyperglycinemia and -uria; long-chain ketonuria; methylmalonicacidemia and -uria	Methylmalonyl-CoA mutase
	Methylmalonic aciduria (B_{12}-responsive)	Feeding difficulty, vomiting, lethargy	(See B_{12}-unresponsive form)	Defective conversion of vitamin B_{12} to

	Methylmalonic aciduria and homocystinuria	Feeding difficulty, lethargy, coma	Methylmalonic aciduria; cystathioninemia; homocystinuria; hypomethioninemia	Defective conversion of vitamin B_{12} to deoxyadenosyl-B_{12} and methyl-B_{12}
Urea cycle	Hyperammonemia	Feeding difficulty, vomiting, lethargy, coma	Respiratory alkalosis; hyperammonemia	Ornithine transcarbamylase
	Citrullinemia	Feeding difficulty, vomiting, coma	Respiratory alkalosis; hyperammonemia; elevated blood and urine citrulline	Argininosuccinate synthetase
	Arginosuccinicaciduria	Ataxia, seizures	Hyperammonemia; argininosuccinicacidemia and -uria	Argininosuccinate lyase
	Argininemia	Spastic diplegia, seizures	Hyperammonemia; elevated blood and urine arginine	Arginase
Sulfur-containing	Methionine malabsorption (oast-house syndrome)	Hypotonia, seizures, musty urine odor	α-Hydroxybutyricaciduria; elevated urine methionine (?)	Gut transport of methionine
	Sulfituria and thiosulfaturia	Pyramidal tract signs, blindness, dislocated lenses	Elevated urine sulfite, thisulfate and S-sulfo-cysteine	Sulfite oxidase
Glycine	Hyperglycinemia (nonketotic)	Developmental failure, seizures	Elevated blood and urine glycine	Glycine decarboxylase (?)
Aromatic	Tyrosinemia	Cirrhosis, rickets, Fanconi syndrome	Hyophosphatemia; tyrosinemia and tyrosyluria; generalized aminoaciduria	*p*-Hydroxyphenylpyruvic acid oxidase (?)
β-Amino	β-Alaninemia	Lethargy, seizures	Elevated blood and urine β-alanine; γ-aminobutyricaciduria	β-Alanine: α-ketoglutarate transaminase (?)
Dipeptide	Carnosinemia	Seizures	Elevated blood and urine carnosine	Carnosinase

Differentialdiagnosis [24]

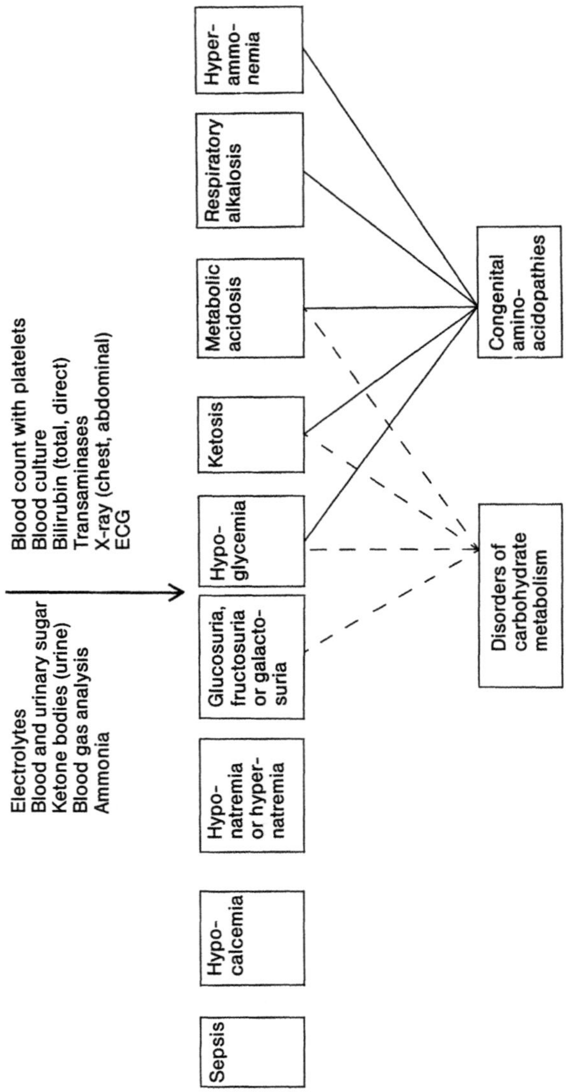

Fig. 31. Differential diagnostic procedure for suspected acute metabolic disease (modified from Duran, 1974 [12])

13.4 Acute Metabolic Disorders

Our discussion is limited to defects of enzymatic activity in the intermediary metabolism which may result in

1. An accumulation of metabolites which are toxic in high concentrations, and
2. A change in metabolism due to the utilization of unusual metabolic pathways.

These are essentially genetically transmitted defects in the metabolism of certain amino acids, organic acids and the urea cycle, which can lead to life-threatening disease in the neonatal period (Tab. 58).
However, marked clinical symptoms or a typical clinical aspect may also suggest disorders of the carbohydrate, fat, and mucopolysaccharide metabolism as well as various other disease syndromes (e. g., adrenogenital syndrome, renal tubular acidosis, congenital lactate acidosis, α_1-antitrypsin deficiency). A description of all metabolic disorders which are manifest in the early neonatal period would exceed the scope of this study. For this the reader is referred to the survey work of Burton and Nadler [7].

Differential Diagnosis [12] (Fig. 31)
The supervision and treatment of affected neonates require cooperation with experienced specialists and a well-equipped laboratory [4, 15]. The task of neonatal intensive medicine in this regard is two-fold:
1. Supervision and diagnosis if a severe metabolic disorder is anticipated (family history, prenatal diagnostics).
2. Supervision and treatment in the presence of a manifest severe metabolic disease.

Suggestive Signs
Family history
Prenatal diagnostics
Marked odor
Gradual appearance of neurologic symptoms after start of feeding regime (protein intake)
Persistent metabolic acidosis or respiratory alkalosis
Decreased bicarbonate level
Hypoglycemia
Ketonuria
Hyperammonemia
Neutropenia
Thrombocytopenia

Clinical Features

Poor feeding	Muscular weakness
Vomiting	Failure to thrive
Apathy	Hepatomegaly
Apneic spells	Respiratory difficulties
Convulsions	Diarrhea
Coma	Dehydration

Diagnosis [9, 12, 26]

1. If severe metabolic disease is expected:
   Within the first 24 h of life:
   a) General diagnosis
      Blood gas analysis
      Daily blood glucose profile
      Blood count including platelets
      Bilirubin (total, direct)
      Transaminases
      Electrolytes (sodium, potassium, chloride, calcium, magnesium, phosphorus)
      Urea, creatinine
      Ammonia
   b) Special tests
      Quantitative determination of amino acids (column chromatography):
      Plasma
      Urine
      Quantitative determination of organic acids (gas chromatography or mass spectroscopy):
      Plasma
      Urine.

If test results are normal, carefully institute a protein-containing feeding regimen over the next 48 h. Repeat the diagnostic procedure at the end of this second 48–h period, or earlier if clinical symptoms appear.

Severe asphyxia (pronounced tissue hypoxia) can sometimes mimic a congenital metabolic disorder by causing increased excretion of ammonia and unusual organic acid patterns in the urine [3].

2. Procedure for manifest severe metabolic disease
   Rapid preliminary tests:
   Ketone bodies (Ketur test)
   MMA test (**m**ethyl**m**alonic **a**ciduria)
   DNPH (**d**i**n**itro**p**henyl **h**ydrazine) test
   $FeCl_3$ (ferric chloride) test.
   Test for reducing substances (galactose, glucose-specific); collect and freeze individual urine batches.

Narrow the diagnosis as much as possible before ordering biochemical tests for congenital metabolic diseases (see above).

The results of each test should be available within 12–24 h if possible. As a rule, most serious metabolic diseases of the newborn can be diagnosed within 48 h by this procedure.

Therapy [9, 15, 17, 26]

1. Symptomatic
   a) Correction of
      acidosis,
      hypoglycemia,
      electrolyte disturbance
   b) Controlled ventilation if required
   c) Anticonvulsive therapy if required.
2. Special
   a) Avoidance or withdrawal of protein intake.
   b) High-caloric nutrition (120–150 calories/kg) to avoid catabolism:
      - 5–10 ml tea with 5% glucose hourly by mouth, increased gradually to 7% glucose and 5%–10% polysaccharide (e. g., maltodextrin)
      - parenteral infusion of 10%–15% glucose, 100 ml/kg/day.
   c) If there is clinical and biochemical deterioration or failure to improve:
      - blood exchange transfusion or
      - peritoneal dialysis [15].
   d) After the diagnosis is established:
      - institution of special diet
      - high intake of special cofactors
      - vitamins.

References

1. AMENDT, P.: Neugeborene diabetischer Mütter II. Makrosomie, Glukosehomeostase und innere Sekretion, Kinderärztl. Prax. *46*, 349 (1978)
2. AMENDT, P.: Neugeborene diabetischer Mütter I. Pathophysiologie und Klinik. Kinderärztl. Prax. *46*, 299 (1978)
3. BAKKEREN, J. A., SENGERS, R. C., TRIJBELS, J. M., ENGELS, P. H.: Organic aciduria in hypoxic premature newborns simulating an inborn error of metabolism. Eur. J. Pediatr. *127*, 41 (1977)
4. BICKEL, H.: Methoden und Resultate des Neugeborenen-Screenings auf Aminoacidopathien. Mschr. Kinderheilk. *124*, 650 (1976)
5. BLUNK, W.: Endokrine Erkrankungen in der Neugeborenenperiode. In: Handbuch der Kinderheilkunde, Bd. 1/2 OPITZ, H., SCHMID, F. (Hrsg.) S. 257. New York, Berlin-Heidelberg: Springer 1971
6. BOSSI, E.: Neonatale Hypoglykämie. Schweiz. Rundschau Med. (Praxis) *64*, 1214 (1975)
7. BURTON, B. K., NADLER, H. L.: Clinical diagnosis of the inborn errors of metabolism in the neonatal period. Pediatrics *61*, 398 (1978)
8. CORNBLATH, M., SCHWARTZ, R.: Disorders of carbohydrate metabolism in infancy. Philadelphia-London: Saunders 1976
9. DANKS, M. D.: Plan of management for newborn babies in whom metabolic disease is anticipated or suspected. Clin. Perinatol. *3* (1), 251 (1976)
10. DAY, R. E., INSLEY, J.: Maternal diabetes mellitus and congenital malformation. Survery of 205 cases. Arch. Dis. Child. *51*, 935 (1976)

11. DORCHY, H., OOMS, H., LOEB, H.: Permanent neonatal diabetes mellitus: A case report with plasma insulin studies. Z. Kinderheilk. *118*, 271 (1975)
12. DURAN, M.: A contribution of the study of organic aciduria. Dissertation, Utrecht 1974 (Wadman)
13. FLECHTER, A. B.: The infant of the diabetic mother. In: Neonatology. AVERY, G. B., (ed.). p. 203. Philadelphia-Toronto: Lippincott 1975
14. FLUGE, G.: Clinical aspects of neonatal hypoglycemia. Acta Paediatr. Scand. *63*, 826 (1974)
15. FRANCOIS, B., CORNU, G., de MEYER, R.: Peritoneal dialysis and exchange transfusion in a neonate with argininsuccinic aciduria. Arch. Dis. Child. *51*, 228 (1976)
16. GUTBERLET, R. L., CORNBLATH, M.: Neonatal hypglycemia revisited 1975. Pediatrics, *58*, 10 (1976)
17. HAMMERSEN, G., WILLE, L., SCHMIDT, H., LUTZ, P., BICKEL, H.: Maple syrup urine disease: Treatment of the acutely Ill newborn Eur. J. Pediatr. *129*, 157 (1978)
18. KALHAN, S. C., SAVIN, S. M., ADAM, P. A. J.: Attenuated glucose production rate in newborn infants of insulin-dependent diabetic mothers. N. Engl. Med. *296*, 375 (1977)
19. LINDSTEN, J., ZETTERSTRÖM, R., FERGUSON-SMITH, M.: Prenatal diagnosis of genetic disorders of the foetus. Conference, Stockholm, June 12–13, 1975, Acta Scand. Paediatr., Suppl. *259*, 1976
20. MAYER, J. B.: Die Embryopathia diabetica. Z. Kinderheilk. *71*, 183 (1952)
21. MILLER, H. C.: The effect of diabetic and prediabetic pregnancies on the fetus and the newborn infant. J. Pediatr. *26*, 455 (1946)
22. PAGLIARA, A. S., KARL, I. E., KIPNIS, D. B.: Transient neonatal diabetes: Delayed maturation of the prancreatic beta cell. J. Pediatr. *82*, 97 (1973)
23. POLAND, R. L., WALTHER, L. J., CHANG, Ch.-H.: Hypertrophic cardiomyopathia in infants of diabetic mothers. Pediatr. Res. *9*, 269/75 (1975)
24. REID, M. McC, REILLY, B. J., MURDOCK, A. I., SWYER, P. R.: Cardiomegaly in association with neonatal hypoglycaemia. Acta Paediatr. Scand. *60*, 295 (1970)
25. ROWLAND, Th. W., HUBELL, J. P., NADAS, A. S.: Congenital heart disease in infants of diabetic mothers. J. Pediatr. *83*, 815 (1973)
26. SCRIVER, Ch. R., ROSENBERG, L. E.: Amino acid metabolism and its disorders. p. 126. Philadelphia-London-Toronto: Saunders 1973
27. SCHRÖTER, W.: Die idiopathische transitorische Neugeborenenhyperglykämie in: Handbuch der Kinderheilkunde Bd. 1/2 OPITZ, H., SCHMID, F. (Ed.). S. 268. New York, Berlin-Heidelberg: Springer 1971
28. STERN, L.: Disturbances in glucose, calcium, and magnesium homeostasis. In: Neonatology. AVERY, G. B. (Ed.). p. 423. Philadelphia-Toronto: Lippincott 1975
29. SWYER, P. R.: The intensive care of the newly born. p. 167. Basel-München-Paris-London-New York-Sydney: Karger 1975
30. WAY, G. L., WOLFE, R. R., PETTETT, G. P., MERENSTEIN, G. B., SIMONS, M. A., SPANGLER, R. D., NORA, J. J.: Echocardiographic assessment of ventricular dimensions and myocardial function in infants of diabetic mothers. Pediatr. Res. *9*, 273/101 (1975)

14 Disturbances of the Electrolyte Balance

L. Wille

14.1 Hyponatremia < 130 mEq/l

Neonates and preterm infants in particular have a low tolerance to sodium retention and excretion during the 1st week of life, especially in the early neonatal period [2, 14, 32] (Table 60)

Remarks on Table 60

1. A daily requirement of 2–3 mEq/kg/day is insufficient for very immature preterm infants (< 1250 g, < 30 weeks gestation). Often 4–8 mEq/kg/day is necessary to maintain sodium homeostasis.
2. Differentiation between the Schwartz-Bartter syndrome and increased sodium demand or increased natriuresis is important from a therapeutic standpoint. Clinical separation: Weight gain (edema) – weight loss (loss of turgor). The adrenogenital syndrome, aldosterone deficiency, and adrenal insufficiency are rare in the newborn infant. However, they may figure in the differential diagnosis and require elucidation which goes beyond the electrolyte disturbance.

Diagnosis

Hematocrit

Serum. Osmolality, sodium, potassium, cloride, urea, creatinine

Urine. Osmolality, sodium, potassium, chloride, creatinine.

Clinical Features. Preterm infants < 30 weeks gestation are particularly susceptible. Besides the symtoms listed in Table 60, the infants often show signs ranging from hypotonia to apathy, hyperexcitability, tremor, convulsions, and apneic spells.

Therapy

1. Schwartz-Bartter syndrome
   Fluid restriction to reduce the excessive extracellular volume: Reduce to the basic requirement (20 ml/kg/day). This is generally sufficient to achieve a normal sodium level.
   Note. Cardiac, renal and hypoproteinemic edema must be excluded.
2. Very immature preterm infants
   Estimate sodium requirement at 4–8 mEq/kg/day starting on the 2nd day of life.

Table 60. Forms of hyponatremia

Pathogenesis	Etiology	Clinical, laboratory findings
Schwartz-Bartter syndrome [16, 24, 25]	Inappropriate ADH secretion (asphyxia, hemorrhage, hydrocephalus, sepsis, meningitis, IPPV)	Nonphysiologic weight gain with initially unremarkable state of hydration. Persistent hyponatremia, hypochloremia, metabolic alkalosis, decreased hematocrit, decreased serum osmolality, increased urine osmolality, increased natriuresis
Increased natriuresis [13, 18, 32]	a) Sodium reabsorption defective due to immaturity of angiotensin-renin-aldosterone system and dissociated maturation of glomerular and tubular functions b) Pseudohypoaldosteronism: diminished response of renal tubules to aldosterone	Very immature preterm infants, weight loss, hyponatremia, elevated hematocrit, increased sodium loss. Diminished skin turgor. Loss of weight and turgor may also appear with normonatremia
Inadequate sodium intake	a) Delay of oral feeding b) Parenteral nutrition	Weight loss, dehydration, hyponatremia, increased hematocrit
Increased sodium demand	Coprecipitation with calcium during postnatal bone formation	Very immature preterm infants, weight loss, dehydration, hyponatremia, increased hematocrit
Maternal hypernatremia	Dilution effect in infant plasma	Hyponatremia
Salt-losing adrenogenital syndrome [22]	21-Hydroxylase-, 3-hydroxysteroid-dehydrogenase-, 20,22-desmolase defect	a) External genitalia *masculine:* pigmented, normal or hypospadiac, cryptorchidism
		b) External genitalia *feminine:* pigmented, clitoral hypertrophy, medial labial fusion, pseudohermaphroditism
		Vomiting, weight loss, apathy, exsiccosis, hyponatremia, hyperkalemia
Aldosterone deficiency [22]	18–Dehydrogenase defect	Weight loss, dehydration, hyponatremia, hyperkalemia, increased hematocrit
Adrenal insufficiency [22]	Trauma, congenital defects of steroid biosynthesis	Shock, peripheral hypoperfusion, convulsions, intermittent fever, hypoglycemia, hyponatremia, hyperchloremia, hyperkalemia
Cystic Fibrosis		Pulmonary or gastrointestinal involvement, hyponatremia

3. Manifest hyponatremia. Calculate deficit by the formula:

$$\frac{(Na_{ideal} - Na_{actual}(mEq) \times kg\ body\ weight)}{3} = sodium\ replacement\ (mEq)$$

The replacement volume can be given as 10% NaCl into parenteral infusion or can be spaced evenly over the 24–h oral feeding regime.

14.2 Hypernatremia > 150 mEq/l

Etiology

1. Restricted fluid intake during the first days of life
2. Excessive Na intake during parenteral infusion therapy
3. Administration of excessive sodium bicarbonate for treatment of acidosis
4. Faulty selection or composition of the milk regime (powder-to-water ratio to high)
5. Accidental sodium chloride replacement instead of glucose in the milk regime
6. Hypernatremic dehydration (diarrhea)
7. Nephrogenic or neurohormonal diabetes insipidus.

Clinical Features. Clinical presentation varies with the underlying disease. In some cases hypernatremia is not apparent until routine electrolyte determinations are done. Hypertonic dehydration: Apathy, hyperexcitability, sunken fontanel, dehydration, convulsions; advanced stage of shock, hypotension, peripheral cyanosis, cold extremities. Diabetes insipidus: Unexplained fever, dehydration, failure to thrive. Hyperelectrolytemia and low urine osmolality are typical.

Therapy (According to Etiology)

For 1. Adequate fluid intake during the first days of life: 65–100 mg/kg on 1st day; on 2nd and following days, supplement daily electrolyte requirement by infusion.

For 2. Adjust the parenteral feeding regime to the fluid and electrolyte requirements of term and preterm infants (see p. 48).

For 3. Giving sodium bicarbonate in excess of 10 mEq/kg/4 h requires monitoring of sodium levels! A sudden rise of plasma osmolality can cause cerebral hemorrhage! [28].

For 4. Correct feeding regime to a fully adapted milk formula (low-sodium).

For 5 and 6. Prolonged reduction of hypernatremia and hyperosmolality or gradual rehydration over 48 h [6]: 125 ml/kg/24 h. *Composition:* 0.9% NaCl (1 part), 5% glucose (3 parts) with 2 mEq/kg/day KCl and 10 ml calcium gluconate/day. Peritoneal dialysis may be required in case of sodium intoxication.

For 7. Adequate fluid replacement is necessary for normal hydration; treatment with hydrochlorothiazide, 1 mg/kg/day, or carbamazepine, 400–600 mg/1.7 m^2/day orally, may also be beneficial. Curative therapy [3, 4] is achieved by replacement with I-deamino-8-D-arginine vasopressin (DDAVP): 100–250 ng in two doses IV, later 1.25–2.5 μg/day intranasally.

14.3 Hypokalemia < 3.8 mEq/l (Table 61)

Table 61. Hypokalemia

Pathogenesis	Etiology	Clinical features
1. Inadequate intake	Daily requirement not met	Common to all forms: symptoms range from muscular weakness to apathy, abdominal distension secondary to paralytic ileus. Hypertension (Liddle syndrome). ECG changes: ST depression, low or negative T wave, prominent U wave, prolonged PR interval, prominent P. Severe cases may show ventricular extrasystole or fibrillation. Therapy: 1. Meet daily requirement: 2 mEq/kg/day 2. Adequate potassium replacement according to deficit Replacement: a) Deficit (mEq) × kg body wt. × 0.5 = K replacement in mEq/day or b) Set daily requirement at 4 (−6) mEq/kg
2. Extensive small bowel resection	Diminished absorption area	
3. Pseudohyperaldosteronism (Liddle syndrome)	Increased potassium and sodium exchange in the distal tubule	
4. Familial hypokalemia and -magnesemia [30]	Potassium- and magnesium-losing nephropathy	
5. Congenital chloride-losing diarrhea	Defect of intestinal chloride absorption	
6. Schwartz-Bartter syndrome	Inappropriate secretion of ADH	
7. Loss of gastrointestinal secretions (fistula, drainage)	General electrolyte losses	
8. Diuretic therapy	Increased tubular potassium secretion	
9. Conn syndrome (primary hyperaldosteronism)	See 3	

14.4 Hyperkalemia > 7 mEq/l (Table 62)

Table 62. Hyperkalemia

Etiology	Pathogenesis	Clinical picture	Therapy
1. Exchange transfusion with ACD blood > 4 days	Loss of potassium from red cells	Monitor screen shows spiked T-waves, increasing ST-depression, widened QRS complex, prolonged R-R interval	Discontinue exchange immediately, give 10% calcium gluconate, 1 ml/kg slowly IV, 10% calcium gluconate, 5 ml/kg/24 h by continuous infusion. In severe cases, calcium-resonium enema, 1 g/kg. Threat to life: 3 ml/kg Na bic. IV, even with normal pH (max. 7.5, glucose infusion with insulin; 4 g glucose: 1 IU insulin).
2. Salt-losing adrenogenital syndrome	Disturbance of steroid synthesis	Vomiting, abdominal distension, weight loss, diarrhea, apathy, hypotension, tachycardia, cyanosis, dyspnea, hyperkalemia, hyponatremia, ECG abnormalities, elevated urea and hematocrit	Correct sodium deficit by infusion therapy. Sodium replacement: 1–2 g/day as 10% NaCl by infusion or with feeds. Causal therapy with deoxycorticosterone acetate (DOCA): 2–4 mg/day in one to two doses
3. Functional renal failure	Acute renal failure (prerenal, renal)	Oliguria or anuria, possibly edema or dehydration. Elevated urea and creatinine	Correct prerenal factors (dehydration, infection) a) Shock symptoms: 20–25 ml human albumin/kg IV. After BP is stabilized (RR systolic 70–80), gradual rehydration with 150 ml/kg/24 h with daily electrolyte requirement. Beware: edema, weight. b) Antibiotic therapy if infection persists (sepsis) c) After adequate rehydration, give osmotic therapy if anuria persists: 20% mannitol, 2.0 ml/kg/dose, furosemide 1 mg/kg/dose. d) Severe hyperkalemia: calcium-resonium enema, 1g/kg e) Indication for dialysis depends on clinical signs, inc. urea > 100 mg, potassium > 6.5 mEq/L
4. Cyanotic congenital defect	Disturbance of cell membrane permeability with loss of potassium	Cyanotic neonate with refractory acidosis (pH < 7.30)	Correct acidosis a) Bicarbonate replacement b) 0.3 molar THAM replacement per infusion c) Administration of O_2
5. Excessive intake	Parenteral infusion therapy	Observed during routine electrolyte tests or from ECG changes on the monitor screen	Correct potassium intake

14.5 Hypocalcemia

Definition

Term infants	<4.0 mEq/l
Preterm infants	<3.5 mEq/l
after 2nd week of life	<4.25 mEq/l [26, 27, 35]

Etiology [15, 33]

Early onset (1st–3rd day of life)

1. Birth trauma
2. Perinatal asphyxia
3. Prematurity
4. Premature infants with RDS
5. SGA infants
6. Infants of diabetic mothers
7. Iatrogenic
   a) Sodium bicarbonate therapy (alkalosis)
   b) Exchange transfusion with ACD blood
   c) Increased free fatty acids (Intralipid)

Late onset (end of 1st and 2nd week of life)

1. Congenital hypomagnesemia with secondary hypocalcemia
2. Transient congenital hypoparathyroidism
   a) After operation or in severe infection
   b) Maternal hyperparathyroidism
   c) Maternal osteomalacia
   d) High phosphate intake (cow's milk formula)
3. Persistent idiopathic hypoparathyroidism
   a) Parathyroid hypoplasia or aplasia
   b) Thymic aplasia
4. Di George syndrome
5. Intestinal malabsorption of calcium

Pathogenesis. Neonatal hypocalcemia results from a disturbance of extrauterine calcium homeostasis due to various factors. Implicated are inadequate dietary calcium and magnesium intake, deficient gastrointestinal absorption, dietary and endogenous increase of phosphate, diminished response of renal tubules to parathormone, diminished parathyroid response to hypocalcemia, elevated calcitonin levels, and stimulation from perinatal asphyxia, as well as defects in the hydroxylation of vitamin D (liver: 25-hydroxy-vitamin D; kidney: 1.25-dehydroxy-vitamin D) [7, 9, 26, 31, 34,].

Clinical Features. General hyperexcitability: tremor, increased myoclonic activity, and hyperreactivity to external stimuli. The classic tetanic signs (Chvostek, Trousseau) are unreliable. Carpopedal spasm and laryngeal stridor are rare. Focal or generalized convulsions may be present; cardiac failure develops in some cases [12, 17].
ECG: Prolonged Q-T interval [12].
Clinical symptoms are due to the decrease in ionized calcium. Thus, hypocalcemia may occur after ACD exchange transfusion despite a normal or elevated calcium level.

Diagnosis

1. Early onset: Daily checks of calcium levels (determination of ionized calcium fraction if possible).
2. If clinical symptoms appear, also check: phosphorus, magnesium, total protein, ECG (Q-T interval)

Therapy

1. In presence of clinical symptoms: 10% calcium gluconate, 2 ml/kg over 10 min intravenously monitoring of EKG is desirable (risk of asystole; beware: digitalis therapy). Prior diagostic blood sampling.
2. In hypocalcemia without clinical symptoms or after immediate treatment: 10% calcium gluconate, 5 ml/kg/day, given slowly intravenously or spaced evenly over oral feeding regime [26]. In newborns with perinatal asphyxia, calcium can also be administered prophylactically by mouth or intravenously in the dosage indicated.
3. Persistent hypocalcemia: 10% calcium gluconate, 5 ml/kg/day, given slowly intravenously or 10% calcium gluconate or calcium chlorate, 0.5–1 (−2) g/day, given orally with feeds (hyperchloremia, risk of acidosis!).
   Change partly or completely to breast milk if circumstances warrant (reduction of phosphate intake).
   The therapeutic use of 1–25 $(OH)_3$ vitamin D_3 in neonatal hypocalcemia still requires further investigation in terms of safety and effectiveness.
4. Primary hypomagnesemia: Magnesium replacement (see p 188).

	mg calcium/1 g salt
Calcium gluconate	89
Calcium chlorate	360

14.6 Hypomagnesemia <1,2 mEq/l

Definition (atomic absorption): <1.2 mEq/l (1.2–2.1 mEq/l is normal) [5, 19]

Etiology [14, 21, 24 30, 33,]

1. Hypoparathyroidism
   a) Maternal hyperparathyroidism
   b) Familial hyperparathyroidism
   c) Parathyroid aplasia
2. Hyperphosphatemia
3. Maternal diabetes mellitus
4. Specific magnesium malabsorption
5. Extensive small bowel resection with malabsorption
6. Intrauterine dystrophy

7. Maternal hypomagnesemia
8. Exchange transfusion
9. Neonatal hepatitis, congenital biliary atresia
10. Insufficient magnesium replacement (parenteral nutrition)
11. Chlorothiazide or diphenylhydantoin therapy
12. Infusion therapy
13. Hyperthyroidism.

Pathogenesis. The biologic control of magnesium is not entirely understood. Parathormone and aldosterone are directly involved in this process, and a special tubular reabsorption mechanism has been discussed. It is also known that a complex relationship exists between magnesium and calcium [1, 20, 29].

Clinical Features. The symptoms correspond to those of hypocalcemia, and edema may also be present [10].
ECG: T-wave inversion and ST depression as opposed to the prolonged Q-T interval in hypocalcemia.

Therapy. Hypomagnesemia should be suspected whenever an infant with hypocalcemia does not respond to adequate calcium replacement. More than half of newborns with clinical symptoms (convulsions) of hypocalcemia also have hypomagnesemia [11]. Hypomagnesemia without hypocalcemia is exceptional.
Hypomagnesemia is treated with 50% magnesium sulfate, 0.1 ml/kg. The dose is repeated every 6 h. Two doses are usually sufficient to relieve the condition. The magnesium level must be checked after the second dose is given! Danger of hypermagnesemia: peripheral neuromuscular blockade with extreme muscular weakness and central depression (apnea) [8].
Long-term therapy [33]: Magnesium ascorbicum, 10–20 mg/kg/day orally (magnesium ascorbicum = 65 mg magnesium). Clinical symptoms and serial magnesium levels must be monitored during treatment.

References

1. Anonym, Neonatal calcium, magnesium and phosphorus homoeostasis, Lancet *1*, 155 (1974)
2. Aperia, A., Broberger, O., Thodenius, K., Zetterström, R.: Developmental study of the renal response to an oral salt load in preterm infants. Acta Paediatr. Scand. *63*, 517 (1974)
3. Aronson, A. S., Anderson, K. E., Berstrand, C. G., Mulder, J. L.: Treatment of diabetes insipitus in children with DDAVP, a synthetic analogue of vasopressin. Acta Paediatr. Scand. *61*, 133 (1973)
4. Aronson, A. S., Svenningsen, N. W.: DDAVP test for estimation of renal concentrating capacity in infants and children. Biol. Neonate *25*, 230 (1974)
5. Bachmann, K. D., Feenders, O., Dominick, H. Chr.: Die klinische Bedeutung des Magnesiums in der Neugeborenenperiode. Geburth. Frauenheilkd. *36*, 308 (1976)

6. Banister, A., Matin-Siddiqi, S. A., Hatcher, G. W.: Treatment of hypernatraemic dehydration in infancy. Arch. Dis. Child. *50*, 179 (1975)
7. Bergman, L.: Studies on early neonatal hypocalcemia. Acta Paediatr. Scand. suppl. 248 (1974)
8. Brandy, J. P., Williams, H. C.: Magnesium intoxication in a premature infant. Pediatrics, *40*, 100 (1967)
9. Chan, G. M., Tsang, R. C., Chen, I.-W., DeLuca, H. F., Steichen, J. J.: The effect of 1,25 (OH), vitamin D_3 supplementation in premature infants. J. Pediatr. *93*, 91 (1978)
10. Chiswick, M. L.: Association of oedema and hypomagnesaemia with hypocalcaemic tetany of the newborn. Brit. Med. J. *2*, 15 (1971)
11. Cockburn, F., Brown, J. K., Belton, N. R., Forfar, J. O.: Neonatal convulsions associated with primary disturbance of calcium, phosphorus, and magnesium metabolism. Arch. Dis. Child. *48*, 99 (1973)
12. Coletti, R. B., Pan, M. W., Smith, M. S. E., Genel, M.: Detection of hypocalcemia in susceptible neonates. N. Engl. J. Med. *290*, 931 (1974)
13. Day, G. M., Raddem, I. C., Balfe, J. W., Chance, G. W.: Electrolyte abnormalities in very low birht weight infants. Pediatr. Res. *10*, 522 (1976)
14. Engelke, St. C., Shah, B. L., Vasan, U., Raye, J. R.: Sodium balance in very lowbirth-weight infants. J. Pediatr. *93*, 837 (1978)
15. Fanconi, A.: Hypoparathyreodismus im Kindesalter. Ergebnisse d. inn. Medizin, N. F. *28*, 54 (1969)
16. Feldman, W., Drummond, K. N., Klein, M.: Hyponatremia following asphyxia neonatorum. Acta Paediatr. Scand. *59*, 52 (1970)
17. Gellis, S. S.: Editor-note. The Year Book of Pediatrics 1975, p. 57. Chicago: Year Book Medical Publishers 1975
18. Honour, J. W., Valman, H. B., Shackleton, C. H. L.: Aldosterone and sodium homeostasis in preterm infants. Acta Paediatr. Scand. *66*, 103 (1977)
19. Jukarainen, E.: Plasma magnesium levels during the first five days of life. Acta Paediatr. Scand., suppl. 222 (1971)
20. Lealman, G. T., Logan, R. W., Hutchison, J. H., Kerr, M. M., Fulton, A. M., Brown, C. A.: Calcium, phosphorus, and magnesium concentrations in plasma during first week of life and their relation to typ of milk feed. Arch. Dis. Child. *51*, 377 (1976)
21. Lombeck, I., Ritzl, F., Schnippering, H. G., Michael, H., Bremer, H. J., Feinendegen, L. E., Kosenow, W.: Primary Hypomagnesemia. Z. Kinderheilkd. *118*, 249 (1975)
22. Moshang, Th., Bongiovanni, A. M.: Endocrine disorders in the newborn. In: Neonatology, Avery, G. B. (ed.), p. 945, Lippincott: Philadelphia-Toronto 1975
23. Müller, M. U., Bierich, J. R.: Zerebraler Salzverlust als Schwartz-Bartter-Syndrom des Kindesalters. Mschr. Kinderheilk. *124*, 66 (1976)
24. Papageorgios, A. N., Moffatt, M.: Bilateral pneumonia and inappropriate secretion of antidiuretic hormone in a premature infant. CMA J. *114*, 1119 (1976)
25. Reynolds, D. W., Dweck, H. S., Cassady, G.: Inappropriate antidiuretic hormone secretion in a neonate with meningitis. Am. J. Dis. Child. *123*, 251 (1972)
26. Rösli, A., Fanconi, A.: Neonatal hypocalcaemia. „Early type" in low birth weight newborns. Helv. Paediatr. Acta *28*, 443 (1973)
27. Schweizer Neonatologie Gruppe, Diagnostische Kriterien, Bern 28. 11. 72
28. Simmons, M. A., Adcock, E. W., Bard, H., Battaglia, F. C.: Hypernatriemia and intraventricular hemorrhage in neonates. N. Engl. J. Med. *291*, 6 (1974)
29. Snodgrass, G. J. A. I., Stimmler, L., Went, J., Abrams, M. E., Will, E. J.: Interrelations of plasma calcium, inorganic phosphate, magnesium, and protein over the first week of life. Arch. Dis. Child. *48*, 279, (1973)
30. Spencer, R. W., Voyce, A.: Familial hypokalaemia and hypomagnesaemia. Acta Paediatr. Scand. *65*, 505 (1976)
31. Stern, L.: Disturbances in glucose, calcium, and magnesium homeostasis. In: Neonatology, p. 423, Avery, G. B., (ed.), Philadelphia-Toronto: Lippincott 1975

32. Thodenius, K.: Renal control of sodium homeostasis in infancy. Acta Paediatr. Scand., Suppl. 253 (1974)
33. Tsang, R. C.: Neonatal magnesium disturbances. Am. J. Dis., Child. *124*, 282 (1979)
34. Tsang, R. C., Steichen, J. J., Brown, D. R.: Perinatal calcium homeostasis: Neonatal hypocalcemia and bone demineralization. Clin. Perinatol. *4* (2), 385 (1977)
35. Usher, R. H.: The special problems of the premature infant. In: Neonatology, p. 157. Avery, G. B. (Ed.): Philadelphia-Toronto: Lippincott 1975

15 Icterus Gravis Neonatorum and Hemolytic Disease of the Newborn

L. Wille

Hyperbilirubinemia and blood group incompatibility are frequent problems in neonatology. They are of particular importance in intensive care with regard to transfusion therapy.

15.1 Definitions

a) Icterus precox
   Total bilirubin <24 h of life >7 mg%
b) Icterus gravis
   Term infants: Total bilirubin >14 mg% [28]
   Preterm infants: Total bilirubin >10 mg% [29]
c) Prolonged jaundice
   Jaundice persisting beyond the 2nd week of life

15.2 Differential Diagnosis and Diagnostic Procedure for Neonatal Jaundice [19] (Fig. 32)

15.3 Hemolytic Disease of the Newborn

This encompasses various forms of hemolytic disease in the fetus or newborn which have a similar immunologic pathogenesis [4]. The mother becomes sensitized by fetal erythrocyte antigens and manufactures antibodies (IgG) against them; these antibodies cross the placenta, causing injury to the fetus and disease in the newborn [32]. Hemolytic disease is classified, as follows, according to severity:
Mild: Anemia neonatorum (Hb <14 g%)
Moderate: Icterus gravis (bilirubin >14 g%)

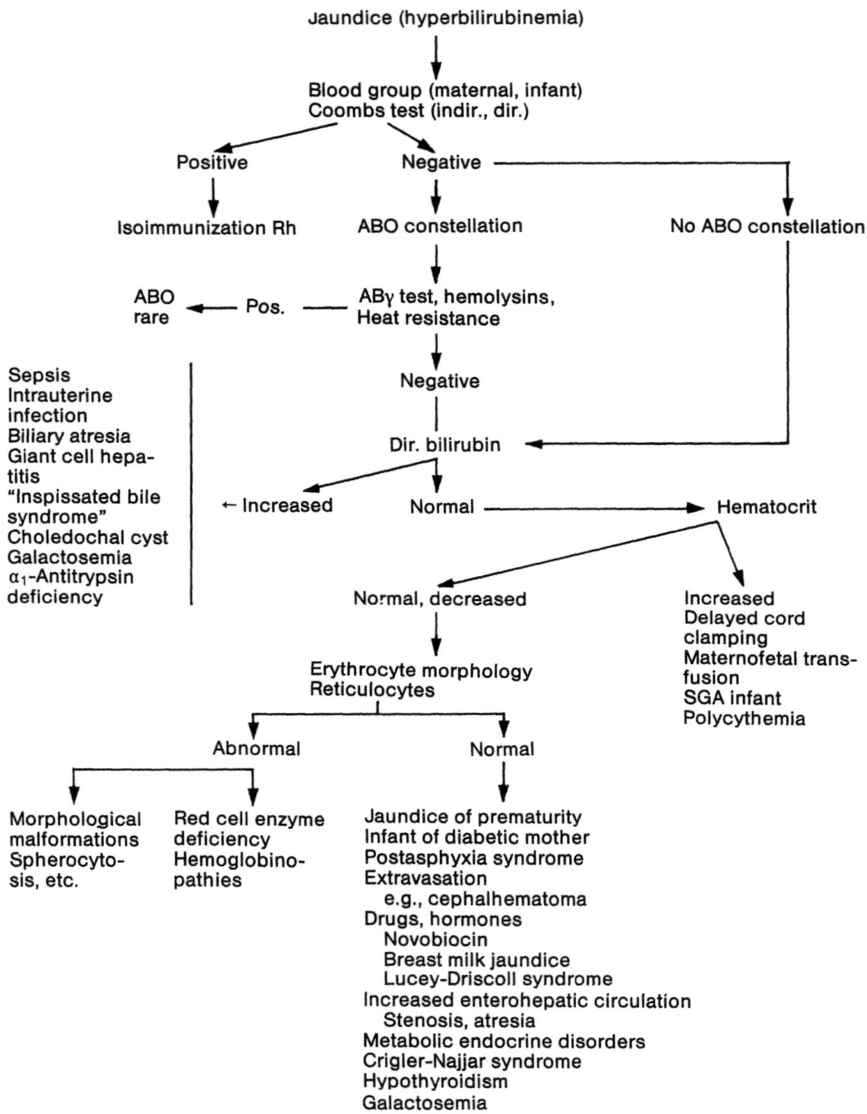

Fig. 32. Differential diagnosis of neonatal jaundice. (Modified from Maisels, 1975 [19])

Severe: Hb <9 g%

a) Anemia gravis (no edema, no ascites)

b) Prehydrops (mild edema and/or mild ascites)

c) Hydrops fetalis (severe edema, gross ascites)

In its most severe form, hemolytic disease can cause intrauterine death, kernicterus and irreversible cerebral damage. The danger lies in the development of bilirubin encephalopathy, marked by hyperexcitability, screaming, somnolence, extreme rigidity, opisthotonos, and convulsions. Mild signs of brain damage in infancy may not become apparent until the 2nd year of life or later [10].

15.3.1 Rh Erythroblastosis (Anti-D)

Diagnosis

Mother. Blood group, Rh factor, demonstration of Rh antibodies (titer).

Infant. Blood group, Rh factor, direct Coombs test, bilirubin (total, direct), blood count (Hb, erythrocytes, reticulocytes, hematocrit, platelets), total protein (albumin, globulin).

Therapy

a) Phototherapy

Considered as a primary measure only in mild cases (bilirubin <24 h <10 mg%, Hb >14 g%) [13, 17, 18], since it does not substantially reduce the number of early exchange transfusions [21, 26]. However, its use immediately after an early exchange can significantly reduce the frequency of repeat exchanges.

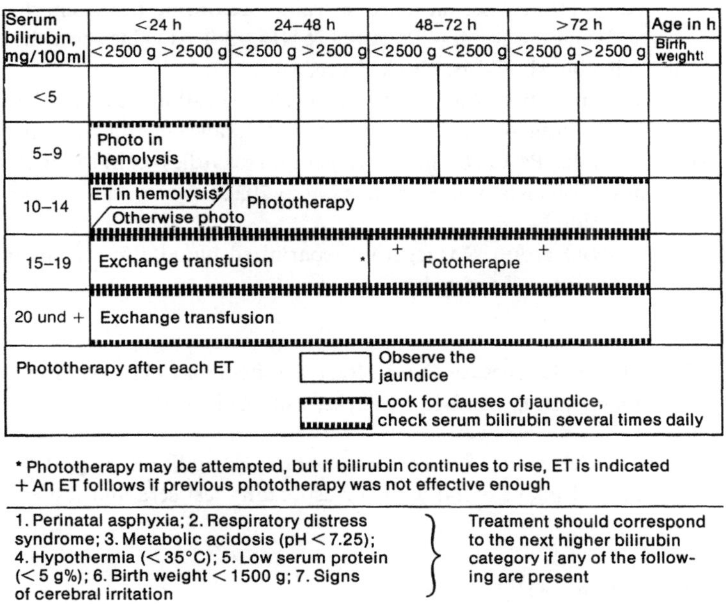

Fig. 33. Guide for the treatment of hyperbilirubinemia by phototherapy and exchange transfusion. (From Maisels, 1972 [18])

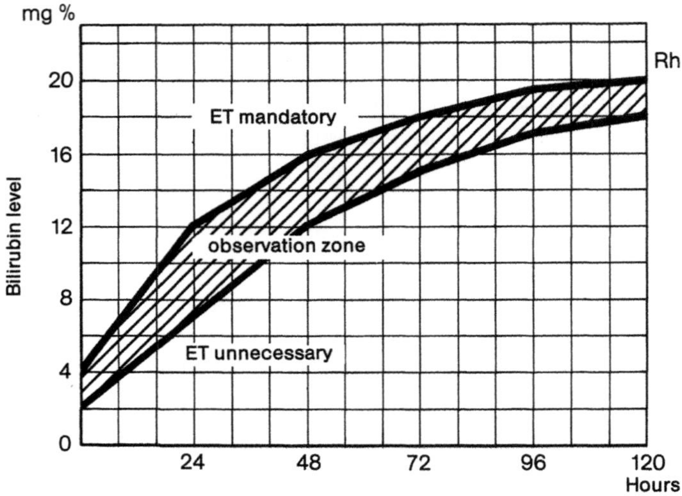

Fig. 34. Guide for assessing the need for exchange transfusion in mature infants with Rh incompatibility (from [25])

b) Indication for exchange transfusion
   Based on indirect serum bilirubin values according to the chart of Maisels [18] (Fig. 33) and the graph of Polacek [25] (Fig. 34). At values near the exchange limit, the bilirubin should be checked every 4 h

In severe form: Hb < 14 g%, immediate exchange within the first 24 h of life, preferably after the 6th hour of life due to improved tolerance (cardiorespiratory adaptation). Hydrops fetalis: Partial exchange transfusion regardless of bilirubin level immediately after initial life-sustaining measures (see p 202).

c) Donor blood
   Same ABO group, Rh negative heparinized blood, if not available ACD blood, citrate-reduced if necessary.

15.3.2 Hemolytic Disease Due to Rare Sensitizations to Blood Group Factors Other than A, B, D (Anti-C, -c, -E, -e, Anti-Kell, -Duffy)

Diagnosis. See under Rh Erythroblastosis; in addition, special serologic tests of maternal and infant blood with corresponding test sera and test eryhtrocytes.

Therapy

See under Rh Erythroblastosis.

Selection of donor blood: Selection is made by the regional blood bank based on the results of the special tests.

15.3.3 ABO Erythroblastosis

Diagnosis

Mother. Blood group, Rh factor, exclusion of Rh antibodies, ABγ test, hemolytic titration, heat resistance test.

Infant. Blood group, Rh factor, direct Coombs test, bilirubin (total, direct), blood count (Hb, erythrocytes, hematocrit, reticulocytes, platelets, microspherocytes). None of these tests excludes ABO incompatibility by a negative outcome!

Therapy

a) Phototherapy
   The treatment of choice. It is administered according to the Maisels chart [26] in Fig. 33 and the Schellong graph [27] in Fig. 35. We avoid exchange transfusions in mature newborns with a bilirubin < 14 mg% during the first 24 h of life owing to the efficacy of phototherapy. Due to the less pronounced hemolysis, early and repeat exchange transfusions can often be avoided.
b) Indications for exchange transfusion
   Based on indirect serum bilirubin according to the charts of Maisels [18] and Schellong [27]. At values near the exchange limit, the bilirubin should be checked every 4 h.

Selection of Donor Blood (Table 63):

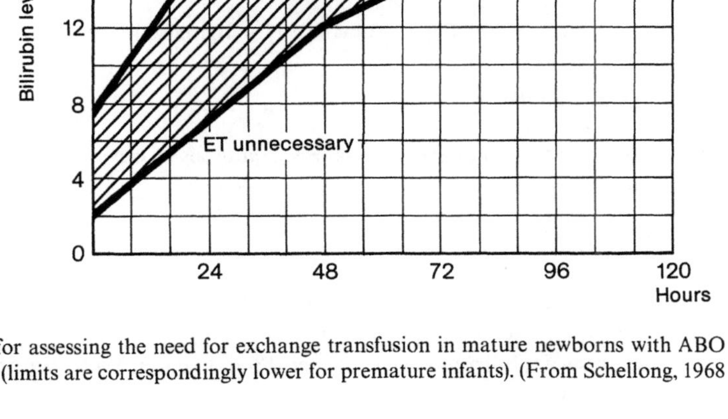

Fig. 35. Guide for assessing the need for exchange transfusion in mature newborns with ABO incompatibility (limits are correspondingly lower for premature infants). (From Schellong, 1968 [27])

Table 63. Selection of donor blood in ABO incompatibility [14]

		Mother-infant constellation		
Common		O–A	O–B	
(Rare)		B–A	A–B	A/B–AB
		Donor blood, same Rh factor		
Antigen-poor whole blood		A_2	–	–
Mixed blood	Packed red cells	O	O	A_2 or O
	Fresh plasma	A or AB	B or AB	AB
Universally or ABO-compatible whole blood (less than 5–7 days old)		O A-lysin-free, weakly A-agglutinating	O B-lysin-free, weakly B-agglutinating	Not recommended due to presence of two antibodies

15.4 Hemolytic Diseases Without Isoimmunization

(E.g., Morphological Anomalies, Hemoglobinopathies, Enzyme Defects, and Drug-Induced Defects)

Diagnosis. In addition to standard diagnostic procedures: Price-Jones curve, determination of erythrocyte osmotic fragility, hemoglobin electrophoresis, red cell enzyme studies.

Therapy. The indications for phototherapy and exchange transfusion depend on the indirect serum bilirubin level and follow the Maisels guidelines [18 (see p 193).

15.5 Hyperbilirubinemia Without Hemolysis

(Defect of Conjugation: Direct Bilirubin Not Increased)

15.5.1 Term Infants

Diagnosis. By exclusion of erythroblastosis, hemolysis of other etiology, and metabolic-endocrine disorders.

Therapy

a) Phototherapy
   In accordance with the Maisels chart [18].
b) Indication for exchange transfusion
   Based on serum bilirubin level between 18 and 20 mg% with consideration for the overall situation:

Postnatal age
Predisposing risk factors [18].

Prematurity	Hypalbuminemia
Hemolysis	Infection
Asphyxia	Drug interactions
Acidosis (pH <7.30)	Starvation
Cold stress (<36.5° C)	Elevated free fatty acids
Hypoglycemia	Cerebral alteration
Respiratory distress syndrome	

c) Selection of donor blood
Same ABO group, Rh factor.

15.5.2 Preterm Infants

Diagnosis (see 15.5.1)

Therapy

a) Phototherapy
Hyperbilirubinemia (total bilirubin >10 mg%) can be expected to appear between the 3rd and 6th day of life. In accordance with the time correlation of the indirect bilirubin level with the exchange limit, phototherapy is initiated 4 mg% below the exchange limit (Table 64). Phototherapy reduces the risk of kernicterus and the number of exchange transfusions needed [11].
b) Indication for exchange transfusion
Based on the indirect serum bilirubin, taking into account postnatal age and predisposing risk factors. Kernicterus can occur in very small preterm infants even at low bilirubin levels [1, 9].
c) Selection of donor blood
Same ABO group and Rh factor; heparinized blood, if not available citrated or citrate-reduced blood.

Table 64. Serum bilirubin levels (mg%) at which phototherapy (Photo) and exchange transfusion (ET) are indicated in nonhemolytic jaundice of prematurity [a]

	1st Day of life		2nd Day of life		From 3rd day on	
Birth weight	Photo	ET	Photo	ET	Photo	ET
2000–2500 g	10 mg%	14 mg%	11 mg%	16 mg%	12 mg%	17 mg%
1500–200 g	6 mg%	12 mg%	8 mg%	15 mg%	10 mg%	16 mg%
100–1500 g	6 mg%	10 mg%	6 mg%	13 mg%	8 mg%	15 mg%
<1000 g	4 mg%	9 mg%	6 mg%	11 mg%	6 mg%	13 mg%

[a] The indication is lowered by one level if risk factors are present (see above)

15.6 Hyperbilirubinemia in Hepatocellular or Obstructive Jaundice

(E. g., Sepsis, Intrauterine Infections, Metabolic-Endocrine Disorders, Liver Disease)

Diagnosis. By exclusion of erythroblastosis and hemolysis of other etiology. Look for congenital infection, metabolic-endocrine disorders, cystic fibrosis, α_1-antitrypsin deficiency. Determine bilirubin level (total, direct).

Therapy

a) Indication for exchange transfusion
   Based on the indirect (unconjugated) bilirubin level in accordance with the procedure for mature term and preterm infants (see p 196, 197).
b) Selection of donor blood
   Same ABO group, Rh factor.
c) Phototherapy
   Cannot be recommended due to possible complex side effects (bronze baby syndrome, hemolysis, anemia) [15, 17, 23, 27, 31].

15.7 Technique of Exchange Transfusion

1. Apparatus: Baxter-type single-use exchange transfusion set with closed cycle.
2. Route of exchange: Umbilical vein, catheterized under sterile conditions (see p 229). The catheters supplied with the exchange transfusion set have reference marks at 6, 7, and 8 cm.
   Length of catheter insertion until free blood flow is achieved:

Weight class	Catheter length	Catheter selection
>2500 g	Approx. 8 cm	Ch 8
2000–2500 g	Approx. 7 cm	
1500–2000 g	Approx. 6 cm	Ch 5
<1500 g	Approx. 5 cm	

   If the umbilical vein is unavailable, the catheter is inserted by cutdown in the femoral triangle from the great saphenous vein into the inferior vena cava.
3. Volume of exchange: The transfusion is performed with three times the infant blood volume (3 × 85 ml/kg body wt.). In this way more than 90% of the infant's blood is replaced [30].
4. Individual exchange portions:

Mature term and preterm infants	2500–2000 g:	20 ml
Preterm infants	2000–1200 g:	10 ml
Preterm infants	<1200 g:	5 ml

5. Rate of exchange: 150 ml/kg/hr = 2.5 ml/kg/min. A slow transfusion rate reduces the circulatory load, enhances the elimination of bilirubin, and avoids the side effects of citrated donor blood.
6. Calcium administration for citrated blood: 10% calcium gluconate, 3 ml/100 ml donor blood. If hypocalcemic symptoms are present, temporarily give an ad-

Table 65. Complications of exchange transfusion (modified from [22])

Vascular
Embolism (air, blood clot)
Thrombosis, portal vein stenosis
Hemorrhagic infarction of the colon
Cardiac
Arrhythmias
Hypervolemia (anemia, overload)
Asystole
Biochemical
Citrated blood (ACD)
Hypocalcemia
Acidosis
Hypochloremia
Hypomagnesemia
Hyperkalemia
Hypoglycemia
Oxygen release in tissues ↑
Heparinized blood
Hypoglycemia
Increased free fatty acids
Coagulative
Thrombopenia
Heparin overdose
Infectious
Syphilis
Cytomegaly
Transfusion hepatitis
Miscellaneous
Perforation of umbilical vein
Mechanical damage to erythrocytes
Hypothermia
Necrotic ileocolitis
Myocardial infarction

ditional 0.5–1.0 ml/100 ml donor blood. Administer by slow injection, preferably under monitor control (danger of asystole).

7. Protamine administration for heparinized blood: Roche Protamine 1000 is injected by umbilical vein catheter at the end of the transfusion (1 ml neutralizes 1000 USP units heparin): Term infant 2,5 ml, preterm infant 1,5 ml
8. Warming the blood: Frekatherm (Fresenius Co.).
9. Donor blood: Three different types of blood may be used:
   a) Heparinized blood: Maximum storage life, 24 h; for safety, should be used within 12 h after preparation if possible. Fresh blood risk! Add 100 000 U penicillin G/100 ml blood.

b) Citrated blood: Ordinary type with 20 vol.% stabilizer, with or without adenine [16]. Should be used within 5 days (hyperkalemia, diphosphoglycerate loss).

c) Citrate-reduced blood: Ordinary citrated blood with 100–150 ml supernatant plasma-stabilizer mixture removed. If more than 100 ml removed, add 20 ml 5% human albumin and 30 ml 5% glucose to balance the hematocrit.

15.8 Phototherapy

Principle. Photodegradation of indirect bilirubin in the skin and capillaries by exposure to intense light, especially at wavelengths between 420 and 480 nm (absorption peak, 460 nm; blue range of spectrum), aided by the action of singlet oxygen. The resulting bilirubin degradation products, di-, tri-, and tetrapyrroles as well as biliverdin, are nonneurotoxic, do not pass the blood-brain barrier, and are excreted in the bile as diazo-positive-reacting products and in the urine as urobilin bodies [2]. Phototherapy also enhances bilirubin excretion via the bile [24]. The efficacy of phototherapy depends upon the dose-response relationship [20]. The light energy in $\mu W/cm^2$ emitted in the blue range of the spectrum is the decisive factor. Blue fluorescent tubes (Westinghouse F20 T 12 BB) are two to three times as effective as white fluorescent tubes (Osram 20 W/10).

Indications. Phototherapy is no substitute for an indicated exchange transfusion! The points at which phototherapy is initiated and discontinued must be decided for each individual case.

a) Hyperbilirubinemia without incompatibility (see p 196)
b) Rh erythroblastosis (see p 193)
c) ABO erythroblastosis (see p 195).

Contraindications. Hemolytic disease of the newborn (Rh, ABO) with severe hemolysis (see above).
Sepsis
Hepatocellular or obstructive liver disease.

Procedure. The infant is placed unclothed into the incubator with only a diaper cloth underneath and is repositioned at 4–h intervals (supine to prone). The eyes must be well covered during phototherapy (danger of retinal damage!). Duration of treatment: 12 h of phototherapy alternating with intervals of 8 h until there is a significant fall in the indirect bilirubin (3–4 mg% below the indication limit for phototherapy). Continuous exposure is given if the values are critical or continue to rise. Phototherapy is discontinued when the indication limit for exchange transfusion is reached.
Phototherapy is done mainly with white fluorescent tubes, but blue lamps are used in severe and critical cases (monitors are required in this case due to the difficulty of visual observation). The combination of four special blue-light fluorescent tubes (Westinghouse F 20 T-BB) with four broad-spectrum fluorescent tubes (Verd-A-Ray F

20 T 12–cc) allows good clinical assessment of the infant with no significant energy loss ($\mu W/cm^2$) [8].

Special Problems

- Phototherapy reduces the degree of visible skin jaundice. The bilirubin level can no longer be estimated from the infant's appearance.
- Four-to 6-hourly checks of the bilirubin level are indicated, depending on the proximity to the exchange limit.
- The nature of the jaundice should be clarified prior to treatment.
- At least 8 h phototherapy is needed to produce a fall of bilirubin.
- A maculopapular rash may appear but is no reason to discontinue treatment.
- Loose, green stools are sometimes observed.
- Hyperthermia is possible; hence frequent checks of body temperature are required.

Complications and Risks (Table 66)

Table 66. Complications and risks of phototherapy (5, 7, 12, 22)

Humans
Diagnostic difficulties
Sepsis (blood cultures!)
Hemolysis (Hb, reticulocytes)
Cyanosis (temporarily discontinue blue light phototherapy, supervise by monitor)
Jaundice (plot bilirubin levels)
Bronze baby syndrome (in hepatic disease)
Ocular damage (cornea)
Water loss (stool, insensible perspiration)
Increased secretion of growth hormone
Development of folic acid deficiency
Hyper- or hypothermia
Absence of lactase activity
UV damage
Animals
Ocular damage (retina)
Delayed onset of sexual maturity
Abnormalities of ovulation
Increase in liver glycogen content
Increase in early bilirubin
Biorhythm disturbances
Malnutrition (shorter transit time through bowel, increased metabolism)
In vitro experiments
Decrease in bilirubin-albumin binding capacity
Differences in the in vivo and in vitro degradation products
Unknown effects on certain medications
Vitamins
Antibiotics
Reduction of oxygen
Increase in membrane permeability

15.9 Hydrops Fetalis

Differential Diagnosis (Table 67)

Table 67. Causes of hydrops fetalis (modified from [6])

1. Severe chronic intrauterine anemia
Erythroblastosis
Homozygous α-thalassemia
Chronic fetomaternal or fetofetal transfusion
2. Cardiac failure
Severe congenital defect
Premature closure of foramen ovale
Large A–V fistula (hemangioma)
3. Hypoproteinemia
Renal disease
Congenital nephrosis (renal vein thrombosis)
Congenital hepatitis
Hepatic hemangioma (Kasabach-Merritt)
4. Intrauterine infections
Syphilis
Toxoplasmosis
Cytomegalovirus
5. Miscellaneous
Maternal diabetes mellitus
Parabiotic syndrome
Sublethal umbilical or chorionic vein thrombosis
Fetal neuroblastoma
Chagas' disease
Cystic adenomatoid pulmonary malformation
Pulmonary lymphangiectasis
Dysmaturity
Cardiopulmonary hypoplasia with bilateral hydrothorax
Gaucher's disease
In situ chorionic carcinoma
Turner syndrome

Therapy

I. First minutes of life

Hypoxia	→	Central respiratory paralysis
Pulmonary edema	→	Impaired gaseous exchange
Cavitary effusion	→	Impaired diaphragmatic respiration
Hypervolemia	→	Cardiac overload.

1. Immediate section of umbilical cord
2. Suctioning, intubation (tracheal edema), controlled ventilation

3. Umbilical vessel catheterization.
4. Normalization of umbilical venous pressure to 8–10 cm H_2O (umbilical vein catheter held vertically) by initial letting of 50–70 ml blood as required (diagnostic blood sample!).
5. In life-threatening emergencies (pronounced hydrops, very severe anemia), there is no time to await the results of blood group determination and cross-matching. Immediate partial exchange transfusion with 0 Rh-neg packed red cells in AB plasma, initiated after blood-letting.
6. Buffering: 8.4% sodium bicarbonate, 3 mEq/kg/dose.
7. Digitalization: digoxin, 0.03 mg/kg/day IV in three doses.
8. Puncture of abdominal ascites, followed by slow, fractionated drainage.
9. Glucocorticoid: prednisolone, 1–2 mg/kg/dose.

II. First hours of life

Hypervolemia	→	Pulmonary edema
Impaired diuresis	→	Pulmonary edema
Hemolysis	→	Fall of Hb and erythrocytes, rise of bilirubin.

1. Check: Hb, erythrocytes, hematocrit, bilirubin (total, direct), umbilical venous pressure, blood gas analysis, thrombocytes.
2. Chest X-ray
3. If necessary, second blood-letting to normalize umbilical venous pressure
4. Continuous phototherapy with blue fluorescent tubes
5. Repeat exchange transfusion: Hb <14 g%, bilirubin level (Polacek graph)
6. Forced diuresis: Furosemide, 1 mg/kg/dose, four to six times daily
7. Adjustment of acid-base balance in accordance with blood gas analysis
8. Controlled ventilation as required.

III. 2nd-5th Day of life

Parenchymatous hemorrhage

Hemolysis

1. Replacement with plasma coagulation factors (fresh frozen plasma).
2. Repeat packed cell transfusion as required.

References

1. ACKERMAN, B. D., DYER, G. Y., LEYDORF, M. M.: Hyperbilirubinämie and kernicterus in small premature infants. Pediatrics *45*, 918 (1970)
2. BALLOWITZ, H.: Hyperbilirubinämie bei Neu- und Frühgeborenen. Paediatr. Prax. *13*, 213 (1973/74)
3. BRÜSTER, H., WIRTZ, P.: Indikation zum Blutaustausch bei Frühgeborenen. Bibl. haemat., No. 32, 324. Basel-New York, Karger 1969
4. Bundesärztekammer, Richtlinien und Informationen zur Blutgruppenbestimmung und Bluttransfusion. Wissenschaftliche Schriftreihe, Bd. 1. Köln-Berlin: Ärzte-Verlag 1968
5. DREW, J. H., MARRIAGE, K. J., BAYLE, V. V., BAJRASZEWSKI, J. M.: Phototherapy: short and long-term complications. Arch. Dis. Child. *51*, 454 (1976)
6. DRISCOLL, Sh. G.: Hydrops fetalis. N. Engl. J. Med. *275*, 1432 (1966)

7. ENTE, G., KLEIN, S. W.: Hazards of phototherapy. N. Engl. J. Med. *283*, 544 (1970)
8. FURST, E., STINTON, V. D., MOORE, F. A., HARRIS, Th. R.: An alternative phototherapy light combination. J. Pediatr. *93*, 102 (1978)
9. GARTNER, L. M., SNYDER, R. N., CHABON, R. S., BERNSTEIN, J.: Kernikterus: high incidence in premature infants with low serum bilirubin concentrations. Pediatrics *45*, 906 (1970)
10. GRÜTTNER, R.: Leberpathophysiologische Ikterusformen. In: Handbuch der Kinderheilkunde, Opitz, H., Schmid, F. (Ed.) Bd. I/2, S. 270. Berlin-Heidelberg-New York: Springer 1971
11. HOHENAUER, L., HASCHKE, F., GERSTL, J. W.: Fototherapie der Neugeborenengelbsucht. Ergebnisse der klinischen Anwendung. Klin. Pädiat. *188*, 314 (1976)
12. KALZ, M., CARIO, W.-R.: Die Phototherapie der Neugeborenen-Hyperbilirubinämie. Kinderärztl. Prax. *46*, 251 (1978)
13. KLUGE, A., GHANDI, M., WILLE, L.: Direkter Coombstest und klinische Relevanz beim Rh-Mhn. Fortschr. Trans. u. Immunhäm. *3*, 423 (1976)
14. KLUGE, A.: Persönliche Mitteilung, 1977
15. KOPELMAN, A. E., BROWN, R. S., ODELL, G. B.: The „bronze" baby syndrom: A complication of phototherapy. J. Pediatr. *81*, 466 (1972)
16. KREUGER, A. O.: Exchange transfusion with ACD-Adenin blood. A follow-up study. Transfusion, *11*, 69 (1973)
17. LUCEY, J. F.: Neonatal jaundice and phototherapie. Pediatr. Clin. North Am. *19*, 827 (1972)
18. MAISELS, M. J.: Bilirubin: On understanding and influencing its metabolism in the newborn infant. Pediatr. Clin. North Am. *19*, 447 (1972)
19. MAISELS, M. J.: Neonatal jaundice, In: Neonatology. AVERY, G. B. (ed.) p. 335. Philadelphia-Toronto: Lippincott 1975
20. MIMS, L. C., ESTRADA, M., GOODEN, D. S., CALDWELL, R. R., KOTAS, V.: Phototherapie for neonatal hyperbilirubinemia – a dose: response relationsship. J. Pediatr. *83*, 658 (1973)
21. MOLLER, J., EBBSEN, F.: Phototherapy in newborn infants with severe rhesus hemolytic disease. J. Pediatr. *86*, 135 (1975)
22. v. MURALT, G.: Neuere Aspekte der Pathogenese und Behandlungsmethoden der Hyperbilirubinämie des Neugeborenen. Paediatr. Fortbild K. Praxis *41*, 274 (1975)
23. ODELL, G. B., BROWN, R. S., KOPELMAN, A. E.: The photodynamic action of bilirubin on erythrocytes. J. Pediatr. *81*, 473 (1972)
24. ODELL, G. B., SCHAFFER, R., SIMOPOULUS, P. (ed.): Phototherapy in the newborn: An overview. National Academy of Science. Washington D. C. 1974
25. POLACEK, K.: Unser Verfahren bei der Indikationsstellung zur Austauschtransfusion. Paediatr. Paedol. *1*, 313 (1965)
26. ROTH-MAINZ, G., SCHELLONG, G.: Phototherapie bei Rh-bedingtem Morbus hämolyticus neonatorum. Mschr. Kinderheilkd. *121*, 467 (1973)
27. SCHELLONG, G.: Indikationen zur Austauschtransfusion. 2. Bremer Bluttransfusionsgespräch: 1967. „Biotest Mitt." *25*, 31 (1968)
28. SCHRÖTER, W.: Die transitorische Neugeborenenhyperbilirubinämie und ihre biochemischen Grundlagen. Ergebnisse d. inn. Medizin, N. F. *29*, 220 (1970)
29. Schweizer Arbeitsgruppe für Neonatologie. Diagnoseliste Neonatologie, August 1973
30. TROSSMAN, Ch. M., ALZOFON, F., MALKIN, H.: An exchange transfusion nomogram. Am. J. Dis. Child. *105*, 449 (1963)
31. WEITZ, R.: Das Bronze-Baby. Paediatr. Prax. *16*, 173 (1975/76)
32. WILKEN, H., ROEWER, J., EGGERS, H.: Morbus haemolyticus beim Fetus und Neugeborenen. Leipzig: Barth 1971

16 Infections

L. Wille

16.1 Prevention of Bacterial Infections [5, 14, 15, 20]:

Strict observance of hygiene:
- Delivery room
- Premature and full-term nursery
- Intensive care unit.

Appropriate measures:
Thorough hand washing, disinfection of hands and forearms
- when starting work
- when hands are dirty
- after using bathroom
- after wiping nose
- when entering or leaving a patient's room
- after attending to a patient
- after working with contaminated material.

Clean room air (air filters, laminar air flow unit)
Frequent disinfection of room
Frequent disinfection of incubator (formalin)
Incubator hygiene
Frequent change of incubator
Thorough disinfection and sterilization of instruments and equipment
Use of disposable equipment
Daily change of: humidifiers, aspiration vessels, ventilator tubing, incubator water, forceps, resuscitation instruments
Aseptic tracheal toilet with disposable catheters and gloves
Sterile preparation of infusion solutions (gown, gloves, mask, laminar air flow unit); infusion change q. 12 h
Frequent change of gown
Strict indication and sterile performance of surgical measures (intubation, umbilical vein catheterization, pleural and ascitic drainage)
Unannounced bacteriologic inspections according to specified guidelines (incubator, wash basin, infusion sets, ventilator, etc.)

Skin care
Motivation, instruction, use of specially trained personnel (hygienic nurses)
Restrictive, specific antibiotic therapy
Periodic checks of environmental microflora.

16.2 Bacteriologic Diagnosis

A thorough diagnostic study is needed to establish a bacterial infection in the neonatal period.

a) Mandatory examination on admission: Bacteriologic smears from the ear, nose, axilla, umbilicus, anus.
   In our experience the histology of the umbilical cord rarely contributes to the diagnosis.
b) Additional tests if risk factors are present:
   Blood cultures
   Differential blood count with thrombocytes
   Quantitative determination of immunoglobulins (IgG, IgA, IgM)
   Gastric aspirate: microscopic examination for leukocytes and (phagocytosed) bacteria.
c) When initial suggestive signs appear (clinical symptoms, leukopenia, leukocytosis, thrombopenia): several venous *blood cultures* are taken under sterile conditions (not from long-indwelling umbilical vessel catheters due to possible contamination and false positive results!).

Lumbar Puncture. Pandy, total protein, protein curve, differential cell count, Gram stain, culture. Cerebrospinal fluid and blood sugar simultaneously!
Bladder Puncture. Leukocytes, bacteria, culture
Stool Culture. Demonstration of enterogenic organisms
Tracheal smear on intubation (routinely twice a week)
Differential blood count with thrombocytes
Counterflow immunoelectrophoresis
Buffy-coat blood smear
Coagulation status
Bilirubin: total, direct

16.3 Sepsis [7, 11, 21, 24, 30]

Predisposing Factors
Maternal infection during last weeks of pregnancy (pyelonephritis)
Toxemia

Placenta previa
Infection of placenta, chorion
Premature membrane rupture >24 h
CTG electrode >8 h
Amnionitis
Vaginitis
Subpartal fever
Asphyxia
Umbilical vessel catheterization of long duration
Prematurity
Functional immaturity of inflammatory response (phagocytosis, opsonins, immunoglobulins).

Bacteriology

Gram-negative organisms
E. coli
Klebsiella-Aerobacter group
Serratia marcescens
Proteus mirabilis
Pseudomonas aeruginosa
Salmonellae

Fungi
Candida species

Gram-positive organisms
Staphylococcus aureus, albus
Streptococcus A–D
Diplococcus pneumoniae
Enterococcus
Listeria

Viruses
Cytomegalovirus
Rubella
Herpes simplex
Coxsackie
Echo

Clinical Features

Hyper- or hypothermia
Apathy or hyperexcitability
Respiratory difficulties (apnea, tachypnea)
Abdominal distension
Cyanosis
Jaundice, hepatosplenomegaly
Purpura, bleeding tendency
Dyspepsia or vomiting
Diarrhea and dehydration

In infections by group B streptococci, a distinction is made between a fulminant sepsis within the first 24 h of life and meningitis appearing after the 1st week of life [29]. The early form is manifested by respiratory difficulties, apneic spells, and development of pronounced shock symptoms a few hours after birth [9]. Due to the nonspecific nature of the clinical symptoms, the following must be clarified:

Respiratory distress syndrome
Pneumothorax
Developmental defect of CNS
Cerebral hemorrhage
Acidosis
Hyponatremia
Hypoglycemia
Gastrointestinal obstruction

Diagnosis (see p 206)

Typical Laboratory Findings. In early stage: Leukocytosis with left shift, followed by rapid leukopenia $<10\,000/mm^3$ [23] with polymorphonuclear neutropenia $<4500/mm^3$ [4].
From 3rd day on: Leukocytosis with or without left shift.
Thrombopenia $<100\,000/mm^3$
Normochromic anemia
Rise of direct bilirubin

Prophylaxis. Precise knowledge of maternal history during pregnancy and delivery. Assessment of existing risk factors, consideration of possible sources and avenues of infection.
Generally we do not favor antibiotic prophylaxis. However, we consider immediate antibiotic therapy to be indicated for premature rupture of membranes >24 h, subpartal fever, amniotic fluid infection syndrome as well as ascitic and pneumothoracic drainage.

Therapy
General Measures. Maintenance of neutral body temperature, antipyresis (reduction of incubator temperature, water bath, ice bag, medication)
Correction of acid-base balance
Adequate oxygenation
Production and maintenance of adequate peripheral circulation
Full oral or parenteral nutrition
Systematic incubator care
Immunglobulin (IgM): 1 ml/kg IM q. 8 days
For pronounced symptoms of shock: Exchange transfusion
For persistent hypotension: Dopamine, 4–8 γ/kg/min
Exchange transfusion with fresh blood [2].

Specific Treatment
a) When pathogen is unknown
   Ampicillin, 100 mg/kg/day IV in three doses
   Oxacillin, 50 mg/kg/day IV in three doses
   Tobramycin, 4 mg/kg/day IM in two doses
   Alternatives:
   Mezlocillin, 150 mg/kg/day IV in two doses
   Oxacillin, 50 mg/kg/day IV in three doses
   Tobramycin, 4 mg/kg/day IM in two doses
   or Cefamandol, 100 mg/kg/day IV in two to three doses
   Tobramycin, 4 mg/kg/day IM in two doses
   For severe course:
   Chlormaphenicol: For preterm infants, 25 mg/kg/day; for term infants, 50 mg/kg/day (with serum level determination where possible).

To avoid promoting the growth of "hospitalism" strains in the intensive care unit, we always employ two different antibiotic regimes concurrently in different patients.

b) After pathogen has been identified:
Treatment is administered in accordance with the sensitivity patterns. A combination of two antibiotics is preferred owing to their synergistic effect. The selection of the sensitivity patterns depends in some circumstances on the development of regional resistances in certain organisms.
Duration of treatment: 14–21 days (criteria for discontinuing therapy: absence of clinical signs, normal blood sedimentation rate).

Prognosis
Depends on organism; overall mortality is 13%–45%, incidence of late sequelae is about 22%.

16.4 Meningitis

Life-threatening disease. Mortality from coliform infections is as high as 75% [10,11,22], with frequent complication in up to 30% of cases in the early phase; about 64%–85% of survivors are left with permanent residual damage [27].

Predisposing Factors [10, 12, 27]
Prematurity
Postmaturity
Prolonged delivery
Premature membrane rupture >24 h
Subpartal fever
Toxemia
Asphyxia.

Time of Onset. The peak frequency during the neonatal period as a whole is within the first 6 days of life. The disease may appear on the 1st or 2nd day of life [12, 27].

Clinical Features. Typical symptoms (tense fontanel, screaming, opisthotonos) do not appear until the advanced stage.
The following signs are suggestive:

Respiratory difficulties
Hypo- or hyperthermia
Paucity of spontaneous movement
Reluctance to feed
Vomiting,
Sensitivity to touch
Pallor
Cyanosis
Syncope
Convulsions
Diarrhea and dehydration
Splenomegaly
Hyperbilirubinemia
Failure to gain weight

Etiologic Agents

Common gram-negative organisms:

E. coli	
Klebsiella-Aerobacter group	Shigella
Pseudomonas	Serratia
Proteus	Neisseria
Salmonellae	Bacteroides

Common gram-positive organisms:
Streptococcus A–D
Listeria
Enterococcus
Staphylococcus

Diagnosis (see p 206). By lumbar puncture (Table 68).

Therapy

a) General measures (see p 208)
b) Specific treatment (Table 69)

Adjust antibiotic therapy in accordance with the antibiogram. The advantage of treatment with two drugs lies in their syngergistic effect.

Continue treatment for at least 3–4 weeks. After 2 weeks change to Cotrimoxazol

Table 68. Cerebrospinal fluid findings in mature, healthy newborns [3]

	Age: 0–24 h	1 day	7 Days
Color	Clear or xanthochromic	Clear or xanthochromic	Clear or xanthochromic
Erythrocytes/mm^3	9 (0–1070)	23 (6–630)	3 (0–48)
Granulocytes/mm^3	3 (0–70)	7 (0–26)	2 (0–5)
Lymphocytes/mm^3	2 (0–20)	5 (0–16)	1 (0–4)
Protein (mg/100 ml)	63 (32–240)	73 (40–148)	47 (27–65)
Glucose (mg/100 ml)	51 (32–78)	48 (38–64)	55 (48–62)

In meningitis accompanied by ventriculitis, pleocytosis $\geq 200/mm^3$ [17, 19]

Table 69. Scheme for initial treatment of neonatal meningitis.

I. *Immediate treatment* until causative organism has been identified or if organism remains unknown:
   Ampicillin, 200 mg/kg/day
   Oxacillin, 100 mg/kg/day
   Tobramycin, 4 mg/kg/day

If cerebrospinal fluid is turbid, immediately administer 2 mg tobramycin intrathecally (have filled syringe ready during lumbar puncture)

(trimethoprim 7 mg/kg/day) or chloramphenicol (preterm infants: 25 mg/kg/day, term infants: 50 mg/kg/day), taking into account the antibiogram. In the presence of *E. coli* meningitis, initial treatment with chloramphenicol is preferred.

Since aminoglycosides cross poorly into the cerebrospinal fluid, the ventriculitis which usually accompanies meningitis must also be treated by intrathecal medication. Either of two methods may be used for this:

1. Suboccipital puncture and instillation (cisternal administration) [16]: More experience needed; complication rate 11.3% in skilled hands.
2. Implantation of a Salmon-Rickham reservoir (ventricular administration) [6, 19, 25]: Technical difficulties may arise during implantation. Complication rate is unclear; computerized axial tomography and neurologic observation are necessary (Fig. 36).

   We employ intraventricular therapy as an adjunct to systemic therapy.

   Daily intrathecal puncture:

a) To instill the antibiotic
b) To check the cerebrospinal fluid.

Criteria for discontinuing intrathecal therapy:

a) Zero bacterial growth in 5 successive days
b) No bacteria on Gram staining
c) Regression of inflammatory cell response (leukocytes $<200/mm^3$)
d) Ventricular cerebrospinal-fluid protein <100 mg/100 ml.

After cerebrospinal fluid findings are normalized, follow-up punctures are done in intervals of 3–10 days.

It must be noted that while concurrent systemic and lumbar therapy can somewhat reduce the mortality, they also increase the incidence of serious sequelae [18].

A diagnostic ventricular puncture is indicated 24 h after the start of therapy. In the presence of ventriculitis (leukocytes $\geq$ $200/mm^3$ and positive Gram stain and/or culture), the antibiotic should be instilled intraventricularly [6, 19, 25, 31, 32]. This requires drainage of a lateral ventricle by means of the Salmon-Rickham reservoir [26, 31].

Suboccipital and intraventricular instillations are not without risks [8, 31]; however, the high mortality and high incidence of sequelae justify active intervention [13, 25].

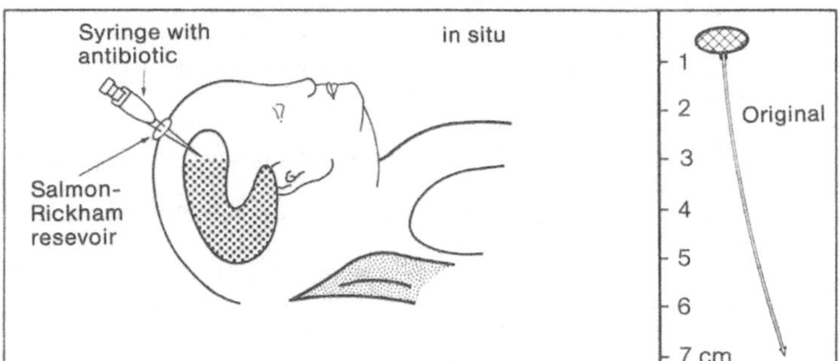

Fig. 36. The Salmon-Rickham reservoir, original and in situ. (From Salmon, 1972 [26])

The efficacy of glucocorticoids in the prevention of hydrocephalus is disputed [10]. We are of the opinion that early intensive antibiotic therapy is decisive and do not employ glucocorticoids.

Residua

Pyocephalus	Statomotor retardation
Hydrocephalus	Spasticity
Subdural hygroma	Epilepsy
Porencephally	Pathologic EEG

16.5 Intrauterine Infections

These may take the course of a severe sepsis, meningitis, or encephalitis [1, 28]. For clinical symptoms see p. 5. The following infections can occur

In utero	At delivery/postpartum period:
Rubella	Herpesvirus hominis
Cytomegalovirus	Coxsackievirus
Toxoplasmosis	Echovirus
Listeriosis	Respiratory syncytial virus
Syphilis	Streptococcus B

References

1. Alford, Ch. A., Stagno, S., Reynolds, D. W.: Diagnosis of chronic perinatal infections. Am. J. Dis. Child. *129*, 455 (1975)
2. Belohradsky, B. H., Muntean, W., Riegel, K., Marget, W.: Austauschtransfusion bei Neugeborenen-Sepsis. Monatsschr. Kinderheilkd. *125*, 590 (1977)
3. Blumenfeld, Th. A.: Appendix: Cerebrospinal fluid of healthy term newborns. In: Neonatal-Perinatal Medicine, Behrman, R. E. (Ed.), p. 940, St. Louis: Mosby 1977
4. Boyle, R. J., Chandler, B. D., Stonestreet, B. S., Oh, W.: Early identification of sepsis in infants with respiratory distress. Pediatrics, *62*, 744 (1978)
5. Daschner, F.: Krankenhauserworbene Infektionen in der Pädiatrie. Mschr. Kinderheilk. *126*, 549 (1978)
6. Davies, P. A.: Neonatal bacterial meningitis. Br. J. Hosp. Med. *18*, 425 (1977)
7. Diekmann, L., Kotzur, J.: Sepsis im Neugeborenen- und Säuglingsalter. Klin. Paediatr. *188*, 135 (1976)
8. Förster, C., Flamm, U.: Komplikationen bei intrathekaler Antibiotica-Therapie im Säuglingsalter. Mschr. Kinderheilkd. *120*, 102 (1972)
9. Hammersen, G., Bartholomé, K., Oppermann, H. C., Wille, L., Lutz, P.: Group B streptococci: A new threat to the newborn. Eur. J. Pediatr. *126*, 189 (1977)
10. Heckmatt, J. Z.: Coliform meningitis in the newborn. Arch. Dis. Child. *51*, 569 (1976)
11. Jährig, K., Dierschke, R.: Neugeborenenmeningitis und Sepsis neonatorum (Vergleichende Untersuchungen zur Ätiologie und Frühsymptomatik). Kinderärztl. Prax. *42*, 295 (1974)

12. Kaiser, E., Fülop, T., Szabo, K.: Purulent meningitis in the newborn infant. Acta. Paed. Acad. Sci. Hung. *16*, 1 (1975)
13. Kerstan, J., Wolf, H.: Die eitrige Meningitis im Neugeborenen- und Säuglingsalter. Dtsch. Med. Wochenschr. *98*, 2060 (1973)
14. Kowalewski, S.: Erreger. In: Symptomatik, Therapie und Prophylaxe der Sepsis in der Neonatologie und pädiatrischen Intensivmedizin – Rundtischgespräch. Pädiatrische Intensivmedizin. Emmrich, P. (Hrsg.) S. 170. Stuttgart: Thieme 1977
15. Kowalewski, S.: Hospitalinfektionen des Neugeborenen. In: Neugeborenen-Infektionen, Simon, C., v. Loewenich, V. (Hrsg.) S. 109. Stuttgart: Enke 1978
16. v. Loewenich, V., Knothe, H., Miething, R., Zichner, R.: Neonatal meningitis: Results of intrathecal treatment. In: Current Chemotherapy: Proceedings of the 10th International Congress of Chemotherapy, Zürich/Switzerland, Sept. 18–23, 1977, Siegenthaler, W., Lüthy, R. (Ed.), Washington: Am Soc. Microbiol. 1978
17. Lorber, J., Kalhan, S. C., Mahgrefe, B.: Treatment of ventriculitis with gentamicin and cloxacillin in infants born with spina bifida. Arch. Dis. Child. *45*, 178 (1970)
18. McCracken, G. H.: Evaluation of intrathecal therapy for meningitis due to Gram-negative enteric bacteria. Pediatr. Res. *9*, 342/516 (1975)
19. McCracken, G. H.: Intraventricular treatment of neonatal meningitis due to gram-negative bacilli. J. Pediatr. *91*, 1037 (1977)
20. Minkowski, A., Fleurquin, N. P.: Prevention of bacterial neonatal sepsis by contamination in an intensive care neonatal unit. Antibiotics Chemother. *21*, 121 (1976)
21. Nicolopoulos, D., Anagnostakis, D., Xanthou, M.: Neonatal Septicemia. Paediatrician *1*, 50 (1972/73)
22. Overall, J. C.: Neonatal bacterial meningitis. J. Pediatr. *76*, 499 (1970)
23. Pohlandt, F., Töllner, U.: Risikofaktoren, Symptome und hämatologische Befunde bei 17 Neugeborenen mit Sepsis durch Gram-negative Keime. In: Pädiatrische Intensivmedizin S. 180. Emmrich, P. (Ed.). Stuttgart: Thieme 1977
24. Quie, P. G.: Neonatal septicemia. Antibiotics Chemother *21*, 128 (1976)
25. Salmon, J. H.: Puncture Porencephaly. Am. J. Dis. Child. *114*, 72 (1967)
26. Salmon, J. H.: Ventriculitis complicating meningitis. Am. J. Dis. Child. *124*, 35 (1972)
27. Steinhoff, M., Ströder, J.: Zur Klinik der bakteriellen Meningitis im Neugeborenen- und Säuglingsalter. Klin. Paediatr. *187*, 189 (1975)
28. Stevenson, R. E.: The fetus and newly born infant: Influences of the prenatal environment. p. 159. St. Louis: Mosby 1973
29. Wannamaker, L. W., Ferrieri, P.: Streptococcal infections – up date. Disease – a – month 1–40 (1975)
30. Wilson, H. D., Eichenwald, H. F.: Sepsis neonatorum. Pediatr. Clin. North Am *21*, 571 (1974)
31. Wolf, H., Kerstan, J.: Neugeborenenmeningitis, kompliziert durch „Ventrikulitis". Mschr. Kinderheilkd. *122*, 402 (1974)
32. Yeung, C. Y.: Intrathecal antibiotic therapy for neonatal meningitis. Arch. Dis. Child. *51*, 686 (1976)

17 Hematologic Disease

L. Wille

17.1 Anemia

Definition [10, 14]
0–48 h postpartum: Hb < 16 g%
49 h–7th day of life: Hb < 14.5 g%
After first week of life: Hb < 10 g%
These determinations are made in capillary blood taken from the warmed heel of newborn infants (> 34 weeks gestation).

Etiology [10]
1. Occult prenatal bleeding
   Fetomaternal transfusion
   Spontaneous
   Traumatic amniocentesis
   Following external cephalic version
   Fetofetal transfusion
2. Obstetric complications
   Umbilical cord rupture
   Precipitous delivery
   Entanglement
   Hematoma of cord or placenta
   Rupture of malformed cord
   Varices
   Aneurysms
   Rupture of anomalous vessels
   Velamentous insertion
   Communicating vessels in multilobed placenta
   Aberrant vessel
   Unusual bleeding from:
   Placental incision during cesarean section
   Placenta previa
   Abruptio placentae
   Internal hemorrhage
      Intracranial

Retroperitoneal
Intraabdominal (rupture of liver or spleen)
Cephalhematoma
Caput succedaneum.

Differential Diagnosis and Diagnostic Procedure [9]. The differential diagnosis of neonatal anemia is often a difficult matter. A systematic procedure is necessary, and rapid treatment is often required.
Before replacement therapy is begun, blood samples (whole, citrated) must be taken and suitably stored for further diagnostic tests (hemorrhagic disease of the newborn, congenital infections, hemoglobinopathies, red cell enzyme defects). In many cases the final diagnosis cannot be made until infancy (e. g., after blood transfusion or exchange).

Clinical Features.
1. Acute hemorrhage
General pallor, tachypnea, or gasping respiration, tachycardia, weak or impalpable peripheral pulse, low or immeasurable blood pressure, low central venous pressure, shock, centralization, no hepatomegaly; occasionally stillbirth from severe intrauterine blood loss, serum iron normal.
2. Chronic blood loss
Pallor with undiminished vitality, occasional cardiac failure with hepatomegaly, hypochromic, microcytic anemia. Normal or raised central venous pressure, serum iron decreased.
3. Internal blood losses
Anemia usually within the 1st day of life, gradual fall of hemoglobin, development of shock symptoms (e. g., rupture of liver).

Therapy. Depends on the degree of anemia and the acuity of the loss.
1. Proper resuscitation postpartum, in particular, good oxygenation.
2. Diagnostic blood sampling (umbilical vein): Hb, erythrocytes, hematocrit, blood typing, cross-matching.
3. Shock or severe anemia: See under Hypovolemic Shock.
4. Mild anemia with no clinical symptoms: Transfusion unnecessary; ferrotherapy (started in 6th week of life): 2 mg/kg in two doses for 3 months.
5. Iatrogenic anemia: Frequent blood samples under intensive care. Correction of anemia is particularly important in infants with respiratory distress. It is possible for a normoxemic metabolic acidosis to develop [2].
   Indications for transfusion: hemoglobin <16 g%
   hematocrit $<45\%$.

Determining the volume of a blood transfusion [8]:
3 ml packed red cells or 6 ml whole blood/kg body wt. raises the hemoglobin concentration by 1 g/100 ml:
Hb deficit (g%) $\times$ 3(ml) $\times$ kg body wt. = replacement volume (packed red cells).

17.2 Hypovolemic Shock

Etiology. Frequently acute perinatal blood losses (see above) or sudden postnatal hemorrhage (e.g., umbilical artery catheter).

Clinical Features. A hemorhage is always an emergency!
Centralization, shock. First, a disturbance of the macrocirculation (failure of vascular regulation), followed by impairment of the microcirculation with metabolic decompensation (cardiac failure) [5].
Tachypnea, pallor, cyanosis, irregular spontaeous breathing, metabolic acidosis, brady- or tachycardia, low central venous pressure. Anemia may be absent initially but develop in time.

Supervision
Blood count, hematocrit
Blood pressure, central venous pressure
Respiration, heart rate
Blood gases

Therapy [5, 6, 11–13]
1. Proper resuscitation and good oxygenation (see p 8). Diagnostic blood samples (umbilical vein): Hb, erythrocytes, hematocrit, blood typing, cross-matching.
2. Volume replacement:
   a) Correction of acidosis: 8,4% sodium bicarbonate (1 ml = 1mEq), 3 ml/kg, with equal amount of 5% glucose IV (peripheral vein, umbilical vein)
   b) Infusion of a rapidly available volume expander: 20 ml/kg over 2–5 min of:
      - Universal blood (O Rh neg. red cells in AB plasma)
      - Plasma
      - 5% human albumin (favorable effect on O_2 transport capacity)
      - Dextran 60 (rapid relief of shock-related metabolic disorders, improvement of O_2 transport capacity and blood flow properties)
      - Dextran 40 Na-free (potent plasma-expanding action, preparation with equal volume of 5% glucose).
3. For bradycardia (< 50/min): 0.1 mg orciprenaline (= 0.2 ml)/dose IV or intracardially as required.
4. Emergency treatment is followed by further volume replacement after hematologic findings are obtained (Hb, erythrocytes, hematocrit) in accordance with serologic studies (blood group, direct Coombs test; watch for blood group incompatibility!).

Formula:
Hb deficit (g%) × 6 (ml) × kg body wt = replacement volume (ml whole blood).

17.3 Polycythemia

Definition

Hematocrit > 65% } venous blood samples
Hemoglobin > 22 g% }

during the 1st week of life.

Etiology [4,9]

Placental hypertransfusion
- Fetofetal
- Maternofetal
- Placentofetal

Placental dysfunction
- SGA infants
- Postmature infants
- Toxemia of pregancy
- Placenta previa

Endocrine or metabolic diseases
- Congenital adrenal cortical hyperplasia
- Neonatal thyrotoxicosis
- Maternal diabetes mellitus
- Trisomy D
- Oligohydramnios
- Beckwith-Wiedemann syndrome

Pathogenesis. A venous hematocrit >65% leads to a considerable increase in blood viscosity, impairs the flow properties of the blood, reduces tissue oxygenation, and can cause microemboli [1, 3, 7].

Clinical Features. Respiratory difficulties, cyanosis, apathy, hyperexcitability, tetany, convulsions, cardiomegaly, cardiac failure, vomiting, oliguria, renal vein thrombosis, priapism.
Laboratory findings: Hyperbilirubinemia, hypocalcemia, hypoglycemia, transient thrombocytopenia, increased blood viscosity, thrombocytopenia, erythroblasts, acidosis, hypoxia.

Therapy. Treatment of hypoglycemia, hypocalcemia, hyperbilirubinemia. Specific therapy is not necessary until clinical symptoms appear, generally at a hematocrit >70%. Exchange transfusion with plasma of infant blood group or 5% human albumin.

Goal. Reduction of the venous hematocrit (HC) to 60%.

Formula [9]: $\frac{\text{Blood volume} \times (\text{actual HC} - \text{desired HC})}{\text{actual HC}} = \text{exchange volume (ml)}$

Blood volume of a newborn infant: (85)–100 ml/kg body wt.
Proceed as in exchange transfusion (see p 198), with individual portions of 10 ml. Normalization of the hematocrit and blood viscocity leads to a regression of symptoms in 8 h–3 days [7]. Fluid supplementation has no effect on clinical symptoms or blood viscosity [7].

References

1. Bergqvist, G.: Viscosity of the blood in the newborn infant. Acta Paediatr. Scand. *63*, 858 (1974)
2. Duc, G.: Behandlung der neonatalen Hypoxie. Peadiatr. prax. *15*, 107 (1975)
3. Gross, G. P., Hathaway, W. E., McGaughey, H. R.: Hyperviscosity in the newborn. J. Pediatr. *82*, 1004 (1973)
4. Kontras, St. B.: Polycythemia and hyperviscosity syndromes in infants and children. Pediatr. Clin. North Am. *19*, 919 (1972)
5. Lemburg, P.: Schockbekämpfung. In: Therapie der Krankheiten des Kindes v Harnack, G.-A. (Ed.). Berlin-Heidelberg-New York: Springer 1976
6. Löwenich, v V.: Volumenersatz beim Neugeborenen. In: Pädiatrische Intensivpflege. 3. Symposium in München 1972. Klin. Pädiatr. Beih. 70, p. 32, Stuttgart: Enke 1973
7. MacIntosh, T. F., Walker, C. H. M.: Blood viscosity in the newborn. Arch. Dis. Child. *48*, 547 (1973)
8. Mollison, P. L.: Blood transfusion in clinical medicine. 3rd ed. p. 614. Oxford: Blackwell 1961
9. Oski, F. A., Naiman, J. L.: Hematologic problems in the newborn, p. 54. Philadelphia-London-Toronto: Saunders 1972
10. Oski, F. A.: Hematologic Problems. In: Neonatology. Avery, G. B. (Ed.) p. 379. Philadelphia-London: Lippincott 1975
11. Paxson, Ch. L.: Neonatal shock in the first neonatal day. Am. J. Dis. Child. *132*, 509 (1978)
12. Ranke, M., Meyer, H., Lemburg, P., Sprock, I.: Veränderungen des zentralvenösen Drucks bei vital gefährdeten Neugeborenen unter Einfluß des Säurebasenhaushalts und der Schocktherapie. In: Pädiatrische Intensivpflege 3. Symposium in München 1972, S. 48. Klin. Pädiatr. Stuttgart: Enke
13. Schöber, J. G.: Pharmaka beim Schock des Neugeborenen. In: Pädiatrische Intensivpflege 3. Symposium in München 1972, S. 35. Klin. Pädiatr. Beih. 70., Stuttgart: Enke 1973
14. Schweizer Neonatologie-Gruppe, Diagnostische Kriterien. Bern, 28. 11. 72

18 Blood Coagulation and Hemorrhagic Diatheses

L. Wille

The various forms of hemorrhage are manifested in 3% of all newborns. They can be severe and are often life threatening. One-third are caused by a defect of blood coagulation [4].

18.1 Blood Coagulation

Blood Coagulation normally occurs more rapidly in infants than in adults. Some factors are present in the cord blood in adequate amounts, while others are deficient (Table 70).

Table 70. Normal values for coagulation factors [11]

	Adults	Term infants (cord blood)	Preterm infants (cord blood)
Fibrinogen (mg%)	200–400	200–250	200–250
Factor II (%)	50–150	40	25
Factor V (%)	75–125	90	60–75
Factor VII (%)	75–125	50	35
Factor VIII (%)	50–150	100	80–100
Factor IX (%)	50–150	25–40	25–40
Factor X (%)	50–150	50–60	25–40
Factor XI (%)	75–125	30–40	–
Factor XII (%) (titer)	75–125	50–100	50–100
Factor XIII (titer)	1 : 16	1 : 8	1 : 8
Time (s)	30–50	70	80–90
Prothrombin time (s)	10–12	12–18	14–20
Thrombin time (s)	10–12	12–16	13–20

Presumably the "fetal" fibrinogen, with its increased thrombin sensitivity, balances out the deficiency of certain coagulation-promoting factors during the clotting process [5, 7, 8]. A similar situation is found in the fibrinolytic system: Increased fibrinolysis with decreased plasminogen and increased activity of the plasminogen activators balances potential deficiencies during the neonatal period. Fibrinogen degradation products can often be demonstrated. The increased activity of the fibrinolytic system appears to represent a logical counterbalance to the hypercoagulability [5, 7, 8].

18.2 Diagnosis [1–3, 10, 13]

History
Family pedigree
Familial bleeding tendency
Known hereditary defect
Maternal disease (e. g., infection, Werlhof's disease)
Drug therapy (maternal, neonatal)
Vitamin K administration

Clinical Features
- Sick neonate: acidosis, hypoxia, hypothermia, sepsis (disseminated intravascular coagulation)
- Severe hepatic disease: hepatomegaly, increase in transaminases and direct bilirubin (production coagulopathy)
- Apparently well neonate: vitamin K deficiency, congenital coagulopathy (hemophilia), thrombocytopenia or -pathy.

Laboratory Findings (Table 71)

An exact diagnosis is essential for specific, effective treatment! Final clarification may require thrombin time, reptilase time, determination of individual plasma factors, TEG, ethanol gel test, latex particle test, euglobulin lysis time, blood smear.

Table 71. Diagnostic procedure for unexplained neonatal bleeding

Outcome of general tests	Differential diagnosis	Further diagnostic procedures
Thrombocytopenia PT normal PTT normal	See under Thrombocytopenia	
Thrombocytes normal PTT normal PT normal	Congenital factor XIII deficiency Platelet dysfunction von Willebrand's disease	Factor XIII determination, bleeding time Thromboelastography; maternal and infant medications?
Thrombocytes normal PT prolonged PTT normal	Congenital deficiency of factors II, VII	Factor determination
Thrombocytes normal PT normal PTT prolonged	Congenital deficiency of factors VIII, IX, XI, XII von Willebrand's disease Heparin therapy	Factor determination

Table 71. (Continued)

Thrombocytes normal PT prolonged PTT prolonged	Vitamin K deficiency Complex defect of production	1 mg/kg Konakion IV; Repeat PT and PTT after 4 h: bleeding stops, PT and PTT normal Diagnosis: vitamin K deficiency
Continued bleeding PT prolonged PTT prolonged	Congenital deficiency of factors V, X Congenital afibrinogenemia Severe hepatopathy	Factor determination Fibrinogen determination
Thrombocytopenia Pt prolonged PTT prolonged	Consumption coagulopathy	Thrombin time, fibrin degradation products, factor V determination, fragmentocytes Factor determination

18.3 Coagulopathies

18.3.1 Congenital Coagulopathies

The coagulation factors are unable to cross the placenta. Nevertheless, genetically determined coagulation defects rarely cause bleeding during the first weeks of life. They are, however, amenable to diagnosis in the neonatal period [1–3, 10].

Suggestive Signs. Family history (hemophilia A, B, von Willebrand's disease, factor XI defect) (Table 72).

Table 72. Genetically determined coagulopathies [10]

Sex-linked recessive
Hemophilia A
Hemophilia B
Autosomal dominant
Factor XI (PTA) deficiency
von Willebrand's disease
Autosomal recessive
Prothrombin deficiency
Factor V (proaccelerin) deficiency
Factor VII (proconvertin) deficiency
Factor X (Stuart-Prower) deficiency
Factor XII (Hageman) deficiency
Factor XIII (fibrin stabilizing factor) deficiency
Afibrinogenemia, congenital

Clinical Features. Prolonged bleeding after capillary puncture or circumcision, bleeding from umbilical cord, cerebral hemorrhage, intramuscular hematoma, rarely hemarthrosis.

18.3.2 Acquired Coagulopathies

Hemorrhagic Disease of the Newborn in the Strict Sense (Vitamin K Deficiency). Can affect newborns with hepatopathy, on breast milk, or on long-term parenteral nutrition (deficient replacement), or the infants of mothers with malnutrition or anticonvulsive therapy (phenytoin, primidone).

Clinical Features. Prolonged bleeding on 2nd or 3rd day of life following capillary puncture or circumcision, cephalhematoma, umbilical-cord or internal bleeding (hematemesis, melena).

Prophylaxis. Phytomenadion (vitamin K_1) 1 mg/kg IM in all high-risk and premature infants.

Therapy

a) Phytomenadion (Vitamin K_1), 2–5 mg IV (beware intramuscular injection).
b) Replacement therapy for extensive bleeding and severe factor deficiency: PPSB (II, VII, IX, X). Dosage: necessary units (factor IX) = $0.6 \times \text{kg} \times$ desired increased (percent of norm). (Concentration of factor IX is preparation and batch dependent.)

Production Coagulopathy in the Broader Sense. In severe liver disease, the coagulation defect goes beyond a deficiency of vitamin K-dependent factors.

Clinical Features. Hepatomegaly, increase of transaminases and direct bilirubin, generalized hemorrhagic diathesis which is unresponsive to vitamin K therapy. Hepatomegaly may be the only early sign.

Therapy. Fresh plasma (frozen) 10 mg/kg body wt.

Consumption Coagulopathy

Etiology

Obstetric complication (e.g., abruptio placentae, dead twin).
Neonatal infections
Various conditions (e.g., acidosis, hypoxia, shock, hemangioma).

Forms [6]

Disseminated intravascular coagulation
Localized thrombosis of large vessels (e.g., renal vein)
Organ-limited intravascular coagulation (hemolytic-uremic syndrome, necrotizing enterocolitis)
Disseminated intravascular thrombocytic microthrombosis.

Clinical Features. Clinical symptoms are not always present. In severe cases, extensive hemorrhage. Seriously ill newborns with symptoms of the primary disease (infection, asphyxia, shock). Petechiae, ecchymoses, skin hemorrhages, pallor, oliguria, peripheral ischemia.
Increased intravascular coagulation, microthromboses in the terminal vessels, exhaustion of coagulation potential.

Therapy

a) General
   Treatment of the primary disease (sepsis, asphyxia, shock)
b) Specific
   Replacement
   Platelet concentrate: 1 (30 ml)–2 q. 12 h
   Fresh plasma (frozen): 10–15 ml/kg q. 8–12 h.
   Based on our experience this will not worsen the consumption coagulopathy. If the primary disease persists, however, these measures will bring only temporary clinical improvement.

Exchange transfusion (see p 198) = fresh blood (ACD, heparinized):
Detoxification (accumulated metabolites, fibrin degradation products, bacteria)
Restoration of coagulation potential (factors, platelets)
Heparin therapy:
Its value in the newborn is disputed [1, 3]. Although the use of heparin is reasonable in theory, the dosage and response vary widely and are difficult to control. Heparin therapy cannot significantly influence the progress of disseminated intravascular coagulation, because often the process has already begun in utero [9]. Furthermore, few studies have been done on the pharmacokinetics of heparin in seriously ill newborns.

Indication. Consumption coagulopathy with predominant thrombosis.

Dosage. Fifty units/kg IV initially, followed by continuous infusion with 350 units/kg/day [9, 12]. Close supervision of the infant's coagulative status is necessary to achieve an optimal therapy adapted to the individual (thrombin time, 50–60 s).

Decrease of the coagulation potential in coagulopathies (Fig. 37).

18.4 Thrombocytopenia

Definition

Platelet count $<100\,000/mm^3$
Most cases of thrombocytopenia are immune-related or are caused by infection. Due to the unavailability of routine serologic tests for diagnosing immune-related disorders, the diagnosis of neonatal thrombocytopenia often remains unclarified.

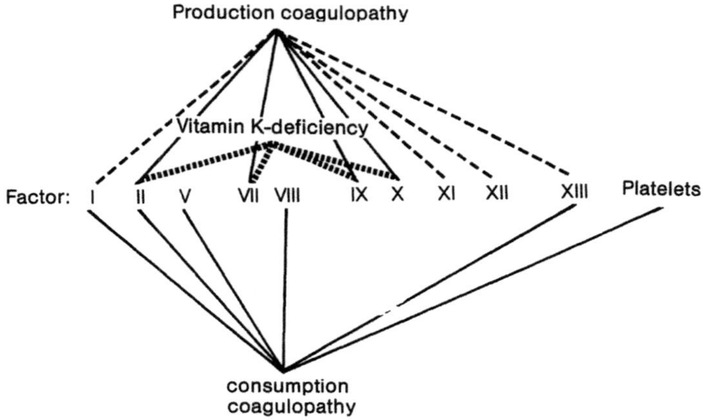

Fig. 37. Decrease of the coagulation potential in coagulopathies

Clinical Features.
Cutaneous petechiae, purpura-like, macular rash of ecchymoses, which are generalized and may run a cyclic course during the first days of life.
Bleeding is seen only in cases of associated coagulopathy or at platelet counts $<30\,000/mm^3$.

Table 73. Differential diagnosis of thrombocytopenia [10]

	Maternal platelet count	
Subnormal 1. Werlhof's disease, SLE 2. Drug-induced purpura Genetically determined thrombocytopenia	Normal	
	Neonatal examination	
a) Normal 1. Isoimmune purpura 2. Thiazide drugs, tolbutamide 3. Genetically determined thrombocytopenia 4. Congenital aplastic anemia 5. Aminoaciduria (e. g., methylmalonic aciduria)	b) Hepatosplenomegaly 1. Infections Bacterial sepsis, congenital syphilis, disseminated herpes, cytomegaly, rubella syndrome, congenital toxoplasmosis 2. Congenital leukemia	c) Congenital anomalies 1. Giant hemangioma 2. Rubella syndrome 3. Radial aplasia 4. Trisomy syndromes (D, E)

18.5 Thrombocytopathy

Etiology
Thrombasthenia
von Willebrand's disease
Thrombopathy of obscure etiology

Diagnosis. Platelet count normal, only the bleeding time is prolonged. In von Willebrand's disease, combined with factor VIII or IX defect. Platelet function test [13].

Clinical Features. Ecchymoses and bleeding in the region of the parenchymatous mucous membranes.

Treatment of Thrombocytopenia and Thrombocytopathy
1. Treatment of primary disease (infection)
2. Active intervention is necessary only if there is a risk of hemorrhage (trauma, operation, intubation, acidosis, hypoxia) or manifestations of hemorrhage.
   a) Immune-related thrombocytopenia: Exchange transfusion followed by transfusion of washed maternal platelets.
   b) Other thrombocytopenias: Transfusion of platelet concentrate:
      Term infants: One platelet concentrate (30 ml)
      Preterm infants: 10 ml/kg body wt.
3. von Willebrand's disease: Replacement of factor XIII or IX. Factor concentration is preparation and batch dependent.
   Formula: Desired blood concentration in % × kg body wt. × 0.6.
4. In less threatening immune-related thrombocytopathies, treat with glucocorticoids: 2 mg/kg orally.

References

1. BUCHANAN, G. R.: Neonate coagulation: normal physiology and pathophysiology, Clin. Haematol. 7 (1), 85 (1978)
2. Editorial: Bleeding in the newborn. Br. med. J. *2*, 915 (1977)
3. GLADER, B. E., BUCHANAN, G. R.: The bleeding neonate. Pediatrics *58*, 548 (1976)
4. GUGLER, E.: Blutgerinnungsstörungen beim Neugeborenen. Paediatr. Fortbild K. Praxis *41*, 262 (1975)
5. HATHAWAY, W. E.: Coagulation problems in the newborn infant. Pediatr. Clin. North Am. *17*, 929 (1970)
6. HATHAWAY, W. E.: The bleeding newborn. Clin. Perinat. *2*, 83 (1975)
7. KÜNZER, W.: Die Blutgerinnung bei Neugeborenen und ihre Störungen. Klin. Wochenschr. *49*, 1 (1971)
8. KÜNZER, W.: Dringliche Therapie beim Neugeborenen. Arch. Gynaekol. *214*, 337 (1973)

9. Maak, B., Frenzel, J.: Ergebnisse der Heparinprophylaxe intervasaler Gerinnungsvorgänge bei mindergewichtigen Neugeborenen. Kinderärztl. Praxis *44*, 56 (1976)
10. Oski, F. A., Naiman, J. L.: Hematologic problems in the newborn. In: Major problems in clinical pediatrics. Schaffer, A. J. (Ed.). p. 236. Philadelphia-London-Toronto: Saunders 1972
11. Oski, F. A.: Hematologic problems. In: Neonatology. Avery, G. B. (Ed.) p. 379. Philadelphia-Toronto: Lipincott 1975
12. Rogner, G.: Untersuchungen zum Heparinspiegel während gerinnungshemmender Therapie bei reifen und unreifen Neugeborenen. Kipra *44*, 193 (1976)
13. Sutor, A. H.: Diagnostik der Blutgerinnungsstörung in Klinik und Praxis. Monatschr. Kinderheilkd. *126*, 588 (1978)

Part IV
Appendix

19 Techniques of Neonatal Intensive Care

L. Wille

General. The techniques described here require a strict aseptic procedure:
1. Wearing of mask, cap, gown, and sterile gloves
2. Thorough washing of hands and forearms
3. Careful cleansing and disinfection of the operative area
4. Covering of other body parts with sterile drapes
5. Aseptic working technique, avoiding contact with unsterile surfaces or instruments.

The use of ready-to-use prepacked catheter material can further reduce the risk of infection.

19.1 Umbilical Vessel Catheterization (Fig. 38)

The introduction of a central catheter through the umbilical vessels is a procedure employed in the intensive management of life-threatened newborns [17]. Its indication must always be weighed against the risk of serious complications. The technical facilities necessary for atraumatic cannulation, catheter supervision, and constant perfusion must be available [18].

The sooner catheterization is undertaken after delivery, the easier it is to cannulate the vessels and the lower the risk of infection. It is advantageous to perform the procedure on a resuscitation table with good lighting, servo temperature control, facilities for oxygen administration and controlled ventilation, and monitoring equipment.

Indications
1. Frequent arterial blood gas determinations ($FiO_2 > 0.21$, CPAP, controlled ventilation). Consider peripheral arterial puncture or cannulation as alternative ($TcPO_2$ adequate?).
2. Exchange transfusion
3. Continuous recording of arterial blood pressure or central venous pressure (hydrops, operation)
4. Angiography.

19.1.1 Umbilical Vein Catheterization

Principle. Introduction of a catheter into the umbilical vein through the ductus venosus and into the inferior vena cava. The umbilical vein is easily accessible during

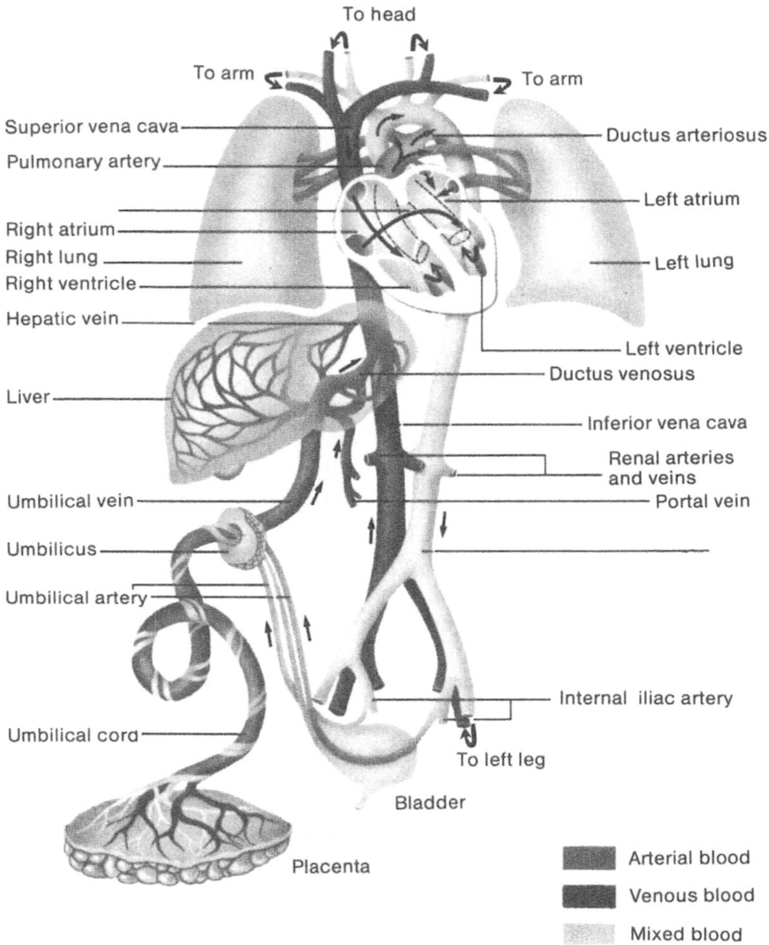

Fig. 38. The fetal circulation

the first 5 days of life, but can sometimes be catheterized up to the 14th day as well, after careful preparation, identification, and removal of intravascular thrombi (beware: thromboembolism).

Technique. Under optimal illumination, place and immobilize the infant in a supine position. Disinfect the cord stump and surrounding abdominal skin. Cut cleanly across the cord 0.5–1.0 cm from the skin. Have dissecting forceps ready in case of bleeding. It can be controlled immediately by grasping the cord stump. Redisinfect the exposed cord remnant. Drape surrounding abdominal skin with slit cloth and other body parts with sterile towels. To expose the vessels, spread the cord stump open with two surgical forceps. If the stump is mummified or badly crushed peripherally, resect until clean tissue is reached.

Localization. The umbilical vein is the largest of the three vessels. It is thin-walled, usually flattened (presenting a slit-shaped lumen), and uncontracted. It is generally located in the sector between 11 : 00 and 2 : 00 on the cut surface of the cord stump (Fig. 39 a–c). Its lumen usually remains open when spread apart. Remove thrombi and residual blood with surgical forceps. Identify the course of the vein by inserting a bulb-headed probe cranialward at an angle of about 60° to horizontal. Insert the umbilical vein catheter, filled with 0.9% NaCl (Argyle Ch 5 for term infants, Ch 3.5 for preterm infants < 1500 g), with syringe attached, applying a slight negative aspiration pressure until blood is obtained. The catheterization proceeds more smoothly if caudal traction is exerted on the cord stump with a surgical forceps. Resistance to advance of the catheter indicates malplacement in the portal fissure. Withdraw the catheter by 1–2 cm, then readvance; this sometimes succeeds in redirecting the catheter into the ductus venosus. If this is unsuccessful, the catheter must be withdrawn to about 2 cm in front of the obstruction.

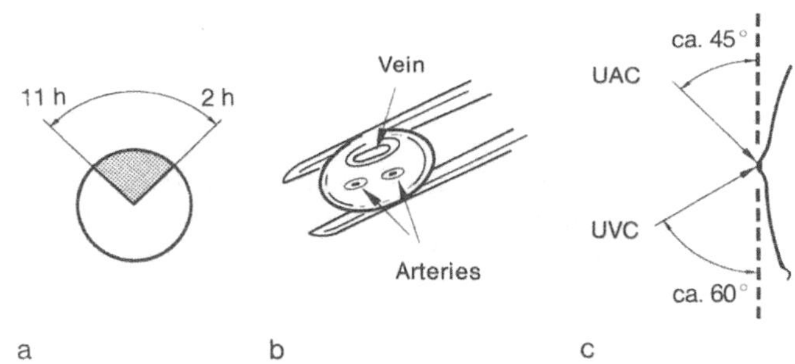

Fig. 39 a–c. Position, characteristics, and angle of insertion of umbilical vein and artery catheters

The correct catheter position is 1 cm above the diaphragm [16]:

Weight class	Length of insertion
< 1000 g	6 cm
1000–1500 g	7 cm
1500–2000 g	8 cm
2000–2500 g	9 cm
> 2500 g	10–12 cm

Advantages. Good dilution of medications and hyperosmolar solutions by the high blood flow. Allows measurement of central venous pressure.

Disadvantage in Case of Malplacement. Infusion of hyperosmolar solution poses risk of hepatic necrosis, portal vein thrombus formation and, eventually, portal hypertension [15, 26]; uncertain measurement of venous pressure [17].

Fixation by purse-string or Z-suture with an extra loop around the catheter. The catheter is marked with *blue* adhesive tape. The placement must be checked by X-ray, since malplacement is common [16, 28].

Removal of Catheter. Fixation is removed, followed by careful withdrawal. Bleeding is stopped by applying a fibrin plate and sterile pressure dressing; suturation may be necessary.

Complications [15, 17, 18, 26, 33]
Inadvertant catheterization of an umbilical artery
Portal hypertension
Functional catheter obstruction
Malplacement in the portal fissure
Liver cell necrosis
Perforation of liver parenchyma
Apnea
Cardiac arrest
Sepsis
Intravascular thrombus formation
Embolism
Esophageal varices
Conduction of stray electric currents (ventricular fibrillation).

Remarks. Due to the risks and complications mentioned, we very rarely perform umbilical vein catheterization. Only the failure of peripheral venous puncture and the urgency of drug infusion and supervision *in the shock phase* are considered grounds for *short-term* umbilical vein catheterization. Long-term parenteral alimentation can be given by the repeated puncture of peripheral veins or the introduction of an Abboven-catheter into a central vein by skilled hands.

19.1.2 Umbilical Artery Catheterization

Principle. Catheterization of an umbilical artery: Cannulation is simple during the first hours of life but becomes more difficult later due to strong arterial spasm. Beyond the 1st day of life, catheterization is often possible for another 4 or 5 days but is very difficult thereafter.

Technique. Preparation as in umbilical vein catheterization. Minimal irritation of the cord stump during preparation (increased arteriospasm) is important for the success of the procedure. If the umbilical vein and artery are both to be catheterized, the artery should be done first.

Localization. The umbilicial arteries are smaller than the umbilical vein, are white in color, circular, thick-walled, and contractile, and present a small central lumen. They are located in the sector between 4 : 00 and 7 : 00 on the cut surface of the cord (Fig. 39

a–c). The catheterization is facilitated by an assistant, who grips the upper and lower edges of the cord stump with surgical forceps. Careful preparation, clean exposure of the proximal arterial stump. Dilate the lumen by inserting a blunt-tipped probe or spreading it open with small dissecting forceps. Grasp the artery wall from the outside and inside with a small dissecting forceps, and with another forceps insert the umbilical artery catheter (Argyle Ch 3.5), which is filled with heparin solution (0.9% NaCl; 1 ml = 5 U heparin). Insert at an angle of about 45° to horizontal in a caudal direction with a slight lateral deviation from the body axis. Meanwhile cranial traction is exerted on the cord stump in order to straighten the course of the artery. Advance the catheter carefully but firmly. Obstructions may be encountered:
After 1–2 cm (downward turn)
After 3–4 cm (outer bladder wall)
After 5–7 cm (junction of internal iliac artery).

Vasospasm: Exert gentle steady pressure for 1–2 min while rotating the catheter slightly. If this is unsuccessful, fill the catheter with 1% mepivacaine and reinsert to the point of obstruction. Inject the local anesthetic, wait for 2–5 min and then try again to advance the catheter. If the arterial spasm cannot be overcome, the catheter may be left in place and another attempt made 30 min to several hours later.
The correct position of the catheter is above the aortic bifurcation (L_4) and can be estimated from the Dunn graph [9] (Fig. 40). We prefer this position because it is below the branches of the great vessels, resulting in fewer intraabdominal complications (Fig. 41) [30]. A randomized prospective study on the frequency of complications associated with low (L_3, L_4) and high (Th_7, Th_8) placement of the catheter tip indicates that pallor and cyanosis of the ipsilateral leg are more frequent

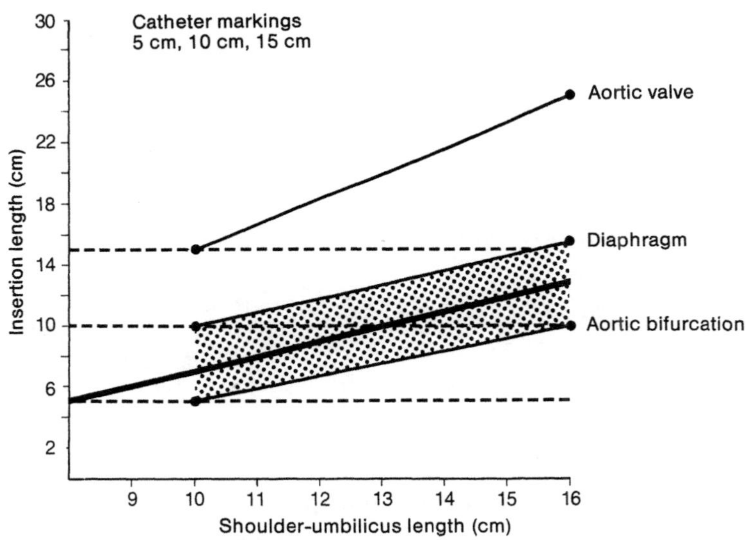

Fig. 40. Guide for determining the position of an umbilical artery catheter. (From Dunn, 1966 [9])

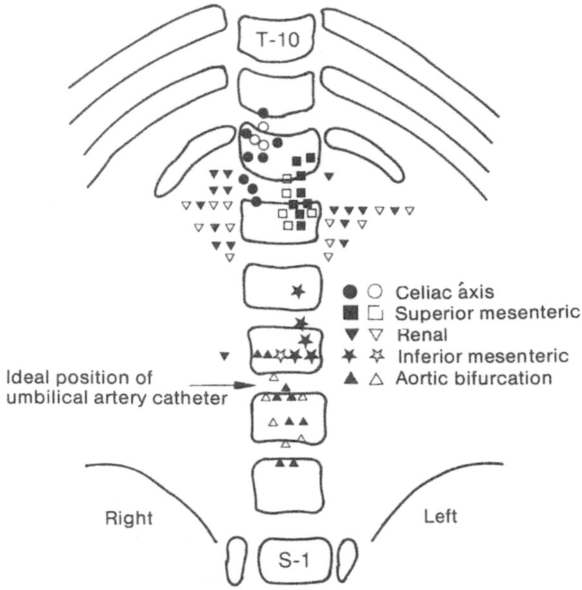

Fig. 41. Location of the major aortic branches in 15 neonates with (*filled symbols*) and without (*open symbols*) cardiac and/or renal anomalies. (From Phelbs et al., 1972 [30])

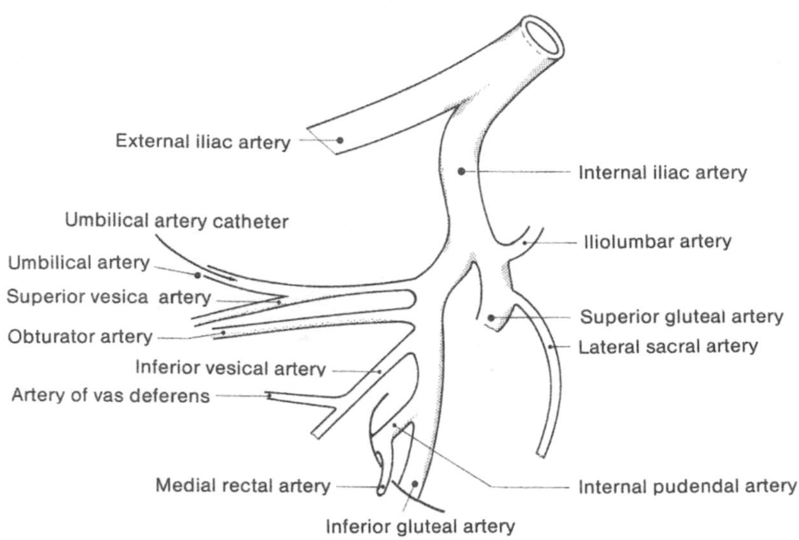

Fig. 42. Branches of the internal iliac artery. (From Hafferl, 1957 [12])

with a low placement [23]. The incidence of thrombosis as demonstrated by X-ray is the same in both groups. As before, we prefer low positioning of the catheter tip, because we have found that pallor and cyanosis of the ipsilateral limb are insignificant complications of umbilical artery catheterization; no serious intraabdominal complications have yet been observed. It should be noted that we use the umbilical artery catheter only for diagnostic blood sampling (blood gas analysis) and not for the injection of drugs or the infusion of solutions. The catheter position should be checked by X-ray [4, 28] and corrected if necessary (Fig. 41).
After insertion, inspect the gluteal area and ipsilateral lower limb and palpate the femoral pulse. Cyanosis, pallor, or absence of the femoral pulse indicates malplacement (inferior gluteal artery, femoral artery, arteriospasm) (Fig. 42). The catheter must be withdrawn as far as necessary until symptoms abate. Catheterization may then be reattempted. If the second attempt fails, removal is necessary.
The catheter is secured as in umbilical vein catheterization and is marked with *red* adhesive tape. The catheter is connected to an infusion system (pump) or is flushed intermittently with heparinized saline (5 U heparin/ml).

Complications [3, 4, 21, 24, 31, 42, 45]
Peripheral ischemia (arteriospasm)
Sepsis
Perforation
Inadvertant catheterization of an abdominal aortic branch
Life-threatening accidental hemorrhage
Intravascular catheter loss
Catheter thrombosis (blockage)
Arterial thrombosis
Embolism
Air embolism
Peripheral necrosis (tissue-irritating drugs, hyperosmolar solutions)
Necrotizing enterocolitis
Renovascular hypertension.

Removal of Catheter. Slowly withdraw the catheter to a point 2 cm from the exit site. Disconnect the attached syringe at intervals to observe the influx of pulsating arterial blood. An arterial spasm will ensue in 2–5 min, stopping the reflux and pulsation in the catheter. The catheter can now be removed without further manipulations. If the onset of arterial contraction is delayed, a purse-string or Z-suture is placed about the vessel, and the catheter is withdrawn while the suture is simultaneously closed.

19.2 Technique of Superior Vena Cava Catheterization [2, 11, 22, 41]

Indications

Emergency situation in shock and centralization
Major operative procedures
Measurement of central venous pressure (CVP)
Long-term parenteral alimentation
Involved diagnostic and therapeutic measures over a prolonged period of time.

Routes of Access

1. External jugular vein
2. Subclavian vein

Topography

1. Posterior external jugular vein: Passes from the angle of the jaw across the sternocleidomastoid muscle into the posterior neck region, where it pierces the superficial fascia, enters the interaponeurotic space, passes through the omoclavicular fascia, and opens into the subclavian or internal jugular vein.
2. Subclavian vein: Continuation of the axillary, located in the deltoid-pectoralis triangle on the medial side of the subclavian artery. From there it passes below the clavicle into the supraclavicular fossa. Here it seperates from the subclavian artery, which runs dorsally through the middle scalene gap. The subclavian vein passes in front of the anterior scalenes muscle through the anterior scalenes gap and joins with the external jugular vein in the angulus venosus to form the brachiocephalic vein.

   Between the clavicle and subclavian vein is the subclavius muscle; it is invested by a strong fascial sheath which unites with the adventitia of the vessel. The connection of the vein with the fascia of the anterior scalenes muscle and the medial cervical fascia also aids in maintaining the caliber of the vessel, thereby preventing its collapse even in shock.

Technique of Puncture

1. External jugular vein: The head is lowered and turned to the opposite side. The vessel is compressed a finger's breadth above the clavicle. The vein is punctured at the middle of the sternocleidomastoid muscle or slightly distal to it. If blood returns through the catheter, it can be advanced. This is often made difficult by venous valves, but the obstruction can usually be overcome by injecting several milliliters of physiologic saline. Deviation of the catheter into superficial veins is not uncommon.
2. Subclavian vein (infraclavicular approach):
   - Sedation: Diazepam 0.25 mg/kg body wt.
     Position: Head is lowered somewhat by placing a roll beneath the shoulders and back of neck (to fill the vein and prevent air embolism). The arms lie loosely on the body.
   - Disinfection

- Local anesthesia: 1 ml 1% mepivacaine. A wheal is raised over the puncture site with a No. 17 cannula, and the anesthetic is infiltrated into deeper tissues.
- Puncture: The needle is inserted infraclavicularly in the middle of the clavicle. It is advanced toward the clavicle at an angle of about 20° to horizontal. Avoid probing! Occlusion of the needle by tissue cylinders can be avoided by injecting small amounts of physiologic saline while the needle is advanced. The advance is continued under constant aspiration. At a depth of 1–3 cm the subclavian vein is pierced, i. e., dark blood is aspirated. If there is no influx of blood, the cannula is slowly withdrawn under careful aspiration. This is often sufficient to obtain a blood influx. Avoid changing the position of the cannula when exchanging the syringe for the catheter by placing the left hand onto the chest. Advance the catheter to the desired location. Once the catheter is in place, withdraw the cannula (caution: withdrawal of catheter through the needle carries risk of catheter embolism!). When the catheter is correctly in place in the vascular lumen, blood can be aspirated.
  Catheter postion: Superior vena cava slightly above its entry into the right atrium. Position must be checked by X-ray! Precautions: Skin suture, daily change of dressing, application of antibiotic powder.
- Technical problems:

1. Venipuncture too steep: Correct the cannula angle so that the catheter can be advanced.
2. Passing the catheter into the superior vena cava may be difficult and require catheter manipulation.
3. No free blood flow: Withdraw catheter or check location by X-ray.
4. Puncture of subclavian artery: Influx of bright red blood into the syringe. Remove the cannula immediately and compromise the artery through pressure on the clavicle.

Several attempts at puncture may be made. If unsuccessful, do not attempt puncture on contralateral side before pneumothorax has been excluded (X-ray film)! Repeated catheterization of the subclavian vein is possible. Due to the technical difficulties of the procedure, subclavian vein catheterization should be reserved for a small circle of physicians.

Complications

1. External jugular vein:
   Faulty puncture
   Air embolism
   Thrombosis
   Infection
2. Subclavian vein:
   a) Acute complications:
      Pneumothorax
      Hemothorax
      Hydrothorax

Catheter breakage, embolism
Catheter malplacement
(mediastinum)
Catheter dislodgement.

b) Long-term complications:
   Thrombosis
   Infection.

19.3 Arterial Puncture and Catheterization

Indications

Hyperoxia test
Monitoring of FiO_2
Impossibility of umbilical artery catheterization.
Both techniques require a certain degree of experience but avoid the potential risks of umbilical catheterization. If the puncture cannot be done within 30 s, the measured PaO_2 may be misleading due to crying and straining of the infant!
The following arteries are suitable for blood sampling:
Radial
(Brachial)
Temporal.

19.3.1 Puncture of the Radial and Brachial Arteries

Both arteries are localized by palpation. The skin is disinfected around the puncture site. Puncture with a no. 14 cannula, which is connected directly to a capillary tube by a short plastic sleeve. An attached plungerless syringe with a capillary tube can also be used [13, 39]. Carefully palpate, puncture vertically, and guide the needle gently but firmly toward the artery. Often the needle will pass through the artery; it is then withdrawn slowly and carefully until a pulsatile blood flow is obtained, indicating that the cannula tip is within the artery. Repeated puncture of the same artery is possible if a 5-min compression is applied after each puncture to avoid perivascular hematoma formation.

Complications

Perivascular hematoma
Arterial spasm
Intravascular thrombosis
Peripheral ischemia
Median nerve injury
Carpal tunnel syndrome.

Due to the danger of median nerve injury with lasting functional impairment, puncture of the brachial artery should be avoided in favor of radial artery puncture [27]!

19.3.2 Percutaneous Catheterization of the Radial Artery [1, 44]

Cannulation of the right radial artery (preductal flow). The hand is passively opened and the radial and ulnar arteries are simultaneously compressed. The ulnar artery is then released to check the blood flow through the blanched hand. If the blood flow to the entire hand is adequate on continued compression of the radial artery, it is safe to catheterize this artery (Allen test).
The wrist is immobilized in extension (45°) and the skin disinfected. The radial artery is palpated under sterile conditions or localized by transillumination [29]. The point of maximum pulsation is noted. An Abbocath-T 22-G is used to make the puncture at an angle of 30° to horizontal. The needle is first passed through the artery. It is then slowly withdrawn until pulsatile blood flow is obtained, showing that the tip lies in the arterial lumen. The catheter is then advanced into the artery and the stylet is withdrawn. The catheter is secured with adhesive tape. It is attached to an extension tubing with a three-way stopcock, and continuous infusion with heparinized 0.9% NaCl (5 units/ml) is started (pump). The hand and forearm are secured on an armboard, leaving the thumbs and fingers exposed. The three-way stopcock can be used at any time for blood sampling or measurement of arterial blood pressure.
Disadvantage. Time- consuming, requires experience.

Complications
Local infection
Hematoma formation
Disturbance of peripheral blood flow
Arterial spasm.

19.3.3 Percutaneous Catheterization of the Temporal Artery [2, 32, 35, 38, 43]

Anatomy. The temporal artery can be palpated anterior and superior to the ear. It ramifies into the frontal and parietal branches (Fig. 43).

Technique. The area is shaved and disinfected. The artery is located by palpation or by means of a Doppler probe. Skin is punctured horizontally with an Abbocath-T 22-G. The puncture catheter is advanced in the direction of the artery until blood is observed in the rear chamber. Then the stylet is removed, while the catheter is carefully advanced a few millimeters farther. It is secured with tape and connected to an extension tubing with a three-way stopcock. An antibiotic powder is applied to the puncture site and adjacent area. The catheter is flushed hourly with heparinized 0.9% NaCl (5 units/ml).

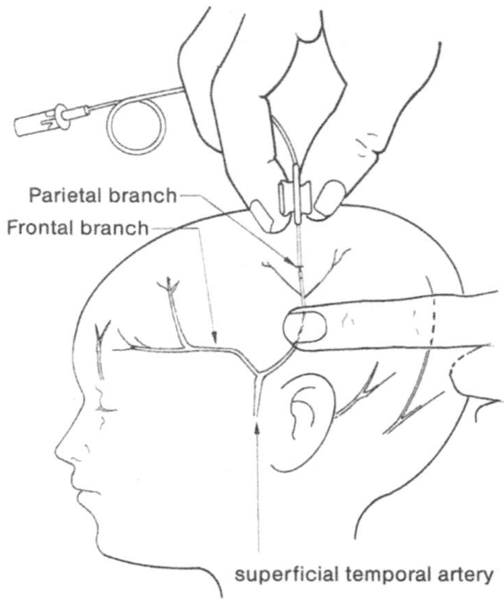

Fig. 43. Puncture of the temporal artery

A pulsating column of blood along the cannula shows that the line is patent and functioning.

Due to the risk of complications (see below), success in the procedure depends upon:

1. Careful instruction of personnel in the handling of the catheter
2. Close clinical observation of the patient
3. Regular flushing of the catheter
4. Removal of catheter in case of blockage
5. No injection or infusion of medications through the catheter.

Advantages

Avoids umbilical artery catheterization
Provides preductal flow for blood sampling.

Complications

Arterial thrombosis
Embolism
Cerebral insult
Hemiplegia
Convulsions
Necrosis of ear or temple
Accidental hemorrhage.

19.4 Venesection [14, 20]

Indications
Failure of percutaneous venipuncture for infusion therapy
Impossibility of umbilical vein catheterization
Measurement of central venous pressure
Angiography.

Site of Procedure
Supramalleolar tibial vein
Basilic or cephalic vein (elbow)
Great saphenous vein (trigonum femorale).

Technique. The field is immobilized and disinfected, an epinephrine-free local anesthetic is administered. Due to swelling of the subcutaneous tissue, it is advisable to mark the precise location of the incision beforehand. The vein is exposed through a transverse incision and is dissected free for a length of 2 cm along its course; an elevator is passed beneath the vein, and it is carefully freed from surrounding fat and connective tissue (permits precise incision, ready location of incision site, and easy introduction of catheter). Two catgut ligatures are passed beneath the proximal and distal segments of the vein and loose loops are tied. A suitable catheter is selected and its tip given a short bevel; it is then filled with 0.9% NaCl. A fine, sharp scissors is used to cut into the vein, which is made tense for this purpose by means of the distal ligature. For incision, the vein is grasped with a forceps, pulled out laterally and at right angles to its course and incised to the center in a longitudinal direction so as to form a V-shaped incision. The incision must be of sufficient depth, lest the catheter be inserted beneath the adventitia. Blood must flow freely from the vein. The vascular lumen can be readily visualized by tightening the ligature or raising the elevator to occlude the flow of blood. The prepared catheter is grasped 0.5 cm from its tip with a forceps and inserted into the vascular lumen, the beveled end pointing toward the vascular center (smoother passage). The catheter tip should ideally be located within the vena cava in front of the right atrium; this prevents wall damage, reduces the risk of thrombosis, and facilitates blood sampling.
Venous spasm. Local anesthetic is injected.
Elastic resistance. Venous valve; catheter is withdrawn by 2 cm and readvanced with a rotary motion while saline solution is simultaneously injected. Catheter patency is checked (by X-ray if catheter is centrally placed).
The proximal segment of the vein is tied around the catheter with the proximal ligature. The distal ligature is removed (later recanalization is possible). The slight oozing of blood is stopped by applying a pressure dressing, followed by wound closure and catheter fixaton.

Localization of the Selected Vein

1. *Great saphenous vein* (*trigonum femorale*)
   Junction of the great saphenous vein with the femoral vein. The latter runs medial and parallel to the femoral artery. The anterior superior iliac spine and pubic tubercle are connected by a straight line; this line is bisected, and a 2-cm incision is made parallel to the inguinal ligament 0.5 cm below the groin crease on the midline of the thigh.
   Disadvantage. Increased risk of infection.
2. *Supramalleolar tibial vein*
   Preferred site for venesection: follows extremely constant course in front of the medial malleolus. A 1-cm transverse incision is made in the skin creases in front of the medial malleolus and directed toward the tendon of the tibial muscle.
   Disadvantage. Increased risk of infection.
3. *Basilic vein and cephalic vein*
   Vascular course is not constant; extension of the incision is often necessary. Congested veins are not always palpable or visible. The basilic vein courses on the ulnar side of the elbow in the lower part of the ulnar groove of the biceps. The cephalic vein passes superiorly along the radial bend of the elbow.
   Disadvantage. Difficulty in advancing the catheter at the junction with the axillary vein.

Frequent Errors

Faulty localization of incision
Inadequate exposure of vein
Inadvertent transection of vein
Inadequate incision
Faulty catheter selection
Inadequate typing or fixation of catheter
Faulty immobilization.

19.5 Drainage of Pneumothorax

19.5.1 Exploratory Puncture

Always done with a 5-ml syringe filled with 0.9% NaCl and a no. 14 needle: aspiration = air bubble. Supine position, rapid disinfection, puncture in fourth intercostal space on the anterior axillary line. Puncture is done at a steep enough angle to ensure intrapleural, rather than subcutaneous, placement of the needle tip.
Suspicion Confirmed. Continuous pleural drainage. There is sample time for this procedure, in as much as the exploratory puncture has removed the air under tension and air from the outside cannot enter the pleural space.

19.5.2 Technique of Pleural Drainage

The infant is immobilized with the arms secured above the head. The skin is disinfected and draped with a sterile perforated towel. Puncture site: fourth intercostal space on anterior axillary line, since most of the air collects here in a supine position. A local anesthetic (about 1 ml 1% mepivacaine) is given. A 4-mm incision is made at the upper edge of the rib which borders on the intercostal space from below. The intercostal muscles are spread apart with Cooper's scissors. The drainage catheter (Argyle, Vygon trocar catheter, Ch 10) is grasped about 2 cm from the tip and introduced into the intercostal space (beware: lung perforation from abrupt penetration of intercostal muscles). Since most of the air collects behind the anterior chest wall at the level of the fourth ICS in the recumbent patient, the catheter tip should be advanced close along the chest wall toward the sternum immediately after it enters the thoracic space. It is connected to an apparatus for continuous drainage (central vacuum unit, large empyema pump). The catheter is secured with skin sutures and its position checked by X-ray.
A water vacumeter should be used for fine adjustment of the drainage suction (setting $= -20$ cm H_2O). Bubble formation signifies that the pleural drain is functioning; absence of bubbles indicates a leak (subcutaneous catheter position, external disconnection).

Prevention of Catheter Occlusion. The catheter is pinched off and "pumped" hourly with the fingers to dilate it. If placement is prolonged, it is recommended that the catheter be flushed with sterile 0.9% NaCl.
Blood coagulum, protein-rich pleural secretions, and pleural adhesions may cause occlusion despite correct placement, with renewed accumulation of pleural air! A second drainage is performed if necessary.
During spontaneous respiration, adhesion of the alveolar rupture can be expected to occur after 48 h; during controlled ventilation, this process often takes several days. The pleural drain may be removed if full lung expansion is confirmed radiologically 6h after the catheter is clamped.

19.6 Drainage of Pneumopericardium

Subxiphoid approach, rapid disinfection of the epigastrium, puncture with Abboven catheter Ch 14 in which a side hole has been cut 1 cm from the tip. In the angle between the xiphoid process and left sternal rib insertion, the catheter is inserted below the sternum and aimed toward the right shoulder [19]. After the catheter has been advanced 2–3 cm with the guide wire, it can be advanced an additional centimeter by itself. Successful pericardial puncture is signified by an immediate improvement of bradycardia, the rapid regression of shock symptoms, good color, and the disappearance of low voltages on the monitor screen. Placement is confirmed by X-ray. It is advisable to leave the pneumopericardial drain in place for the next few days under artificial ventilation. It may be removed after prior clamping and exclusion of any new accumulation (chest film). Setting of drainage suction, -5 cm H_2O.

19.7 Abdominal Paracentesis

Indications
Relief of abdominal distention
Diagnostic examination (air insufflation).

Site of Procedure. Left lower quadrant. The distance between the anterior superior iliac spine and umbilicus is divided into three equal parts. The puncture is made at the junction between the lateral and medial thirds.

Technique. The bladder is evacuated and the patient immobilized in supination. The site is disinfected, local anesthesia is given, and a 0.5-cm incision is made. A trocar catheter (Argyle Ch 12) is inserted through the incision and tunneled through the abdominal musculature with firm pressure and slight rotation. Penetration of the parietal peritoneum is signified by a slight jerk. The trocar catheter should be grasped close to the skin to avoid internal injuries. The trocar is then withdrawn and the catheter connected to a three-way stopcock. The ascitic fluid is fractionally tapped and measured (to avoid shock). The outflow can be slowed by repositioning the catheter or the patient.

Complications
Intestinal perforation with distension
Perforation of filled bladder
Shock (excessively rapid drainage)
Peritonitis (unsterile technique).

19.8 Endotracheal Intubation [8, 40]

Indications
Respiratory insufficiency
Aspiration of meconium-stained fluid.

Preparation
All instruments are held in readiness
Ventilation bag is provided with suitable tube adapter

Aspirator function is checked
Respirator function is checked
Respiratory adapter is held in readiness
Assistant stands ready
Pharynx is thoroughly suctioned and stomach is evacuated
Infant is ventilated briefly with oxygen by mask and bag (exception: aspiration).

19.8.1 Orotracheal Intubation

Position. The shoulders are elevated slightly with a folded towel; the head is in the mid-position and partially extended (e. g., position on Draeger intubation mattress). Grasp the laryngoscope with the left hand distal to the handle-blade angle, with the fourth and fifth fingers around the infant's chin. This fixates the head and raises the angle of the jaw slightly. Insert the blade at the right corner of the mouth, moving the tongue to the left. Advance the blade until the glottis comes into view. The tip of the blade may be guided either over the epiglottis or into the vallecula. With the little finger of the left hand, press on the larynx externally to aid the blade tip in opening the entrance to the larynx. The epiglottis is now in full view, and the rima glottidis is visible dorsalward (Fig. 44).
Advance the endotracheal tube along the laryngoscope guide into the larynx. There may be difficulty in passing the vocal cords. A further obstruction at the level of the cricoid can be overcome by carefully rotating the tube. If the rima glottidis is closed, it is necessary to await the next inspiratory movement. After the tube is introduced, carefully remove the laryngoscope. The tube is held in place until it can be secured. To save time, orotracheal intubation is preferred during primary resuscitation.

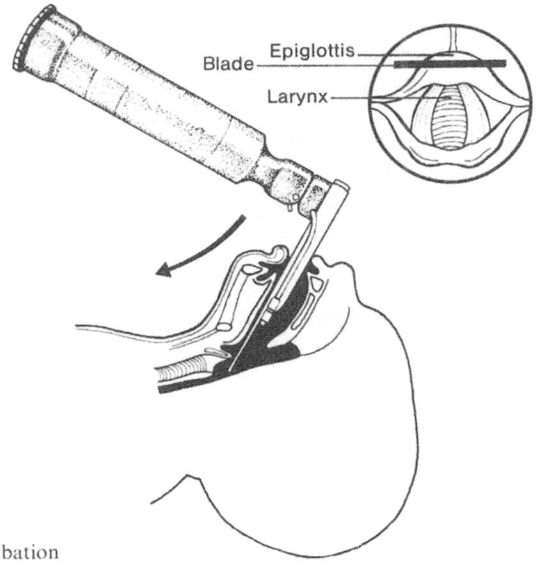

Fig. 44. Field of vision during intubation

19.8.2 Nasotracheal Intubation

The tube is connected to a Dangel fixation plate [37] and the proper tube length is established (see below). To facilitate nasal passage, the tip of the tube is coated with 0.1% Xylocaine gel and carefully inserted. Obstructions in the nasal passage can usually be overcome by rotating the tube slightly. The rest of the procedure is like that in orotracheal intubation. When the tube becomes visible in the pharynx, its tip is grasped with Magill infant forceps under laryngoscopic vision and guided into the trachea. The tube is repeatedly grasped and advanced until it has reached its final position. The advantages of nasotracheal intubation are:
More stable fixation
Better oral and pharyngeal hygiene.

19.8.3 Confirmation of Tube Placement

Mask and Bag Ventilation
Symmetrical movements of chest wall
Uniform aeration of the lungs (auscultation).
We regard radiologic confirmation of endotracheal tube placement as absolutely necessary. If this is not possible, the uniform aeration of both lungs must be established beyond question. The correct tube placement is midway between the medial ends of both clavicles [5].
Unsuccessful attempts should be discontinued and the infant reventilated with oxygen by mask and bag! Intubation under monitor control allows better clinical supervision (bradycardia, arrhythmia).

Tube Selection

1000–2000 g	Ch 2.5
2000–3000 g	Ch 3.0
>3000 g	Ch 3.5

Curved, plastic endotracheal tubes with a uniform diameter (Vygon, Portex) are excellent. Flow resistance and turbulence are reduced to a minimum. The main advantage of the soft tubes is that they are atraumatic to the nasal passage, laryngeal entrance, vocal cords, and trachea.

19.8.4 Tube Lengths

Oral Intubation

Distance from dental lamina of upper jaw to tracheal bifurcation:
Term infant: 10.5–11 cm
Preterm infant: 9 cm.
The tubes are correspondingly marked at 8, 9, or 10 cm and introduced for the length required.

Nasotracheal Intubation

Formula: body length × 0.21 = length of tube in cm.

Body length	Tube length
28 cm	6.0 cm
30 cm	6.5 cm
32 cm	6.8 cm
34 cm	7.2 cm
36 cm	7.6 cm
38 cm	8.0 cm
40 cm	8.5 cm
42 cm	9.0 cm
44 cm	9.3 cm
46 cm	9.7 cm
48 cm	10.0 cm
50 cm	10.5 cm
52 cm	11.0 cm
54 cm	11.5 cm

19.8.5 Fixation of Tube

Oral Intubation. Secure with crossed adhesive strips starting from the jaw angle on one side and passing once around the tube to the other side. Prior to this the skin is degreased with ether for better adhesion.

Nasotracheal Intubation. The selected tube is pushed through the Dangel fixation plate [37] prior to intubation. This plate has a hole on each side through which a cloth strap can be threaded. After intubation, this strap is passed around the back of the head, threaded through the hole on the other side, and loosely knotted. Caution: Overtightening the strap can cause cerebellar hemorrhage. The strap is secured with adhesive tape, completing the fixation of the tube.

19.8.6 Most Frequent Sources of Error During Intubation

Incomplete or nonfunctioning instruments
Inadequate tube size
Injury to upper jaw
Field of vision obstructed by secretions.

19.9 Technique of Peritoneal Dialysis [10, 25, 34]

Indications

Acute renal failure
Acute metabolic disease

Fluid and electrolyte imbalance with no response to conservative treatment
Chronic renal failure (special indications).

Principle. Dialysis of the blood through the peritoneal membrane against an artificially produced ascites, which is continuously renewed during the treatment period.

Placing the Peritoneal Catheter

The bladder is evacuated and a bladder catheter is placed.

The patient's baseline weight is determined

Sedation. Diazepam, 0.25 mg/kg body wt.

Position. Supine.

Puncture Site. In upper third of umbilical symphysis. If midline insertion is not possible, puncture at the junction of the second and third thirds of the distance between the umbilicus and the anterior iliac spine (left) (Fig. 45).

Local Anesthesia. 1 ml of 1% mepivacaine with epinephrine added (to decrease the bleeding tendency). A wheal is raised over the puncture site with a No. 17 needle and infiltrated down to the peritoneum.

Dialysis Fluid. 30 ml/kg warmed physiologic saline (to avoid trauma to abdominal organs).

The *skin* is incised for a length of about 2 mm with a sharp scalpel to obtain a snug catheter fit (reduces tissue hemorrhage).

The stylet catheter is inserted perpendicularly with a rotary motion into the abdominal cavity. It should be grasped close to the incision. Penetration is clearly felt as the abdominal resistance is overcome. After the catheter tip has passed the peritoneum, the stylet is withdrawn a short distance, and fluid enters the catheter.

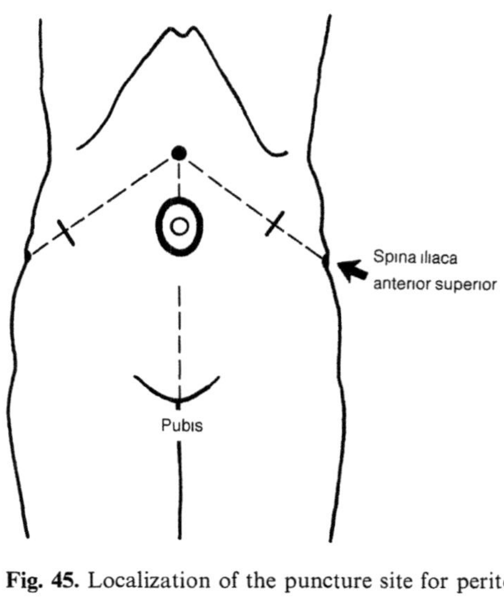

Fig. 45. Localization of the puncture site for peritoneal catheterization

Catheter Position. With the stylet withdrawn about 1 cm, the catheter is advanced at an angle of 45° caudal into the abdominal cavity toward Douglas' space; it bypasses the bladder on the right or left. The stylet is removed (Fig. 46).
A skin suture is placed if necesarry to secure the catheter. The area is treated with Polybactrim powder, and sterile compression is applied. The catheter is connected to the dialysis system.

Technical Problems. If an obstruction is met while the catheter is being advanced, it is likely that the catheter has become lodged in the greater omentum. It must then be repositioned to ensure good dialysis.

Procedure. We perform the dialysis with the Peritocomb III automatic dialysis unit.
Volume of dialysate: 30 ml/kg.
The dialysis begins with drainage of the physiologic saline administered transcutaneously.
The first cycles of instillation and drainage are done with a short dwell time (3–5 min) in order to check for difficulties. During the first two or three cycles, the retention of a small volume of dialysate in the abdominal cavity can be tolerated. Thereafter the amount of fluid drained must be greater than the amount of dialysate instilled. Effective dialysis requires the free in- and outflow of fluid through the catheter. Catheter displacement (bowel, omentum) or occlusion (fibrin) must be corrected.
Short dwell times of 5–15 min allow rapid fluid withdrawal, while long dwell times of 20–30 min provide more effective clearance (electrolytes, urea, creatinine).
Dialysis is maintained for 24–36 h. If indications persist, it may be repeated every 48 h.
Dialysis solutions: Peritosteril G I or G IK with 100 units heparin/L added (stable for 6h).

Dialysis Record and Patient Supervision

Volume of fluid instilled
Volume of fluid drained
Fluid balance (individual and overall)
Weight after drainage (bed scales)
Dialysate (clear, bloody, turbid)
Change of dialysate (time)

Skin turgor, fontanel
Pulse rate, respiratory rate
Blood pressure
Abdomen: tenderness, tension, redness
Blood glucose (Dextrostix)
Electrolytes
Urea, creatinine
Total protein
Culture dtainage once daily

Removal of the Peritoneal Catheter. The last drainage is tested bacteriologically. Physiologic saline (5 ml) is rapidly injected to irrigate the catheter, which is then withdrawn from the abdomen with a slight rotary motion. No resistance must be encountered (beware: eventration of the omentum!). If resistance is met, an attempt must be made to overcome it by further rotary movements of the catheter.

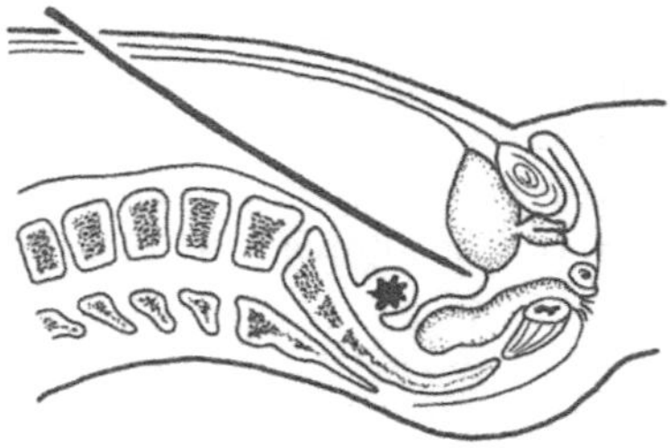

Fig. 46. Position of the peritoneal catheter

Complications

1. *Mechanical*
   Pain
   Intraabdominal hemorrhage
   Inadequate drainage
   Leakage
   Perforation of the bowel
2. *Inflammatory*
   Abscess at puncture site
   Intraabdominal infection
   Sterile peritonitis
3. *Pulmonary*
   Basal atelectasis
   Pleural effusion
   Respiratory effort
4. *Cardiovascular:*
   Volume overload
   Hypo- or hypertension
   Arrhythmia
   Cardiac arrest
5. *Metabolic*
   Hyperglycemia, coma
   Postdialysis hypoglycemia
   Protein loss
   Electrolyte imbalance.

Table 74. Solutions for peritoneal dialysis

Peritosteril G I K		*Peritosteril G III K*	
Total osmolarity: 363 mosmol/l		Total osmolarity: 515 mosmol/l	
Composition:		*Composition:*	
1 l contains:		1 l contains:	
Na^+	132.0 mmol = 132.0 mEq	Na^+	132.0 mmol = 132.0 mEq
K^+	4.0 mmol = 4.0 mEq	K^+	4.0 mmol = 4.0 mEq
Ca^{++}	1.7 mmol = · 3.5 mEq	Ca^{++}	1.7 mmol = 3.5 mEq
Mg^{++}	0.7 mmol = 1.5 mEq	Mg^{++}	0.7 mmol = 1.5 mEq
Cl^-	106.0 mmol = 106.0 mEq	Cl^-	106.0 mmol = 106.0 mEq
Lacate$^-$	35.0 mmol = 35.0 mEq	Lactate$^-$	35.0 mmol = 35.0 mEq
Glucose monohydrate 16.5 g/l		Glucose monohydrate 46.75 g/l	

In hyperkalemia, Peritosteril G (potassium-free), with a total osmolarity of 355 mosmol/l, can be used initially.

19.10 Ventriculopuncture

Principle. Blind transcortical puncture of the right lateral ventricle through the anterior fontanel.

Indications

Cerebrospinal fluid analysis (ventriculitis)
Meningitis therapy (intraventricular instillation of antibiotics)
Ventriculography (air insufflation) (6).

Position. Horizontal, head in midposition, crown of the head at the table edge. The assistant steadies the head bilaterally in the temoral and buccal region, placing one index finger on the infant's nose to facilitate position checks in all planes during puncture.
The physician is seated at the infant's head, with the anterior fontanel before him.

Instrumentarium

As in lumbar puncture.
Puncture is done with spinal needle (Becton-Dickinson)

Preterm infants < 1500 g	20 G 1 $^{1}/_{2}$
Preterm infants > 1500 g	20 G 3 $^{1}/_{2}$
Term infants	20 G 3 $^{1}/_{2}$

Localization of Puncture Site. Slightly in front of the right lateral angle of the anterior fontanel, which can be readily located by the hiatus of the coronal suture. The needle is inserted at the edge of the anterior fontanel, which is bounded anteriorly by the frontal bone. The puncture site thus lies 1–1.5 cm from the parietal midline. A needle inserted in this region remains outside the central convolutions of the cerebral cortex and precludes injury of the superior sagittal sinus.

Procedure. The fontanel area is shaved, the skin is disinfected, and the head is draped. The free hand is braced and holds the infant's head in the mid position. The other hand grips the puncture needle like a pencil or between the index and middle finger with the thumb pressing on the head of the stylet. A bayonet stab is made through the scalp and external dura; it is important that the needly be guided perpendicular to the cranial surface with no directional deviations ot rotation during insertion (brain injury!). Since the thickness of the dura varies and the width of the ventricles is usually unknown, the needle should be stopped after each centimeter or so and the stylet withdrawn to check for cerebrospinal fluid. As a rule, the lateral ventricle will be reached after the following distances:

Preterm imfants of	1000–1500g	2–3 cm
Preterm infants of	1500–2500 g	3–4 cm
Preterm infants	> 2500g	~4 cm

The procedure is used to obtain cerebrospinal fluid for diagnostic purposes, for the instillation of antibiotics, and for the insufflation of air.

The puncture is completed by slowly and carefully withdrawing the puncture needle with the stylet reinserted. The area is immediately redisinfected. The puncture site is covered with a sterile compress, and a pressure dressing is applied.

Sources of Error. Puncture too far laterally into the dura.

Aftercare
Slight elevation of head
Monitoring of pulse and respiration
Clinical observation

Complications
Subdural hemorrhage
Piercing of superior sagittal sinus
Vascular injury
Intracerebral abscess
Porencephaly.

References

1. ADAMS, J. M., RUDOLPH, A. J.: The use of indwelling radial artery catheters in neonates. Pediatrics *55*, 261 (1975)
2. AU-YEUNG, Y. B., SUGG, W. M., KANTOR, N. M., CHIU, TH. T., GARRISON, R. D.: Percutaneous catheterization of scalp arteries in sick infants. J. Pediatr. *91*, 106 (1977)
3. AZIZ, E. M., ROBERTSON, A. F.: Paraplegia: a complication of umbilical artery catheterization. J Pediatr. *82*, 1051 (1973)
4. BAKER, D. H., BERDON, W. E., JAMES, S. ST.: Proper localization of umbilical arterial and venous catheter by lateral roentgenograms. Pediatrics, *43*, 34 (1969)
5. BEDNAREK, F. J., KUHNS, L. R.: Endotracheal tube placement in infants determined by suprasternal palpation: A new technique. Pediatrics *56*, 224 (1975)
6. BLIESENER, J. A., KELLERMANN, K.: Ventriculography with positive contrast medium in early infancy Pediat. Radiol. *8*, 133 (1979)
7. BURRI, C., GASSER, D.: Der Vena Cava-Katheter. Berlin-Heidelberg-New York: Springer 1971
8. DICK, W., AHNEFELD, F. W.: Primäre Neugeborenen-Reanimation. Berlin-Heidelberg-New-York: Springer 1975
9. DUNN, P. M.: Localization of the umbilical catheter by post-mortem measurement. Arch. Dis. Child. *41*, 69 (1966)
10. GILLI, G.: Persönliche Mitteilung 1979
11. GROFF, D. B., AHMED, N.: Subclavia vein catheterization in the infant. J. Pediatr. Surg. *9*, 171 (1974)
12. HAFFERL, A.: Lehrbuch der topographischen Anatomie. S. 542. Berlin-Göttingen-Heidelberg: Springer 1957
13. HUCH, A., HUCH, R.: New method for arterial blood sampling in infants and adults. Arch. Dis. Child. *48*, 982 (1973)
14. HUGHES, Jr., W. T.: Pediatrie procedures. Philadelphia-London: Saunders 1964
15. JUNKER, P., EGEBLAD, M., NIELSON, O., KAMPER, J.: Umbilical vein catheterization and portal hypertension. Acta Paediatr. Scand. *65*, 499 (1976)

16. KEUTH, U., CONTER, C., WILHELMI, J.: Zur Position des Nabelvenenkatheters (Röntgenanalyse von 200 Fällen aus dem klinischen Routinebetrieb). Mschr. Kinderheilk. *120*, 175 (1972)
17. KITTERMAN, J. A., PHIBBS, R. H., TOOLEY, W. H.: Catherization of umbilical vessels in newborn infants. Pediatr. Clin. North Am. *17*, 895 (1970)
18. KOCH, H.: Katheterisierung der Nabelgefäße. In: Pädiatrische Intensivbehandlung. v. LOEWENICH, V., KOCH, H. (Ed.). S. 29. Stuttgart: Thieme 1974
19. KOCH, H.: Komplikationen bei der Beatmung – Prophylaxe und Therapie. In: Pädiatrische Intensivbehandlung. v. LOEWENICH, V., KOCH, H. (Ed.) Stuttgart: Thieme 1974
20. KÖBLER, H.: Die Venae sectio. Dtsch. Ärztebl., *68*, 1246 (1971)
21. KRISHNAMOORTHY, K. S., FERNANDEZ, R. J., TODRES, I. D., DE LONG, G. R.: Paraplegia associated with umbilical artery catheterization in the newborn. Pediatrics *58*, 443 (1976)
22. LITTMANN, K., MEDRANO, J., BRACHT, H.: Methodik und Ergebnisse der Vena subclavia-Katheterung bei Früh- und Neugeborenen. Monatsschr. Kinderheilkd. *126*, 324 (1978)
23. MOKROHISKY, St. T., LEVINE, R. L., BLUMHAGEN, J. D., WESENBERG, R. L., SIMMONS, M. A.: Low positioning of umbilical-artery catheters increases associated complications in newborn infants. N. Engl. J. Med. *299*, 361 (1978)
24. NEAL, W. A., REYNOLDS, J. W., JARVIS, CH. W., WILLIAMS, H. J.: Umbilical artery catheterization: demonstration of arterial thrombosis by aortography. Pediatrics *50*, 6 (1972)
25. NOLPH, K. D.: Peritoneal dialysis. In: Replacement of renal function by dialysis. DRUKKER, W., PARSONS, F. M., MAHER, J. F. (Eds.), p. 277. The Hague-Boston-London: Martinus Nighoff Medical Clinicum Division 1978
26. OBLADEN, M., ERNST, D., FEIST, D., WILLE, L.: Portal hypertension in children following umbilical disorders. J. Perinat. Med. *3*, 101 (1975)
27. PAPE, K. E., ARMSTRONG, D. L., FITZHARDINGE, P. M.: Peripheral median nerve damage secondary to brachial arterial blood gas sampling. J. Pediatr. *93*, 852 (1978)
28. PASTER, St. B., MIDDLETON, Ph.: Roentgenographic evaluation of umbilical artery and vein catheter. JAMA *231*, 741 (1975)
29. PEARSE, R. O.: Percutaneous catheterization of the radial artery in newborn babies using transillumination. Arch. Dis. Child. *53*, 549 (1978)
30. PHELBS, D. L., LACHMAN, R. S., LEAKE, R. D., OH, W.: The radiologic localization of the major aortic tirbutaries in the newborn infant. J. Pediatr. *81*, 336 (1972)
31. PLUMER, L. B., KAPLAN, G. W., MENDOZA, ST. A.: Hypertension in infants – a complication of umbilical arterial catheterization. J. Pediatr. *89*, 802 (1976)
32. PRIAN, G. W., WRIGHT, G. B., RUMACK, C. M., O'MEARA, O. B.: Apparent cerebral embolization after temporal artery catheterization. J. Pediatr. *93*, 115 (1978)
33. RUBALTELLI, F. F., ZANARDO, V., SAIA, O. S., D'ELIA, R., AUDINO, G., LARGAJOLLI, G., CANTARUTTI, F.: Umbilical vessel catheterization. The immediate risks with the venous route. Paediatr. Paediol. *13*, 39 (1978)
34. SCHÄRER, K., CHANTLER, C., DONCKERWOLCKE, R. A.: Paediatric Dialysis. In: Replacement of renal function by dialysis. DRUKKER, W., PARSONS, F. M., MAHER, J. F. (Eds.), p. 444. The Hague-Boston-London: Martinus Nighoff Medical Clinicum Division 1978
35. SCHLUETER, M. A., JOHNSON, B. B., WANG, L. Y., NAMKUNG, P., HEASLEY, S. V., HADDOCK, S. A., TOOLEY, W. H.: Blood sampling from scalp arteries in infants. Pediatrics *51*, 120 (1973)
36. SCHMID, F., DANGEL, P. H., DUC, G. V.: Nasale Anwendung von CPAP. In: Pädiatrische Intensivmedizin, Bd. 3 P. Emmrich (Ed.) S. 33. Stuttgart: Thieme 1977
37. SIMMONS, M. A., LEVINE, R. L., LUBCHENCO, L. O., GUGGENHEIM, M. A.: Warning: Serious sequalae of temporal artery catheterization. J. Pediatr. *92*, 284 (1978)
38. SMITH, A. D.: Arterial blood sampling in neonates. Lancet *1*, 254 (1975)
39. STOLL, W.: Die primäre Reanimation des Neugeborenen. Stuttgart: Enke 1975
40. STOPFKUCHEN, H., ECKERT, H.-G., EMMRICH, P.: Subclavialkatheter im Neugeborenen- und Säuglingsalter. Monatsschr. Kinderheilk. *126*, 325 (1978)
41. SYMANSKY, M. R., FOX, A.: Umbilical vessel catheterization: indications, management and evaluation of technique. J. Pediatr. *80*, 820 (1972)

42. Tiller, R., Frey, G.: Schläfen- und Ohrnekrose als Folge versehentlicher Infusion hyperosmolarer Lösungen in die rechte Schläfenarterie eines Frühgeborenen. Z. Ärztl. Fortbild. (Jena) *71*, 716 (1977)
43. Todres, I. D., Rogers, M. C., Shannon, D. C., Moylan, F. M., Ryan, J. F.: Percutaneous catheterization of the radial artery in the critically ill neonate. J. Pediatr. *87*, 273, (1975)
44. Tooley, W. H.: What is the risk of an umbilical artery catheter? Pediatrics *50*, 1 (1972)

20 Instrumentarium for Procedures in Neonatal Intensive Medicine

L. Wille

20.1 Intubation Set

One Negus laryngoscope, ∅ 18 cm
One Negus blade, length 105 mm
One Negus blade, length 75 mm
One Magill infant forceps
Three Vygon endotracheal tubes, Ch 2.5, 3.0, 3.5
Three standard adapters, No. 2.0, 2.5, 3.0
Two suction catheters with mucus trap
One Penlon bag
Two Rendell-Baker masks, sizes 0, 1
One stethoscope
Three Dangel fixation plates, Ch 2.5, 3.0, 3.5

20.2 Pneumothorax Set

One disposable scalpel, No. 15 (Feather Industries)
One slender dissecting forceps, length 13 cm
One slender surgical forceps, length 13 cm
One slender, curved scissors (sharp-blunt), length 12 cm
Two tube clamps, length 14 cm
One ophthalmic needle holder (Boynton), length 12.5 cm
One Portex Y-connector, order no. 700/140/002
One Portex connecting piece, order no. 700/110/200
One Portex connecting piece, order no. 700/150/634
Four slit swabs, 5 × 5 cm
Four slit swabs, 8 × 8 cm
Two sterile towels
Two hand towels
One Argyle trocar catheter, Ch 10.

20.3 Abdominal Paracentesis Set

One slender dissecting forceps, length 13 cm
One slender surgical forceps, length 13 cm
One slender curved scissors (sharp-blunt), length 12 cm
One steel vaccination lancet, length 13 cm
One ophthalmic needle holder (Boynton), length 12.5 cm
Two tube clamps, length 14 cm
One catheter nozzle, size 3: 2.5×9.0 mm $\varnothing$, Luer-Lok, female, order no. 1365 (Volzer Medizintechnik)
One flowthrough stopcock, Luer-Lok, male, order no. 5505 (Volzer Medizintechnik)
Four slit swabs, 5×5 cm
Four slit swabs, 8×8 cm
Two sterile towels
One slit towel
Two hand towels.

20.4 Umbilical Catheter Set

One dissecting forceps, length 13 cm
One delicate curved scissors (sharp-blunt), length 13 cm
One straight Halstead mosquito forceps, length 12.5 cm
Two fine surgical forceps (Semken), length 12.5 cm
Two ophthalmic dissecting forceps (0.8 mm), length 10 cm
Two ophthalmic surgical forceps (0.8 mm), length 10 cm
Four double bulb-headed probes, diameter: 1.0, 1.2, 1.5 mm, length 13 cm
One metal rule (flexible, rustproof), length 14 cm
One ophthalmic needle holder (Boynton), length 12.5 cm
One delicate straight scissors (sharp-blunt), length 13 cm
Eight compresses, 5×5 cm
Eight compresses, 8×8 cm
Two sterile towels
One slit towel
Two hand towels
Two strongly curved ophthalmic forceps (0.8 mm), length 10 cm
Two Argyle umbilical catheters, Ch 3.5, 5.0

20.5 Venesection Set

One disposable scalpel, No. 15 (Feather Industries)
One curved micro-Halstead mosquito forceps, length 12.5 cm
One curved Halstead mosquito forceps, length 14.0 cm
Two fine blunt wound retractors (Achsenfeld), length 14.5 cm (three-toothed)
Two fine blunt wound retractors (Achsenfeld), length 14.5 cm (two-toothed)
Two lid retractors (Desmares)
Two straight micro-Halstead mosquito forceps, length 12.5 cm
Two straight Halstead mosquito forceps, length 12.5 cm
One straight vascular scissors (sharp-sharp), length 9.5 cm
One guide, length 14 cm
Two bulb-headed probes, diameter: 1.5 mm, length 14.5 cm
Two bulb-headed probes, diameter: 1.2 mm, length 14.5 cm
Two introduction cannulas, diameter: 1.5 mm
Two introduction cannulas, diameter: 1.2 mm
One strongly curved ophthalmic forceps (0.8 mm), length 10 cm
One ophthalmic dissecting forceps (0.8 mm), length 10 cm
One ophthalmic surgical forceps (0.8 mm), length 10 cm
One slender surgical forceps, length 13 cm
One slender dissecting forceps, length 13 cm
One curved scissors (blunt-blunt), length 12 cm
One ophthalmic needle holder (Boynton), length 12.5 cm
One Luer-Record metal adapter
One Record-Luer metal adapter
One Luer connecting stopcock
One grain forceps.

20.6 Peritoneal Dialysis Set

One disposable scalpel, No. 15 (Feather Industries)
One slender dissecting forceps, length 13 cm
One slender surgical forceps, length 13 cm
One slender curved scissors (sharp-blunt), length 12 cm
One ophthalmic needle holder (Boynton), length 12.5 cm
Four slit swabs, 5 × 5 cm
Four slit swabs, 8 × 8 cm
Two sterile towels
Two hand towels
One stylet catheter, 1.5 × 2.7 × 200 mm with connecting piece (Braun-Melsungen)
One tubing system for Peritocomb III (Fresenius)
One dual puncture system for Peritocomb III tubing (Fresenius).

21 Neonatal Drug Therapy

L. Wille

The general immaturity of newborn infants, especially prematures, as well as the rapid postnatal changes and continuous maturation of bodily and organ functions must be taken into account when administering drugs to neonates [2, 3]. The pharmacokinetic peculiarities of the neonatal period must be considered [5]:

Absorption	Subcutaneous, intramuscular, vasomotor instability
	Oral ↓ Intestinal motility ↓ Gastric acidity Delayed intestinal enzyme development
Distribution	Relative organ mass, fat content, blood flow
	"Leaky" blood-brain barrier
	Alteration in body water compartments
	↓ Serum albumin
	↓ Albumin drug binding
Metabolism	Enzyme immaturity
	↑ Relative hepatic size
Excretion	↓ Glomerular filtration rate
	↓ Tubular function

By applying general pharmacologic principles (clearance, distribution volume, protein binding, half-life, steady state) in the neonatal period, the drug dosage for term and preterm infants can be calculated on a pharmacokinetic basis [7].
Questions on the testing of drugs in neonates are covered by the Helsinki Declaration (7), the WHO report on "Guidelines for the Evaluation of Drugs for Human Use", and the latest german drug regulations (1).

A drug is considered suitable for general use only after adequate experience has been gained in its pediatric use, and systematic studies have been done on its pharmacodynamics, pharmacokinetics, and toxicology in term and preterm infants. Often such studies are lacking, and the manufacturer's information may not cover this age group, i. e., the drug has not been certified safe in every case for use in newborn infants. Rarely are such variables as gestational age (immaturity) and postnatal age (maturity) incorporated into dosage guidelines. It must also be noted that certain disease situations (e. g., renal and cardiac failure) and modern intensive care treatments (e. g., giving albumin in perinatal shock) can alter the behavior of a drug.

An important task of neonatal intensive medicine is to explore and develop new therapeutic possibilities [6]. In some cases this requires the use of new pharmacologic agents or known pharmaceutical products for other indications. Such therapy may be administered only if the parents have given their informed consent, adequate records are kept, and means are available for observing the patient's progress. The critical testing of new medications (e. g., prostaglandin E, indomethacin, tolazoline) in term and preterm infants should be conducted only in regional centers under the direction of a clinical pharmacologist! The following pharmaceutical products are used in our intensive care unit in the dosages indicated; all information is based on the current state of the literature (Table 75).

Table 75. Dosage guidelines for drug therapy in term and preterm infants

Generic name	Adminis-tration	Dosage	Dose distrib.	Remarks
Acetazolamide	IV p. o.	5 mg/kg/day 15–35 mg/kg	3 q. 8 h	
Albumin	Slowly IV	1 g/kg/day		Avoid circulatory overload
Amikacin	IM IV over 20'	15 mg/kg/day	2	
Amphotericin B	Slow infusion over 4–6 h	0.1–1.0 mg/kg/day		Increase gradually to full dose over course of a week. Side effects: anemia, hypokalemia, nephrotoxicity! Dilution for infusion: 0.1 mg/1 ml
Amoxicillin	p. o.	50 (–100)mg/kg/day	3 (–4)	
Ampicillin	IV	50–200 mg/kg/day	3–4	

Table 75. (Continued)

Generic name	Adminis-tration	Dosage	Dose distrib.	Remarks
Alcuronium chloride	IV	Initial: 0.3 mg/kg Maintenance: 0.1 mg/kg	about q. 4–6 h as needed	Duration of action about 30′; up to 12 h in preterm infants
Atropine sulfate	SC	0.01 mg/kg		Side effects: tachycardia, possibly hyperthermia
Azlocillin	IV	100 mg/kg/day	2	
Blood and blood derivatives	IV	10–20 mg/kg	May be repeated	Slow infusion
Packed red cells	IV	5–10 ml/kg	May be repeated	Slow infusion
Human fibrinogen	IV	50 mg/kg	Repeat as needed	Plasma factor determination must be taken into account
IgM–globulin	M	Prophylaxis: 0.2–0.4 ml/kg Therapy: 0.5–1.0 ml/kg		Repeat after 10–14 days Repeat after 1 week
Fresh frozen plasma	IV	10–20 ml/kg	May be repeated	
Carbenicillin	IV over 15–20′	200–400 mg/kg/day	3–4	
Cefamandole	IV	100 mg/kg/day	2–3	
Cefazolin	IV	60 mg/kg/day	2–3	
Cefuroxime	IV	100 mg/kg/day	2–3	
Cefoxitin	IV	100 mg/kg/day	2–3	
Chlor-amphenicol	IV	Preterms: 25 mg/kg/day Term infants ≤2 weeks: 25 mg/kg/day Term infants ≥3 weeks: 50 mg/kg/day	2 2	Determination of serum level necessary for adjusting dosage
Chloral hydrate	Rectally	Convulsions: 50 mg/kg/day Sedation: 25 mg/kg/day	3	
Clonazepam	IM, IV	Convulsions: 0.2–2.0 mg/kg	May be repeated	

Table 75. (Continued)

Generic name	Adminis-tration	Dosage	Dose distrib.	Remarks
Clindamycin	IV	10–15 mg/kg/day	3–4	Not certified safe for use in neonatal period. Concentration: 6 mg/ml. Give by infusion over 10–20 min
	p.o.	8–20 mg/kg/day	4	
Clonidine		0.002 mg/kg	May be repeated	
Calcium gluconate		5 ml/kg/day		Hypocalcemia: 1–2 ml/kg slowly IV. Attempt correction by long-term (24–h) infusion. During digitalization, correct only by long-term infusion!
Dexamethasone	IM, IV	0.5–1.0 mg/kg/day	3–4	
Diazepam	IM, IV	Sedation: 0.1–0.8 mg/kg/day		Avoid use in hyperbilirubinemia
		Convulsions: 0.2–2.0 mg/kg	May be repeated	
Diazoxide	IV	2–5 mg/dose	May be repeated	Hyperglycemia
Dicloxacillin		50 (–100) mg/kg/day	4	
Digoxin	IM, IV	Term/preterm infant sat. dose: 0.03 mg/kg/day;	3	During 1st and 2nd week of life
		maint. dose: 0.005 mg/kg/day	2	
		Term/preterm infant sat. dose: 0.04 mg/kg/day; maint. dose: 0.01 mg/kg/day		From 3rd week of life on
Dihydralazine	IV	1–9 mg/kg/day	2–4	
Dihydroergo –cornine -cristine -cryptine	IV	30 μg/kg	May be repeated	
Flucytosine	IV	100 (–150) mg/kg/day	Short-term infusion over 20–30′	

Table 75. (Continued)

Generic name	Adminis-tration	Dosage	Dose distrib.	Remarks
Furosemide	IV p.o.	1 mg/kg 2–3 mg/kg	q. 3–8 h q. 8–12 h	
Glucagon	SC, IM, IV	30–100 µg/kg	q. 6–12 h	
Gentamycin	IM IV 1–2 h	1st week of life: 5 mg/kg/day; from 2d week on: 7.5 mg/kg/day	2 3	Limited use for 7–10 days; nephrotoxicity
	intrathecally, intraventri-cularly	2 mg	Single dose daily	For treatment of ventriculitis
Heparin	IV	Initial dose: 50 USP units/kg Maintenance: 300–400 USP units/kg/day	4; 24-h infusion is preferred	
Insulin	SC, IV	0.1–1.0 units per kg	Initial dose, cont. infusion is preferred	
Indometacin	p.o.	0.2 mg/kg	q. 12 h	No more than 3 doses in all!
Levallorphan	IM, IV	0.1–0.25 mg/kg	May be repeated	Respiratory depression!
Lidocaine	IV, intracardially	Initial: 10 mg/kg, 0.1–0.2 mg/kg/min	May be re-peated Continuous infusion	
Lysine hydrochloride	IV, infusion	BE × kg × 0.3		1 ml contains: 1 mEq L-lysine$^+$ and 1 mEq Cl^-
Mannitol	IV over 20′	200–400 mg/kg	q. 6, 8, or 12 h	
Magnesium ascorbate 20%	IM, IV	0.2 ml/kg	q. 12 h	Indication: hypo-magnesemia; check serum level after 2nd dose!
Mezlocillin	IV	150 mg/kg/day	2	
Neostigmine	IM, IV	0.02–0.04 mg	q. 4–6 h	Beware: bradycardia
Sodium bicar-bonate 8.4%	IV, over 2′	Blind buffering: 3 mEq/kg meta-bolic acidosis: BE × kg × 0.3 Resuscitation	Infusion over 15′	1 ml contains: 1 mEq Na^+ and 1 mEq HCO_3 diluted 1 : 1 with 5% glucose

Table 75. (Continued)

Generic name	Adminis-tration	Dosage	Dose distrib.	Remarks
Orciprenaline	IV, intracardially	0.1 mg	May be repeated	
Oxacillin	IM, IV over 15–20′	50–100 mg/kg/day	2–3	
Pethidine	IM	0.5–1 mg/kg	q. 6 h	
Penicillin G	IM, IV over 15–20′	50 000–75 000 units/kg/day	2	
		Meningitis: 100 000–200 000 units/kg/day	Continuous infusion	
		B streptococci: 250 000 units/kg/day	Continuous infusion	
Procaine Penicillin G	IM	50,000 units/kg/day	2	
Promethazine	p. o.	1 mg/kg	q. 4–6 h	
Prednisolone	IV	1–3 mg/kg/day	4	
Phenobarbital	IM, IV p. o.	Saturation: 15 mg/kg		for convulsions
		Maintenance: term infants in 1st week: 3 mg/kg/day	1	
		Term infants from 2d week on: 4 mg/kg/day	1	
		Preterm infants in 1st week: 2 mg/kg/day	1	
		From 2d week on: 3 mg/kg/day	1	
Polymyxin B	IM	100 000–200 000 units/kg/day	2	
Protamine chloride	IV	1 ml inactivates 1000 USP units heparin		
Sodium polysty-rene sulfonate	p. o., rectally	1.0–1.5 g/kg	May be repeated	1.0 g reduces hyper-kalemia by 1.0 mEq
Sisomycin	IM	4–6 mg/kg/day	2–3	
Spironolactone	p. o.	0.5–1.0 mg	q. 8 hr	

Table 75. (Continued)

Generic name	Adminis-tration	Dosage	Dose distrib.	Remarks
Trometamol (THAM)	IV, infusion	BE × kg × 0.3	Continuous infusion	Dilute each 8 ml THAM with 2 ml of 50% glucose due to hypoglycemia
Theophylline	p. o.	Saturation: 6 mg/kg Maintenance: 2 mg/kg	 q. 12 h	Better: pharmacy preparation, 1 drop = 1 mg
Cefalexin	p. o.	60 mg/kg/day	4	
Trimethoprim-Sulfamethoxazole	p. o., IV	5 mg trimethoprim/kg body wt		Only in lifethreatening situation with no alternative. 1 ml of parent solution per 25–30 ml infusion solution. Infuse over at least 90′
Dopamine	IV	Renal perfusion: 2 γ/min Hypotension: 4–6 γ/min	Continuous infusion	
Tobramycin	IM, IV over 20–60′	4 mg/kg/day	2	Limited use for 7–10 days, nephrotoxicity
Tolazoline	IV	Initial: 1 mg/kg Maintenance: 1–2 mg/kg/hr	In 30 s Continuous infusion	
Verapamil	IV	0.3 mg/kg 0.1–(1.0) mg/h	Continuous infusion	Give total dose in 5 ml of 5% glucose (1 ml/min.)
Propranolol	IV p. o.	0,05–0,15 mg/kg/day 0.5–2 mg/kg/day	 2–4	
Methyldopa	IV p. o.	 5–50 mg/kg/day	 2–4	
Sodium nitroprusside	IV	2.5–5 µg/kg/min		continuous infusion with 5% glucose
Phenytoin	Infusion over 20 min	Loading dose: 15 mg/kg/day Maint. dose: 5 mg/kg/day		Determination of serum level necessary for adjusting dosage. Resorption following oral administration doubtful in the neonate.

Table 75. (Continued)

Generic name	Adminis-tration	Dosage	Dose distrib.	Remarks
Phyto-menandion	IV, IM	1 mg/kg		
Carbamazepine	p.o.	400–700 mg/ 1.7 m^2/day		In diabetes in-sipidus renalis
Hydrochlor-othiazide	p.o.	1 mg/kg/day		In diabetes in-sipidus renalis
Dextran 40, Na free	Infusion	3–4 ml/kg		For shock with peripheral vasoconstriction
Dextran 60	Infusion	5–10 ml/kg		For hypovolemia

References

1. Gesetz über den Verkehr mit Arzneimittel vom 24. 8. 1976 (BGBl. I, S. 2445 (AMG)
2. Giacoia, G. P., Gorodisher, R.: Pharmakological principles in neonatal drug therapy in: Symposium on drug therapy in the neonate Yaffee, S. J. (Ed.). Clin. Perinatol. *2* (1) 125 (1975)
3. McCracken, E. H., Nelson, J. D.: Antimicrobial therapy for newborns. New York-San Franzisco-London: Grune & Stratton 1977
4. Seyberth, H.: Persönl. Mitteilung 1978
5. Udkow, G.: Pediatric clinical pharmacology – a practical review. Am. J. Dis. Child. *132*, 1025 (1978)
6. White, R. D.: Investigation of new drugs in neonates: a problem? Pediatrics *61*, 936 (1978)
7. WHO Chronicle: Biomedical research: a revised code of ethics. 19, 31 (1965)

22 Results of Neonatal Intensive Care

M. Obladen

22.1 Neonatal Mortality

Neonatal and infant mortality is a measure of the quality of the pre-, peri-, and postnatal care of the fetus and newborn. Despite a high level of individual care to critically ill newborns, neonatal and infant mortality of the Federal Republic of Germany compares unfavorably to those of other European nations (Table 76).

Table 76. Comparison of infant mortality rates in various European countries (modified from Ewerbeck, 1977 [5] and the German Statistical Bureau, 1978 [23])

	Perinatal mortality in 1973 (before and during the first 7 days of life, per 1000 live- and stillbirths)	Neonatal mortality in 1973 (in the first 28 days of life, per 1000 live births)	Infant mortality in 1973 (in 1st year of life, per 1000 livebirths)	Infant mortality in 1976 (in 1st year of life, per 1000 livebirths)
Sweden	14,1	7,8	9,9	8,6
Denmark	14,6	8,7	11,5	10,3
Switzerland	15,5	9,4	13,2	10,7
Netherlands	16,4	8,5	11,5	10,5
Norway	16,8	8,5	11,8	11,1
England	21,3	11,1	16,9	14,5
Federal Republic of Germany	23,0	16,6	22,7	17,4
Austria	24,8	17,9	23,8	18,3
Poland	21,3	16,4	25,8	24,4
Greece	25,8	17,3	24,1	22,3
Yugoslavia	23,4	20,6	43,3	38,1
Portugal	33,8	21,2	44,8	38,9

One of the main reasons for a continued unacceptable high neonatal mortality rate has been the lack of regionalization, that is, a lack of well-staffed, well-equipped regional centers to which all high-risk pregnancies and seriously ill neonates can be referred [16]. Figure 47 illustrates the declining trend of neonatal and infant mortality in the Federal Republic of Germany during recent years.

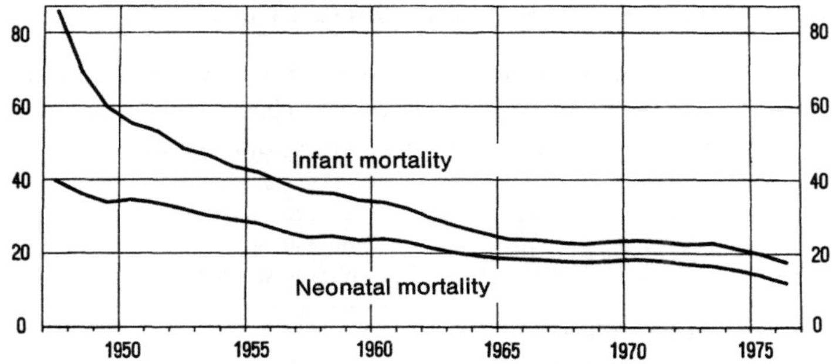

Fig. 47. Neonatal and infant mortality in the Federal Republic of Germany during the last 30 years (German Statistical Bureau, 1978 [23])

22.1.1 Organizational Measures for Reducing Neonatal Mortality

- Establishment of regional centers for perinatal and intensive care.
- Concentration of high-risk deliveries in obstetrical departments with more than 1000 deliveries per year.
- Close association of delivery room and intensive care facilities.
- Expansion of neonatal transport systems.
- Round-the-clock staffing of neonatal intensive care unit with well-trained doctors and nurses.
- Minimum size of neonatal intensive care unit: six beds! Only with constant practice can the technique of artificial ventilation be mastered by all staff.

22.2 Cerebral Handicaps

22.2.1 Incidence

From 6% to 7% of the entire population exhibit cerebral or intellectual handicaps in early childhood [21]. Such a handicap can arise before, during, or after birth. When neonatal intensive care was introduced a decade ago and an increasing number of seriously ill infants survived, the fear was expressed by many that the higher survival rate would mean an increase in the number of neurologically inpaired individuals among the survivors [3]. Numerous follow-up studies around the world indicate that this fear was unwarranted (Fig. 48): Whereas half of former premature infants were assessed as having neurological impairment during the 1950 s [3, 14], studies in the 1960 s showed an incidence of only 35%, and recent studies show only 10%–20% [2, 15]. Even in infants who had respiratory distress syndrome, follow-ups clearly indicate a trend toward improvement (Fig. 48).

22.2.2 Prognostic Value of Neonatal Risk Factors

Even in very seriously ill neonates with neurologic symptoms, brain damage can never be predicted with certainty. In follow-up studies we found the following incidence of permanent handicaps for specific risk factors (total of mild and severe handicaps [17]):

Risk factors	Number of children studied	Percentage with handicaps
Preterm infants without respiratory distress	50	10.0
Small-for-gestational-age infants (without malformations)	23	4.3
Respiratory distress syndrome	78	10.2
Sepsis and meningitis	39	12.8
Severe heart defects	12	25
Severe acidosis	41	19.5

22.2.3 Origin of Perinatal Brain Damage

Key factors are immaturity, birth asphyxia, and placental insufficiency (Fig. 49). Of the numerous factors leading to brain injury, limited evidence suggests that cerebral hemorrhage and infection can presently be prevented. All other factors such as hypothermia, hypoxia, acidosis, shock, and hypoglycemia can be avoided or promptly treated by prenatal monitoring, adequate resuscitation, optimized transport, and neonatal intensive care. The close supervision and treatment of the jeopardized newborn thus contributes significantly to the prevention of perinatal brain damage.

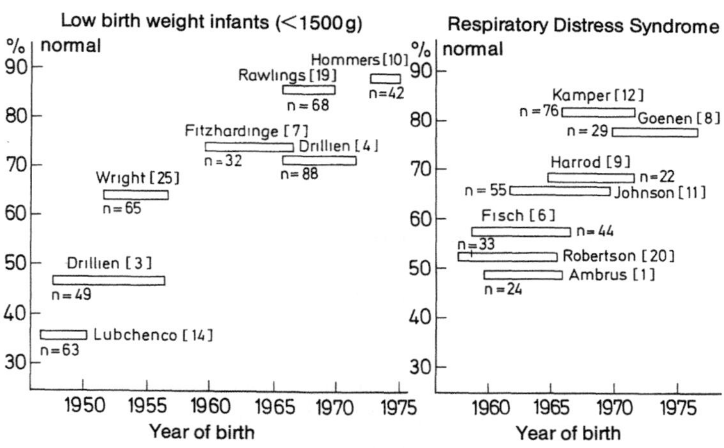

Fig. 48. Literature survey on the long-term prognosis of premature infants. *Left:* Follow-ups of low-birth weight infants (<1500 g). *Right:* Follow-ups after RDS. The *bars* correspond to individual publications. *Abscissa:* Child's year of birth. *Ordinate:* Percentage of children assessed as normal in follow-up

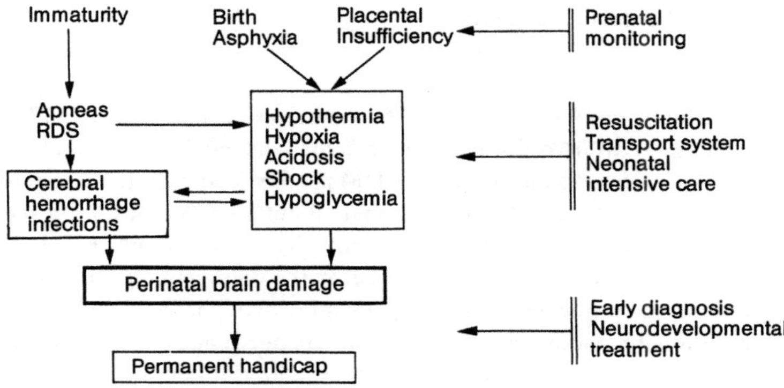

Fig. 49. Pathogenesis (*left*) and prevention (*right*) of perinatal brain damage. (From Obladen, 1979 [17])

22.3 Follow-Up Examination

22.3.1 Timing

Recognized early, a neurologic impairment does not always result in a lasting handicap, but can often be mitigated or even cured by physiotherapy. Impairments of hearing or vision must be recognized before they lead to mental handicap. Funduscopy should always be done before discharge to rule out retrolental fibroplasia. Every seriously ill or immature newborn must be referred to a specialist for a follow-up neurologic examination. Important: Stress the preventive nature of the examination to the parents to avoid aggravating existing fears (see p 272). The follow-up examination is best done after the disappearance of tonic reflexes; This is about 4 months for the mature infant and 4–6 months for the preterm infant

22.3.2 Examination Procedure

Developmental anamnesis: difficulties in sucking or swallowing, sleep disturbances, respiratory difficulties, screaming, rigidity, flaccidity, postural asymmetry, lateral disparities of grasping and kicking, swaddling difficulties, tolerance of prone position, constant closure of fists, developmental retardation.

Examination at 4 months: persistence of tonic reflex activity [13], abnormal muscle tone [21], hyperexcitability, asymmetries.

Examination at 12 months: fine movements, coarse movements, perception, speech, speech comprehension, social behavior, labyrinthine and equilibrium reflexes, observation in high chair, during crawling, during active attempt at standing and, if necessary, during assisted walking.

22.4 Economic Aspects

Neonatal intensive care is costly. The annual cost of operating our 12-bed unit is over 1.5 million DM (two-thirds of which is for salaries). When cost-accounted on a per diem basis this amounts to over 600 DM per day. In the United States, the daily cost of caring for infants < 1000 g birthweight is about $ 450.00; the total cost for managing a newborn infant < 1000 g birthweight until discharge is as high as $ 40 287 [18]. These tremendous costs are entirely justified by the therapeutic goal, however. Besides its personal and medical priority, the prevention of permanent handicaps is important to the national economy: A seriously brain-damaged child receiving governmental social services requires over 1 million DM over a 50-year period. This is equivalent to the gross income of an intensive care nurse during the same period. If even a single serious brain injury is prevented each year by a neonatal intensive care unit with a six-bed capacity, the operation of this unit is "paid for" in an economic sense.

References

1. AMBRUS, C. M., WEINTRAUB, D. H., NISWANDER, K. R., FISCHER, L., FLEISHMAN, J., BROSS, I. D. J., AMBRUS, J. L.: Evaluation of survivors of respiratory distress syndrome at 4 years of age. Am. J. Dis. Child. *120*, 296 (1970)
2. CUKIER, F., AMIEL-TISON, C., MINKOWSKI, A.: Evolution neuro-psychologique d'une groupe d'enfants atteints de détresse respiratoire néonatale traités sous respirateur à pression positive intermittente. Arch. Fr. Pediatr. *33*, 131 (1976)
3. DRILLIEN, C. M.: The incidence of mental and physical handicaps in schoolage children of very low birth weight. Pediatrics *27*, 452 (1961)
4. DRILLIEN, C. M.: Aetiology and Outcome in Low-birthweight Infants. Dev. Med. Child. Neurol. *14*, 563 (1972)
5. EWERBECK, H.: Neue Definition bei der Säuglingssterblichkeit. Mschr. Kinderheilkd: *125*, 674 (1977)
6. FISCH, R. O., GRAVEM, H. J., ENGEL, R. R.: Neurological status of survivors of neonatal respiratory distress syndrome. Pediatrics, *73*, 395 (1968)
7. FITZHARDINGE, P. M., RAMSAY, M.: The Improving Outlook for the Small Prematurely Born Infants. Dev. Med. Child Neurol. *15*, 447 (1973)
8. GOENEN, M., NINANE, J., DUCOFFRE, B., DECLERCK, Y., CLAUS, D., FERRIERE, G., VANMOERBEKE, R. M. T., MOULIN, D., DEMEYER, R., TREMOUROUX, J.: Hyaline Membrane Disease: Prognostic Factors and Medium-Term Follow-Up. Eur. J. Pediatr. *127*, 181 (1978)
9. HARROD, J. R., L'HEUREUX, P., WANGENSTEEN, O. D., HUNT, C. E.: Longterm follow-up of severe respiratory distress syndrome treated with IPPB. J. Pediatr. *84*, 277 (1974)
10. HOMMERS, M., KENDALL, A. C.: The Prognosis of the Very Low-birth-weight Infant. Dev. Med. Child Neurol. *18*, 745 (1976)
11. JOHNSON, J. D., MALACHOWSKI, N. C., BROBSTEIN, R., WELSH, D., DAILY, W. J. R., SUNSHINE, P.: Prognosis of children surviving with the aid of mechanical ventilation in the newborn period. Fet. and Neonat. Med. *84*, 272 (1974)
12. KAMPER, J.: Long term prognosis of infants with severe idiopathic respiratory distress syndrome. I. Neurological and mental outcome. Acta Paediatr. Scand. *67*, 61 (1978)
13. KÖNIG, E., TOBLER, R., BIRO, Z.: Erfassung zerebraler Bewegungsstörungen bei Frühgeborenen. Praxis *44*, 1530 (1968)

14. LUBCHENCO, L. O., HORNER, F. A., REED, L. H., HIX, I. E., METCALF, D., COHIG, R., ELLIOTT, H. C., BOURG, M.: Sequelae of Premature Birth. Am. J. Dis. Child. *106*, 135 (1963)
15. MARRIAGE, K. J., DAVIES, P. A.: Neurological sequelae in children surviving mechanical ventilation in the neonatal period. Arch. Dis. Child. *52*, 176 (1977)
16. MENTZEL, H., MICHAELIS, R.: Die Säuglingssterblichkeit in der Bundesrepublik als Problem der regionalen Neugeborenen- und Säuglingssterblichkeit der Kinderarzt *9*, 303 (1978)
17. OBLADEN, M., WILLE, L., STENZEL, K., KNAPPE, G., KAUFMANN, M.: Der Einfluß neonataler Risikofaktoren auf Mortalität und Spätprognose von Neugeborenen. Med. Tech. *99*, 12 (1979)
18. POMERANCE, J. J., UKRAINSKI, C. T., UKRA, T., HENDERSON, D. H., NASH, A. H., MEREDITH, J. L.: Cost of living for infants weighing 1000 grams or less at birth. Pediatrics, *61*, 908 (1978)
19. RAWLINGS, G., REYNOLDS, E. O. R., STEWART, A., STRANG, L. B.: Changing prognosis for infants of very low birth weight. Lancet *1*, 516 (1971)
20. ROBERTSON, A. M., CRCIHTON, J. U.: Neurological sequelae in children with neonatal respiratory distress. Am. J. Dis. Child. *117*, 271 (1969)
21. SANDER, A.: Die statistische Erfassung von Behinderten in der Bundesrepublik Deutschland. In: Sonderpädagogik I: Gutachten und Studien der Bildungskommission. MUTH, J. (Hrsg.), S. 93. Stuttgart: Klett 1973
22. STAHLMAN, M., HEDVALL, G., DOLANSKI, E., FAXELIUS, G., BURKO, H., KIRK, V.: A six-year follow-up of clinical hyaline membrane disease. Pediatr. Clin. North Am. *20*, 433 (1973)
23. Statistisches Bundesamt: Statistisches Jahrbuch 1978 für die BRD. Stuttgart, Berlin, Köln, Mainz: Kohlhammer 1978
24. TOUWEN, B. C. L.: Frühdiagnose der Zerebralparese. Paediatr. Prax. *16*, 347 (1976)
25. WRIGHT, F. H., BLOUGH, R. R., CHAMBERLIN, A., ERNEST, T., HALSTEAD, W. C., MEIER, P., MOORE, R. Y., NAUNTON, R. F., NEWELL, F. W.: A Controlled Follow-Up Study of Small Prematures Born from 1952 through 1956. Am. J. Dis. Child. *124*, 506 (1972)

23 Parents in the Intensive Care Unit

M. Obladen

23.1 Normal Reaction of Parents to the Birth of a Premature or Sick Infant

With their hopes for a healthy child destroyed, parents normally react with:
- Rejection of the child [4];
- Guilt feelings (Why didn't *I* have a healthy child?);
- Anxiety (Is the child's life in danger? Long-term effects?);
- Overprotectiveness or indifference.

Because premature and seriously ill newborns requiring intensive care are highly vulnerable for a prolonged period of time, it is these infants in particular who are in need of parental care and devotion. Thus, an important therapeutic objective must be to avert or mitigate the above reactions as quickly as possible. An initial, brief conversation of the transport team with the mother or father, before they have been separated from their child, establishes early contact and reduces fears and misunderstandings.

23.2 Consequences of Prolonged Maternal-Infant Separation

- Weakening of emotional bond.
- Impairment of parental consciousness [17]: The child becomes a stranger.
- Incursions into all aspects of family life [12], including the relationship between mother and father.

Normally, the newborn infant actively interacts with the mother at 3 weeks of age, displaying a reproducible pattern of movement in response to facial contact [1]. If maternal-infant contact is prevented during the neonatal period, lasting damage to the child's development may result [2, 9, 18]. Moreover, maternal-infant separation undermines the mother's confidence in her ability to care for the child herself [17]. The maternal anxieties or attitudes of rejection which may have precipitated the premature birth in the first place [13] are reinforced. Many premature infants are later neglected or abused by their parents [10]; this may well be due to the weakened emotional bond or the disturbance of parental consciousness [3].

Conclusion. The "hygienic" visitation rules formerly enforced for sick neonates constitute mental abuse for the child [7].

23.3 Parental Functions in the Intensive Care Unit

A newborn infant belongs to his parents. They must share the responsibility for his welfare. They should be encouraged, rather than instructed, to make frequent visits [2]. If large distances are involved, telephone calls should be encouraged, or travel vouchers issued if circumstances require. No limits are placed upon the time or duration of parental visits (this applies to parents only). Of course the parents must conform to the hygienic rules of the ward with regard to protective clothing, scrubbing, etc. As a rule, though, well-informed parents tend to wash more thoroughly than the staff themselves.

Means of promoting parent-child contact [6, 12, 16]:

- There should be no limitation of visiting privileges.
- Encourage the parents to touch their child and speak to him.
- Parents may hold their child if possible and may photograph him if desired.
- Involve the parents in nursing care (e. g., feeding, diaper change, etc.)
- Even if the infant cannot be nursed, encourage the mother to bring her milk for the child.

It is particularly important that eye contact be established between mother and child [15], possibly necessitating the removal of phototherapy eye patches, and that the mother touch her child [8], which she may be reluctant to do because of the infant's fragile appearance. Physical contact tends to follow a typical, gradual pattern: Fingertips on the extremities, fingertips on the trunk, palm of the hand on the trunk. This contact promotes a lasting response and bond between the parent and child. Besides physical contact, the parents should be given an opportunity to express their concerns. The doctors and nurses must let them know that their presence is helping the child [16]. In particularly difficult situations, the parents should be allowed to spend the night at the intensive care unit, and facilities for this should be provided.

23.4 Informing the Parents

The parents should be informed by the physician as early, as objectively, and as completely as circumstances and reason permit. First try to become acquainted with the parents. Before their first visit to the ICU, prepare them briefly for the technical atmosphere they will encounter there. One way to start conversation at the infant's bedside is to ask the parents for their opinion of the child. They must always feel free to express their fears openly. Serious problems (malformations, unfavorable prognosis, major surgery) should be discussed in the company of both parents if possible. Give no prognosis in the first hours of life! Avoid using such negative terms as "deformity," "incomplete recovery," or "high-risk infant."

Note. Parents are usually very observant. Any change in the infant's condition reported by the mother should be taken seriously by the physician or nurse.

23.5 Conference Following the Death of a Newborn

When conferring with the parents after their child's death, do not try to suppress your own sorrow. Encourage the parents to express their feelings, both to you and to each other. Prepare them for the anticipated mourning response, which also should not be suppressed [1].

Normal mourning response to the death of a newborn [5]:

- Sadness, subjective sorrow
- Somatic disturbances, loss of appetite, sleeplessness
- Guilt feelings
- Irritability and aggressive behavior toward others
- Inability to resume normal activities.

A severe mourning response can usually be expected for 1–6 weeks; it then subsides gradually over the next 6 months or so [14].

An autopsy approval should be obtained if possible, in order to confirm the diagnosis, ascertain the effects of therapy, and to obtain information for a possible genetic consultation. Always schedule another conference after the autopsy, preferably after several weeks, to discuss the results with the parents and answer any questions that remain.

23.6 Atmosphere of the Intensive Care Unit

Unless the parents are properly informed, the sterile, technical ambience of the intensive care unit with its beeping monitors, blinking lights, ventilators and so forth can heighten their fears and further compromise the already tenuous bond between parent and child. The physicians and nurses must exercise discipline in their conversations and develop an awareness of the fact that parents' fears often stem from different observations than the staff's fears. For example, parents are often alarmed to observe that:

- The baby is so small;
- Its eyes are covered by phototherapy eye patches;

- A stomach tube is in place: the child is getting "nothing to eat";
- Its elbows or heels bear puncture marks;
- A "rash" or jaundice is developing.

Usually the overriding concern is whether the child will develop normally. A prompt, patient, and frank explanation of the signs of the disease and the necessary treatment will help to allay parental fears, characterize the intensive care apparatus as a safety factor in the child's interests, and make the parents valuable partners in the treatment of their child.

References

1. BRAZELTON, T. B., TRONICK, E., ADAMSON, L., ALS, H., WEISE, S.: Early mother-infant reciprocity. In: Parent-Infant Interaction. Amsterdam-Oxford-New York: Elsevier 1975
2. FANAROFF, A.: Follow-up of low-birthweight infants – the predictive value of maternal visiting patterns. Pediatrics *49*, 287 (1972)
3. GALDSTON, R.: Dysfunction of parenting: The battered child, the neglected child, the emotional child. In: Modern Perspectives in International Child Psychiatry. HOWELLS, J. G. (Ed.). New York: Brunner/Mazel 1971
4. KAPLAN, D. M., MASON, E. A.: Maternal reactions to premature birth viewed as an acute emotional disorder. Am. J. Orthopsychiatry, *30*, 539 (1960)
5. KENNELL, J., SLYTER, H., KLAUS, M.: The mourning response of parents to the death of a newborn. N. Eng. J. Med. *283*, 344 (1970)
6. KENNELL, J. H., KLAUS, M. H.: Care of the mother of the high-risk infant. Clin. Obstet. Gynaecol. *14*, 926 (1971)
7. KEUTH, U.: Das Kind im Krankenhaus. Besuchsregelung, Mitaufnahme der Mutter. Pädiatr. Prax. *18*, 3–6 (1977)
8. KLAUS, M. H., KENNELL, J., PLUMB, N., ZUEHLKE, S.: Human maternal behaviour at the first contact with her young. Pediatrics *46*, 187 (1970)
9. KLAUS, M. H., KENNEL, J. H.: Care of the mother. In: Neonatology. BEHRMAN, R. E. (Ed.). Saint Louis: Mosby 1973
10. KLEIN, M., STERN, L.: Low birthweight and the battered child syndrome. Am. J. Dis. Child. *122*, 15 (1971)
11. LEIDERMAN, P. H., LEIFER, A. D., SEASHORE, M. J., BARRETT, C. R., GROBSKIN, R.: Mother infant interaction: Effects of early deprivation, prior experience and sex of infant. Research Publications of the Association for Research in Nervous and Mental Disease. *51*, 223 (1973)
12. LEIDERMAN, P. H., SEASHORE, M. J.: Mother-infant-separation: Some delayed consequences. In: Parent-Infant Interaction, p. 213. Amsterdam-Oxford-New York: Elsevier 1975
13. McDONALD, R. L.: The role of emotional factors in obstetric complications: A review. Psychosom. Med., *30*, 222 (1968)
14. PARKES, C. M.: Bereavement and mental illness. Part 2. A classification of bereavement reactions. Br. J. Med. Psychol. *38*, 13 (1965)
15. ROBSON, K.: The role of eye-to-eye contact in maternal-infant attachment. J. Child Psychol. Psychiatry *8*, 13 (1967)
16. SAMEROFF, A.: Psychological needs of the mother in early mother-infant interactions. In: Neonatology. Pathophysiology and management of the newborn. AVERY, G. B. (Ed.), p. 1023. Philadelphia-Toronto: Lippincott 1975
17. SEASHORE, M. J., LEIFER, A. D., BARNETT, C. R., LEIDERMAN, P. H.: The effects of denial of early mother-infant interaction on maternal self-confidence. J. Pers. Soc. Psychol. *26*, 369 (1973)
18. STONE, F. H.: Psychological aspects of early mother-infant relationships. Br. Med. J. *4*, 224–226 (1971)

Subject Index

GPSR Compliance

The European Union's (EU) General Product Safety Regulation (GPSR) is a set of rules that requires consumer products to be safe and our obligations to ensure this.

If you have any concerns about our products, you can contact us on ProductSafety@springernature.com

In case Publisher is established outside the EU, the EU authorized representative is:

Springer Nature Customer Service Center GmbH
Europaplatz 3
69115 Heidelberg, Germany

Batch number: 10584442

Printed by Printforce, the Netherlands